AF449248

Applied Mathematical Sciences
Volume 162

Editors
S.S. Antman   J.E. Marsden   L. Sirovich

Advisors
J.K. Hale   P. Holmes   J. Keener
J. Keller   B.J. Matkowsky   A. Mielke
C.S. Peskin   K.R. Sreenivasan

Applied Mathematical Sciences

1. *John:* Partial Differential Equations, 4th ed.
2. *Sirovich:* Techniques of Asymptotic Analysis.
3. *Hale:* Theory of Functional Differential Equations, 2nd ed.
4. *Percus:* Combinatorial Methods.
5. *von Mises/Friedrichs:* Fluid Dynamics.
6. *Freiberger/Grenander:* A Short Course in Computational Probability and Statistics.
7. *Pipkin:* Lectures on Viscoelasticity Theory.
8. *Giacaglia:* Perturbation Methods in Non-linear Systems.
9. *Friedrichs:* Spectral Theory of Operators in Hilbert Space.
10. *Stroud:* Numerical Quadrature and Solution of Ordinary Differential Equations.
11. *Wolovich:* Linear Multivariable Systems.
12. *Berkovitz:* Optimal Control Theory.
13. *Bluman/Cole:* Similarity Methods for Differential Equations.
14. *Yoshizawa:* Stability Theory and the Existence of Periodic Solution and Almost Periodic Solutions.
15. *Braun:* Differential Equations and Their Applications, 3rd ed.
16. *Lefschetz:* Applications of Algebraic Topology.
17. *Collatz/Wetterling:* Optimization Problems 4th ed.
18. *Grenander:* Pattern Synthesis: Lectures in Pattern Theory, Vol. I
19. *Marsden/McCracken:* Hopf Bifurcation and Its Applications.
20. *Driver:* Ordinary and Delay Differential Equations.
21. *Courant/Friedrichs:* Supersonic Flow and Shock Waves.
22. *Rouche/Habets/Laloy:* Stability Theory by Liapunov's Direct Method.
23. *Lamperti:* Stochastic Processes: A Survey of the Mathematical Theory.
24. *Grenander:* Pattern Analysis: Lectures in Pattern Theory, Vol. II.
25. *Davies:* Integral Transforms and Their Applications, 2nd ed.
26. *Kushner/Clark:* Stochastic Approximation Methods for Constrained and Unconstrained Systems.
27. *de Boor:* A Practical Guide to Splines: Revised Edition.
28. *Keilson:* Markov Chain Models–Rarity and Exponentiality.
29. *de Veubeke:* A Course in Elasticity.
30. *Sniatycki:* Geometric Quantization and Quantum Mechanics.
31. *Reid:* Sturmian Theory for Ordinary Differential Equations.
32. *Meis/Markowitz:* Numerical Solution of Partial Differential Equations.
33. *Grenander:* Regular Structures: Lectures in Pattern Theory, Vol. III
34. *Kevorkian/Cole:* Perturbation Methods in Applied Mathematics.
35. *Carr:* Applications of Centre Manifold Theory
36. *Bengtsson/Ghil/Källén:* Dynamic Meteorology: Data Assimilation Methods.
37. *Saperstone:* Semidynamical Systems in Infinite Dimensional Spaces.
38. *Lichtenberg/Lieberman:* Regular and Chaotic Dynamics, 2nd ed.
39. *Piccini/Stampacchia/Vidossich:* Ordinary Differential Equations in R^n.
40. *Naylor/Sell:* Linear Operator Theory in Engineering and Science.
41. *Sparrow:* The Lorenz Equations: Bifurcations, Chaos, and Strange Attractors.
42. *Guckenheimer/Holmes:* Nonlinear Oscillations, Dynamical Systems, and Bifurcations of Vector Fields.
43. *Ockendon/Taylor:* Inviscid Fluid Flows.
44. *Pazy:* Semigroups of Linear Operators and Applications to Partial Differential Equations.
45. *Glashoff/Gustafson:* Linear Operations and Approximation: An Introduction to the Theoretical Analysis and Numerical Treatment of Semi-Infinite Programs.
46. *Wilcox:* Scattering Theory for Diffraction Gratings.
47. *Hale:* Dynamics in Infinite Dimensions/Magalhães/Oliva, 2nd ed.
48. *Murray:* Asymptotic Analysis.
49. *Ladyzhenskaya:* The Boundary-Value Problems of Mathematical Physics.
50. *Wilcox:* Sound Propagation in Stratified Fluids.
51. *Golubitsky/Schaeffer:* Bifurcation and Groups in Bifurcation Theory, Vol. I
52. *Chipot:* Variational Inequalities and Flow in Porous Media.
53. *Majda:* Compressible Fluid Flow and Systems of Conservation Laws in Several Space Variables.
54. *Wasow:* Linear Turning Point Theory.
55. *Yosida:* Operational Calculus: A Theory of Hyperfunctions.
56. *Chang/Howes:* Nonlinear Singular Perturbation Phenomena: Theory and Applications.
57. *Reinhardt:* Analysis of Approximation Methods for Differential and Integral Equations.
58. *Dwoyer/Hussaini/Voigt (eds):* Theoretical Approaches to Turbulence.
59. *Sanders/Verhulst:* Averaging Methods in Nonlinear Dynamical Systems.
60. *Ghil/Childress:* Topics in Geophysical Dynamics: Atmospheric Dynamics, Dynamo Theory and Climate Dynamics.

(continued following index)

Habib Ammari   Hyeonbae Kang

Polarization and Moment Tensors

With Applications to Inverse Problems and Effective Medium Theory

With 25 Figures

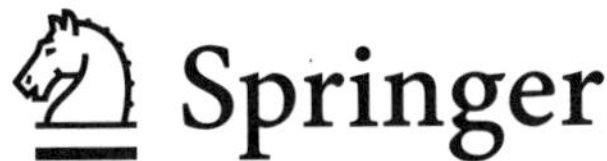 Springer

Habib Ammari
Center of Applied Mathematics
École Polytechnique
91128 Palaiseau Cedex, France
habib.ammari@polytechnique.fr

Hyeonbae Kang
Department of Mathematics
Seoul National University
Seoul 151-747, Korea
hkang@math.snu.ac.kr

Editors:

S.S. Antman
Department of Mathematics
and
Institute for Physical Science
and Technology
University of Maryland
College Park, MD 20742-4015
USA
ssa@math.umd.edu

J.E. Marsden
Control and Dynamical
Systems, 107-81
California Institute of
Technology
Pasadena, CA 91125
USA
marsden@cds.caltech.edu

L. Sirovich
Laboratory of Applied
Mathematics
Department of
Biomathematical Sciences
Mount Sinai School
of Medicine
New York, NY 10029-6574
USA
chico@camelot.mssm.edu

ISBN-13: 978-0-387-71565-0   e-ISBN-13: 978-0-387-71566-7

Printed on acid-free paper.

Library of Congress Control Number: 2007925444

Mathematics Subject Classification (2000): 35R30, 35B27, 35B40, 35R05, 74B05, 78M40, 78M35

www.springer.com   (KeS/MP)

Preface

Recent developments in imaging and effective medium theory reveal that these fields share several fundamental concepts. One of the unifying threads is the use of generalized polarization (GPTs) and moment tensors (EMTs) that depend only on the geometry and the conductivity or the Lamé parameters of the inclusion. These concepts generalize those of classic Pólya–Szegö polarization tensors, which have been extensively studied in the literature by many authors for various purposes. The notion of Pólya–Szegö polarization tensors appeared in problems of potential theory related to certain questions arising in hydrodynamics and in electrostatics.

The study of GPTs and EMTs with applications in imaging and effective medium theory forms the heart of the book. We show that GPTs and EMTs are key mathematical concepts in effectively reconstructing small conductivity or elastic inclusions from boundary measurements as well as in calculating accurate, effective electrical or elastic properties of composite materials.

Due to the character of its topic, this book is of interest not only to mathematicians working in inverse problems and effective medium theory, but also to physicists and engineers who could communicate with mathematicians on these issues. It highlights the benefits of sharing new, deep ideas among different fields of applied mathematics.

This book would not have been possible without the collaborations and the conversations with a number of outstanding colleagues. We have not only profited from generous sharing of their ideas, insights, and enthusiasm, but also from their friendship, support, and encouragement. We feel especially indebted to Graeme Milton, Gen Nakamura, Jin Keun Seo, Gunther Uhlmann, and Michael Vogelius.

Paris and Seoul,
March 2007

Habib Ammari
Hyeonbae Kang

Contents

Preface v

1 Introduction 1

2 Layer Potentials and Transmission Problems 7
    Introduction 7
  2.1 Notation and Preliminaries 7
     2.1.1 Lipschitz Domains 7
     2.1.2 Function Spaces 8
     2.1.3 Poincaré Inequalities 10
     2.1.4 Harmonic Functions 10
     2.1.5 Divergence Theorem and Stokes's and Green's Formulae 12
     2.1.6 Variational Solutions 13
  2.2 Layer Potentials on Smooth Domains 14
     2.2.1 Fundamental Solution 14
  2.3 Layer Potentials on Lipschitz Domains 24
     2.3.1 Jump Relations 24
     2.3.2 Injectivity of $\lambda I - \mathcal{K}_D^*$ 25
     2.3.3 Surjectivity of $\lambda I - \mathcal{K}_D^*$ 26
     2.3.4 Mapping Properties 33
     2.3.5 Concept of Capacity 37
  2.4 Neumann and Dirichlet Functions 39
  2.5 Representation Formula 45
  2.6 Energy Identities 50
  2.7 Anisotropic Transmission Problem 51
  2.8 Periodic Isotropic Transmission Problem 52
  2.9 Periodic Anisotropic Transmission Problem 59
  2.10 Further Results and Open Problems 66

3 Uniqueness for Inverse Conductivity Problems 67
      Introduction 67
      3.1 Uniqueness With Many Measurements 68
      3.2 Uniqueness With One Measurement 71
            3.2.1 Uniqueness in the Monotone Case 72
            3.2.2 Uniqueness of Disks With One Measurement 73
      3.3 Further Results and Open Problems 74

4 Generalized Isotropic and Anisotropic Polarization Tensors 75
      Introduction 75
      4.1 Definition 76
      4.2 Explicit Formulae 81
      4.3 Extreme Conductivity Cases 88
      4.4 Uniqueness Result 90
      4.5 Symmetry and Positivity of GPTs 91
      4.6 Estimates of the Harmonic Moments 94
      4.7 Optimal Bounds for the Polarization Tensor 97
      4.8 Monotonocity 103
      4.9 Estimates of the Center of Mass 104
      4.10 Polarization Tensors of Multiple Inclusions..........106
            4.10.1 Definition 107
            4.10.2 Properties 108
      4.11 Explicit Formulae for the Polarization Tensor
            of Multiple Disks 112
            4.11.1 Representation by Equivalent Ellipses 117
      4.12 Anisotropic Polarization Tensors 119
      4.13 Further Results and Open Problems 127

5 Full Asymptotic Formula for the Potentials 129
      Introduction 129
      5.1 Energy Estimates.....................................131
      5.2 Asymptotic Expansion 135
      5.3 Derivation of the Asymptotic Formula for Closely Spaced
            Small Inclusions 140
      5.4 Derivation of the Asymptotic Formula for Anisotropic
            Inclusions 142
      5.5 Further Results and Open Problems 143

6 Near-Boundary Conductivity Inclusions 145
      Introduction 145
      6.1 Optimal Gradient Estimates 146
      6.2 Asymptotic Expansions 150
            6.2.1 Main Results 150
            6.2.2 Proof of Theorem 6.3 151
            6.2.3 A Numerical Example 157

6.3   Further Results and Open Problems 160

7   Impedance Imaging of Conductivity Inclusions 161
       Introduction 161
7.1   Preliminary...162
7.2   Projection Algorithm — Reconstruction of a Single Inclusion . 163
7.3   Quadratic Algorithm — Detection of Closely Spaced Inclusions 169
7.4   Simple Pole Method 172
7.5   Least-Squares Algorithm 173
7.6   Variational Algorithm...174
7.7   Linear Sampling Method 176
7.8   Lipschitz-Continuous Dependence and Moment Estimations... 182
       7.8.1   Lipschitz-Continuous Dependence 182
       7.8.2   Moment Estimations 185
7.9   Detection of Anisotropic Inclusions 186
7.10 Further Results and Open Problems 192

8   Effective Properties of Electrical Composites 195
       Introduction 195
8.1   Computation of Effective Conductivity 197
8.2   Anisotropic Composites 205
8.3   Further Results and Open Problems 210

9   Transmission Problem for Elastostatics 211
       Introduction 211
9.1   Layer Potentials for the Lamé System 211
9.2   Kelvin Matrix Under Unitary Transformations 215
9.3   Transmission Problem..218
9.4   Complex Representation of the Displacement Field 225
9.5   Periodic Green's Function 230
9.6   Further Results and Open Problems 235

10 Elastic Moment Tensor 237
       Introduction 237
10.1 Asymptotic Expansion in Free Space.......................237
10.2 Properties of EMTs..241
10.3 EMTs Under Linear Transformations 248
10.4 EMTs for Ellipses 251
10.5 EMTs for Elliptic Holes and Hard Ellipses 256
10.6 Further Results and Open Problems 259

11 Full Asymptotic Expansions of the Displacement Field 261
       Introduction 261
11.1 Full Asymptotic Expansions 261
11.2 Further Results and Open Problems 267

12 Imaging of Elastic Inclusions 269
    Introduction 269
    12.1 Detection of EMTs 269
    12.2 Representation of the EMTs by Ellipses 273
    12.3 Detection of the Location 275
    12.4 Numerical Results 277
    12.5 Further Results and Open Problems 283

13 Effective Properties of Elastic Composites 285
    Introduction 285
    13.1 Derivation of the Effective Elastic Properties 286
    13.2 Further Results and Open Problems 289

A Appendices 291
    Introduction 291
    A.1 Compact Operators 291
    A.2 Theorem of Coifman, McIntosh, and Meyer 292
    A.3 Continuity Method 293

References 295

Index 311

1

Introduction

Science and engineering have been great sources of problems and inspiration for generations of mathematicians. This is probably true now more than ever as numerous challenges in science and technology are met by mathematicians. One of these challenges is understanding imaging of complex media such as biological and medical samples and nanostructures.

This book is concerned with recent developments in electrical impedance imaging of small conductivity inclusions, elastic imaging, and the theory of dilute composite materials. The unifying thread is the use of generalized polarization and moment tensors that depend only on the geometry and the conductivity or the Lamé parameters of the inclusion. Our main approach is based on layer potential techniques.

Electrical impedance imaging uses measurements of boundary voltage potentials and associated boundary currents to infer information about the internal conductivity profile of an object. Let Ω be a bounded domain in $\mathbb{R}^d, d \geq 2$. Set σ to be the conductivity distribution in Ω. The steady-state voltage potential u is the solution to

$$\begin{cases} \nabla \cdot \sigma \nabla u = 0 & \text{in } \Omega\,, \\ \left. \dfrac{\partial u}{\partial \nu} \right|_{\partial \Omega} = g\,, \\ \displaystyle\int_{\partial \Omega} g = \int_{\partial \Omega} u = 0\,. \end{cases}$$

Complete information about all voltages u on $\partial \Omega$ and currents g is known to uniquely characterize an isotropic conductivity distribution σ [198, 199, 285, 251, 295, 296, 50]. In its most general form electrical impedance imaging is severely ill-posed and non-linear [1, 4]. These major and fundamental difficulties can be understood by means of a mean value type theorem in elliptic partial differential equations. The value of the voltage potential at each point inside the region can be expressed as a weighted average of its neighborhood potential where the weight is determined by the conductivity distribution. In this weighted averaging way, the conductivity distribution is conveyed to the boundary potential. Therefore, the boundary data are entangled in the global structure of the conductivity distribution in a highly non-linear way. This is the main obstacle to finding non-iterative reconstruction algorithms with limited data. If, however, in advance we have additional structural information about the conductivity profile σ, then we may be able to determine specific features about the conductivity distribution with a satisfactory resolution. One such type of knowledge could be that the body consists of a smooth background containing a number of unknown small inclusions with a significantly different conductivity. The simplest case is a conductivity profile of the body Ω given by $\sigma = 1 + (k-1)\chi(D)$, where D is a small inclusion of constant conductivity k and χ denotes its characteristic function. The inclusions might in a medical application represent potential tumors [89, 49, 40, 282, 209, 93], in a material science application they might represent impurities in the material [117, 67], and finally in a war or post-war situation they could represent anti-personnel mines [129].

Over the last 10 years or so, a considerable amount of interesting work has been dedicated to the imaging of such low volume fraction inclusions [129, 130, 132, 84, 81, 83, 64, 26]. The method of asymptotic expansions of small volume inclusions provides a useful framework to accurately and efficiently reconstruct the location and geometric features of the inclusions in a stable way, even for moderately noisy data [26]. The first-order perturbations due to the presence of the inclusions are of dipole-type.

The new concepts of generalized polarization tensors (GPTs) associated with a bounded Lipschitz domain and an isotropic or anisotropic conductivity are central in this asymptotic approach.

On one hand, the GPTs are the basic building blocks for the full asymptotic expansions of the boundary voltage perturbations due to the presence of a small conductivity inclusion inside a conductor.

Consider B to be a Lipschitz bounded domain in $\mathbb{R}^d, d \geq 2$, containing the origin, and let the conductivity of B be equal to $k, 0 < k \neq 1 < +\infty$. Let H be a harmonic function in $\mathbb{R}^d$, and let u be the solution to the following problem:

$$\begin{cases} \nabla \cdot ((1 + (k-1)\chi(B))\nabla u) = 0 & \text{in } \mathbb{R}^d \, , \\ u(x) - H(x) = O(|x|^{1-d}) & \text{as } |x| \to \infty \, . \end{cases}$$

As shown in Chapter 4, the GPT's, $M_{ij}(k, B)$, can be defined through the following far-field expansion of u:

$$(u - H)(x) = \sum_{|i|,|j|=1}^{+\infty} \frac{(-1)^{|i|}}{i!j!} \partial_x^i \Gamma(x) M_{ij}(k, B) \partial^j H(0) \quad \text{as } |x| \to +\infty \, ,$$

where Γ is a fundamental solution of the Laplacian.

It is then important from an imaging point of view to precisely characterize these GPTs and derive some of their properties, such as symmetry, positivity, and optimal bounds on their elements, for developing efficient algorithms to reconstruct conductivity inclusions of small volume. The GPTs seem to contain significant information on the domain and its conductivity which are yet to be investigated. Indeed, making use of the GPTs allows us to reconstruct the small inclusions with higher resolution and even to identify quite general conductivity inclusions without restrictions on their sizes [43].

On the other hand, the use of these GPTs leads to stable and accurate algorithms for the numerical computations of the steady-state voltage in the presence of small conductivity inclusions. It is known that small size features cause difficulties in the numerical solution of the conductivity problem by the finite element or finite difference methods. This is because such features require refined meshes in their neighborhoods, with their attendant problems [188].

The concepts of higher-order polarization tensors generalize those of classic Pólya–Szegö polarization tensors that have been extensively studied in the literature by many authors for various purposes [81, 38, 84, 115, 225, 222, 132, 195, 202, 266, 105, 106, 107]. The notion of Pólya–Szegö polarization tensors appeared in problems of potential theory related to certain questions arising in hydrodynamics and in electrostatics. If the conductivity is zero, namely, if the inclusion is insulated, the polarization tensor of Pólya–Szegö is called the virtual mass.

The concept of polarization tensors also occurs in several other interesting contexts, in particular in asymptotic models of dilute composites such as biological cell suspensions [128, 48, 262] and brain tissues [294]. The determination of the effective or macroscopic property of a two-phase medium consisting of inclusions of one material of known shape embedded homogeneously in another one, having physical properties different from the former one's, has been one of the classic problems in physics. See [245, 38, 114, 236, 95]. When the inclusions are well-separated d-dimensional spheres and their volume fraction is small, the effective electrical conductivity of the composite medium is given by the well-known Maxwell–Garnett formula.

Despite the importance of calculating the effective properties of composites, there has been very little work addressing the influence of the inclusion shape. Most theoretical treatments focus on generalizing the Maxwell–Garnett formula to finite concentrations. These methods include bounds on the effective properties of the mixtures, and many effective medium-type models have been proposed [236, 173]. Indeed, some effective medium calculations attempt to extend the Maxwell–Garnett formula to higher powers of the volume fraction, but only for the case of d-dimensional spherical inclusions [171, 277].

Until recently, ellipsoids are the only family of inclusions that could be rigorously and accurately estimated [310]. Douglas and Garboczi [115, 134, 225] made an important advance in treating more complicated shape inclusions by formally finding that the leading-order term in the expansion of the effective conductivity (and other effective properties) in terms of the volume fraction could be expressed by means of the polarization tensors of the inclusion. See also, in connection with this, the work of Sánchez-Palencia [276] and its extension to the Navier–Stokes equation by Lévy and Sánchez-Palencia [215].

The study of the GPTs with applications in imaging and effective medium theory forms the heart of the book. We show that the GPTs are a key mathematical concept in effectively reconstructing small conductivity inclusions from boundary measurements as well as in calculating accurate effective electrical properties of composite conducting materials. We study important properties of symmetry and positivity of the GPTs and present certain inequalities satisfied by the tensor elements of the GPTs. These relations can be used to find bounds on the weighted volume of the inclusion. We also provide a general unified layer potential technique for rigorously deriving very accurate asymptotic expansions of electrical effective properties of dilute media for non-spherical Lipschitz isotropic and anisotropic conductivity inclusions. The approach is valid for high contrast mixtures and inclusions with Lipschitz boundaries and allows us to compute higher-order terms in the asymptotic expansion of the effective conductivity. Our result has important implications in imaging composites. It shows that the volume fractions and the GPTs form the only information that can be reconstructed in a stable way from boundary measurements. The volume fraction is the simplest but most important piece of microstructural information. The GPTs involve microstructural information beyond that contained in the volume fractions (material contrast, inclusion shape and orientation).

We then extend this important concept of GPTs to linear elasticity defining generalized elastic moment tensors (EMTs). We confine our study to isotropic elasticity. We investigate some important properties of the EMTs such as symmetry and positive-definiteness. We also obtain estimations of their eigenvalues and compute EMTs associated with ellipses, elliptic holes, and hard inclusions of elliptic shape. These results are applied in elastic imaging of small inclusions and effective properties of dilute elastic composites. We develop a method to detect the first-order EMT and the location of an inclusion in a homogeneous elastic body in a mathematically rigorous way. We then present a simple and rigorous scheme for the derivation of accurate asymptotic expansions of the effective elastic parameters of periodic dilute two-phase composites in terms of the elastic moment tensor and the volume fraction occupied by the elastic inclusions. Our derivations are based again on layer potential techniques and are valid for inclusions with Lipschitz boundaries and even when the phase moduli differ significantly.

The book is intended to be self-contained. Here is an outline of its contents.

In Chapter 2, we introduce the main tools for studying the isotropic and anisotropic conductivity problems and collect some preliminary results regarding layer potentials. This chapter offers a comprehensive treatment of this subject, covering some less well-known results on periodic layer potentials.

Chapter 3 is devoted to inverse conductivity problems. We briefly discuss some uniqueness results. The book by Isakov [166] gives more detailed treatments of this subject.

In Chapter 4, we introduce the GPTs associated with a Lipschitz bounded domain and an isotropic or anisotropic conductivity and provide their main properties. We prove that the knowledge of the set of all the GPTs allows for uniquely determining the domain and its conductivity. We also provide important properties of symmetry and positivity of the GPTs and derive isoperimetric inequalities satisfied by the tensor elements of the GPTs. These relations can be used to find bounds on the weighted volume.

In Chapter 5, we provide a rigorous derivation of high-order terms in the asymptotic expansions of the voltage potentials.

The problem considered in Chapter 6 is of practical interest in many areas such as surface defect detection in the semiconductor industry and optical particle sizing. We shall discuss the case where the conductivity inclusion is at a distance comparable with its diameter apart from the boundary of the background conductor. In this case, a more complicated asymptotic formula should be used instead of the dipole-type expansion, which is only valid when the potential within the inclusion is nearly constant. On decreasing the distance between the inclusion and the boundary of the background medium, this assumption begins to fail because higher-order multi-poles become significant due to the interaction between the inclusion and the boundary of the background medium. We provide some essential insight for understanding this interaction. Since our formula carries information on the location, the conductivity and the volume of the inclusion, it can be efficiently exploited for imaging near-boundary inclusions.

In Chapter 7, we present non-iterative reconstruction algorithms based on asymptotic formulae of the boundary perturbations due to the presence of the conductivity inclusions.

Chapter 8 is devoted to the determination of the effective electrical conductivity of a two-phase composite material using boundary layer potentials.

Chapters 9 through 13 are devoted to the study of the elastic moment tensors. We prepare the way in Chapter 9 by reviewing a number of basic facts on the layer potentials of the Lamé system, which are very useful in the subsequent chapters.

In Chapter 10, we provide in a way analogous to GPTs, mathematical definitions of elastic moment tensors (EMTs) and show symmetry and positive-definiteness of the first-order EMT. The first-order EMT was introduced by Maz'ya and Nazarov [228].

In Chapter 11, we find a complete asymptotic formula of solutions of the linear elastic system in terms of the size of the inclusion. The method of derivation is parallel to that for the conductivity problems, apart from some technical difficulties due to the fact that we are dealing with a system, not a single equation, and the equations inside and outside the inclusion are different. Based on this asymptotic expansion we derive in Chapter 12 formulae to find the location and the order of magnitude of the elastic inclusion. The formulae are explicit and can be easily implemented numerically.

Chapter 13 provides a rigorous derivation of accurate asymptotic expansions of the effective elastic parameters of periodic dilute two-phase composites in terms of the elastic moment tensor and the volume fraction occupied by the elastic inclusions.

The book concludes with three appendices. The first of these recalls a few facts about compact operators. The second states the theorem of Coifman, McIntosh, and Meyer. The third establishes the continuity method.

It is important to note that some of the techniques described in this book can be applied to problems in many fields other than inverse boundary value problems and effective medium theory. In this connection we would particularly like to mention the mathematical theory of of photonic and phononic crystals [205, 256, 270] and topological shape optimization [253, 216, 137, 142, 275].

A preliminary version of some of the material discussed in this book was published as a Springer Lecture Notes [26].

Layer Potentials and Transmission Problems

Introduction

In this chapter we review some well-known results on the solvability and layer potentials for isotropic and anisotropic conductivity problems, which we shall use frequently in subsequent chapters. Our main aim here is to collect the various concepts, basic definitions, and key theorems on layer potentials on Lipschitz domains, with which the readers might not be familiar. This chapter gives a concise treatment of this subject, covering some less well-known results on periodic layer potentials as well. A familiarity with basic concepts and results from linear functional analysis and linear elliptic equations is assumed, but some effort will be made to refresh the reader's memory.

The first three sections of this chapter cover relevant parts of the theory of layer potentials. The reader will need to understand this material at a practical level before proceeding any further. Next, we prove a decomposition formula of the steady-state voltage potential into a harmonic part and a refraction part. We then discuss the anisotropic transmission problem and proceed to establish a representation formula for the solution to this problem. The last two sections of the chapter are devoted to the study of periodic transmission problems. Results in these sections are not completely standard. We will use them when we consider the effective properties of composite materials.

2.1 Notation and Preliminaries

We summarize below some of the less elementary tools we will use in the text.

2.1.1 Lipschitz Domains

We begin with the concept of a Lipschitz domain. A bounded open connected domain D in $\mathbb{R}^d$ is called a Lipschitz domain with Lipschitz character (r, L, N)

if for each point $x \in \partial D$ there is a coordinate system $(x', x_d), x' \in \mathbb{R}^{d-1}, x_d \in \mathbb{R}$, so that with respect to this coordinate system $x = (0,0)$, and there are a double truncated cylinder Z (called a coordinate cylinder) centered at x with axis parallel to the x_d-axis and whose bottom and top are at a positive distance $r < l < 2r$ from ∂D, and a Lipschitz function φ with $\|\nabla\varphi\|_{L^\infty(\mathbb{R}^{d-1})} \leq L$, so that $Z \cap D = Z \cap \{(x', x_d) : x_d > \varphi(x')\}$ and $Z \cap \partial D = Z \cap \{(x', x_d) : x_d = \varphi(x')\}$. Here $L^\infty(\mathbb{R}^{d-1})$ denotes the space of bounded functions on $\mathbb{R}^{d-1}$, with the sup norm. The pair (Z, φ) is called a coordinate pair. By compactness it is possible to cover ∂D with a finite number of coordinate cylinders $Z_1, \ldots, Z_N$. Bounded Lipschitz domains satisfy both the interior and the exterior cone conditions.

2.1.2 Function Spaces

A function u is said to be a $\mathcal{C}^n$-function on D, for $n \in \mathbb{N}$, if all its derivatives of order $\leq n$ exist and are continuous in D. We express higher-order derivatives of a $\mathcal{C}^n$-function u by setting

$$\partial^i u = \partial^{i_1} \ldots \partial^{i_d} u \quad \text{for } i = (i_1, \ldots, i_d) \in \mathbb{N}^d .$$

By $\mathcal{C}^{n+\alpha}(D), 0 < \alpha < 1, n \in \mathbb{N}$, we denote the Hölder space of all functions u defined on the Lipschitz bounded domain D satisfying, for any $i \in \mathbb{N}^d$ with $|i| := i_1 + \ldots + i_d = n$,

$$\left| \partial^i u(x) - \partial^i u(y) \right| \leq C|x - y|^\alpha, \quad \forall\, x, y \in D ,$$

where C is a positive constant depending on u but not on x and y.

For ease of notation we will sometimes use ∂ and ∂^2 to denote the gradient and the Hessian, respectively.

Following the notation in the subsection above, we say that $f \in W_1^2(\partial D)$ if $f \in L^2(\partial D)$, the space of square summable functions on ∂D, and for every cylinder Z with associated Lipschitz function φ, there are $L^2(\partial D \cap Z)$ functions $g_p, 1 \leq p \leq d - 1$, such that

$$\int_{\mathbb{R}^{d-1}} h(x') g_p(x', \varphi(x'))\, dx' = -\int_{\mathbb{R}^{d-1}} \frac{\partial}{\partial x_p} h(x') f(x', \varphi(x'))\, dx'$$

for $1 \leq p \leq d - 1$, whenever $h \in \mathcal{C}_0^\infty(\mathbb{R}^{d-1} \cap Z)$. Here $\mathcal{C}_0^\infty(\mathbb{R}^{d-1} \cap Z)$ denotes the set of infinitely differentiable functions with compact support in $\mathbb{R}^{d-1} \cap Z$. Fixing a covering of ∂D by cylinders $Z_1, \ldots, Z_N$, $f \in W_1^2(\partial D)$ may be normed by the sum of L^2 norms of all the locally defined g_p's together with the L^2 norm of f.

Let $T_1, \ldots, T_{d-1}$ be an orthonormal basis for the tangent plane to ∂D at x, and let $\partial/\partial T = \sum_{p=1}^{d-1}(\partial/\partial T_p)\, T_p$ denote the tangential derivative on

∂D. The space $W_1^2(\partial D)$ is then the set of functions $f \in L^2(\partial D)$ such that $\partial f/\partial T \in L^2(\partial D)$.

We define the Banach spaces $W^{1,p}(D), 1 < p < +\infty$, for an open set D by

$$W^{1,p}(D) = \left\{ u \in L^p(D) : \int_D |u|^p + \int_D |\nabla u|^p < +\infty \right\},$$

where ∇u is interpreted as a distribution, and $L^p(D)$ is defined in the usual way, with

$$\|u\|_{L^p(D)} = \left(\int_D |u|^p \right)^{1/p}.$$

The space $W^{1,p}(D)$ is equipped with the norm

$$\|u\|_{W^{1,p}(D)} = \left(\int_D |u|^p + \int_D |\nabla u|^p \right)^{1/p}.$$

Another Banach space $W_0^{1,p}(D)$ arises by taking the closure of $\mathcal{C}_0^\infty(D)$, the set of infinitely differentiable functions with compact support in D, in $W^{1,p}(D)$. The spaces $W^{1,p}(D)$ and $W_0^{1,p}(D)$ do not coincide for bounded D. The case $p = 2$ is special, since the spaces $W^{1,2}(D)$ and $W_0^{1,2}(D)$ are Hilbert spaces under the scalar product

$$(u, v) = \int_D u\, v + \int_D \nabla u \cdot \nabla v .$$

If D is a bounded Lipschitz domain, we will also need the space $W_{\mathrm{loc}}^{1,2}(\mathbb{R}^d \setminus \overline{D})$ of functions $u \in L_{\mathrm{loc}}^2(\mathbb{R}^d \setminus \overline{D})$, the set of locally square summable functions in $\mathbb{R}^d \setminus \overline{D}$, such that

$$hu \in W^{1,2}(\mathbb{R}^d \setminus \overline{D}), \forall\, h \in \mathcal{C}_0^\infty(\mathbb{R}^d \setminus \overline{D}) .$$

Furthermore, we define $W^{2,2}(D)$ as the space of functions $u \in W^{1,2}(D)$ such that $\partial^2 u \in L^2(D)$ and the space $W^{3/2,2}(D)$ as the interpolation space $[W^{1,2}(D), W^{2,2}(D)]_{1/2}$; see, for example, the book by Bergh and Löfström [66].

It is known that the trace operator $u \mapsto u|_{\partial D}$ is a bounded linear surjective operator from $W^{1,2}(D)$ into $W_{\frac{1}{2}}^2(\partial D)$, where $f \in W_{\frac{1}{2}}^2(\partial D)$ if and only if $f \in L^2(\partial D)$ and

$$\int_{\partial D} \int_{\partial D} \frac{|f(x) - f(y)|^2}{|x - y|^d}\, d\sigma(x)\, d\sigma(y) < +\infty .$$

See [138]. Let $W_{-\frac{1}{2}}^2(\partial D) = (W_{\frac{1}{2}}^2(\partial D))^*$, and let $\langle,\rangle_{\frac{1}{2}, -\frac{1}{2}}$ denote the duality pair between these dual spaces.

2.1.3 Poincaré Inequalities

We recall that, if D is a bounded Lipschitz domain, then the Poincaré inequality [138],

$$\int_D |u(x) - u_0|^2 \, dx \le C \int_D |\nabla u(x)|^2 \, dx \, ,$$

holds for all $u \in W^{1,2}(D)$, where

$$u_0 = \frac{1}{|D|} \int_D u(x) \, dx \, .$$

We also recall that according to [240] and [104] (Theorem 1.10), if D is a bounded Lipschitz domain (with connected boundary), then the following Poincaré inequality on ∂D holds

$$\|f - f_0\|_{L^2(\partial D)} \le C \left\| \frac{\partial f}{\partial T} \right\|_{L^2(\partial D)} , \tag{2.1}$$

for any $f \in W_1^2(\partial D)$, where $f_0 = (1/|\partial D|) \int_{\partial D} f \, d\sigma$. Here the constant C depends only on the Lipschitz character of D.

2.1.4 Harmonic Functions

The results on harmonic functions that we cite here without proofs can be found in [47]. Let D be a domain in $\mathbb{R}^d$ and u a $\mathcal{C}^2$ function on D. The function u is called harmonic in D if $\Delta u = 0$ in D. In the case of the plane, the relationship between harmonic and holomorphic functions is described below. Part (i) of the following lemma may be used to write down many examples of harmonic functions; for example, with $z = x_1 + ix_2$,

$$2x_1 x_2 = \Im z^2, \quad x_1^4 - 6x_1^2 x_2^2 + x_2^4 = \Re z^4, \quad e^{x_1} \cos x_2 = \Re(e^z) \, .$$

Lemma 2.1 (i) *If $w = u + iv$ is holomorphic in a domain $D \subset \mathbb{R}^2$, then u and v are harmonic in D. The function v is called a harmonic conjugate of u.*

(ii) *If u is a harmonic function in a simply connected domain $D \subset \mathbb{R}^2$, then u is the real part of a holomorphic function in D.*

For a harmonic function u, the function value at the center x of the ball $\overline{B_r(x)} \subset D$ of radius r is equal to the integral mean values over both the surface $\partial B_r(x)$ and $B_r(x)$ itself.

Lemma 2.2 *Let u be a harmonic function in D. Then*

$$\begin{aligned}
u(x) &= \frac{1}{\omega_d r^{d-1}} \int_{\partial B_r(x)} u(y) \, d\sigma(y) \\
&= \frac{d}{\omega_d r^d} \int_{B_r(x)} u(y) \, dy \quad \text{whenever } \overline{B_r(x)} \subset D \, ,
\end{aligned} \tag{2.2}$$

where ω_d is the area of the unit sphere in $\mathbb{R}^d$.

This result, known as the mean value property, in fact also characterizes the harmonic functions among all continuous functions in D.

Lemma 2.3 *If $u \in \mathcal{C}^0(D)$ and (2.2) holds, then u is harmonic in D.*

The mean value property leads to the maximum principle for harmonic functions.

Lemma 2.4 *Let u be a harmonic function in D and $x \in D$.*

(i) *If u attains a local maximum at x, then u is constant in some neighborhood of x.*
(ii) *If D is connected and u attains an extremum at x, then u is constant.*
(iii) *If $u \in \mathcal{C}^0(\overline{D})$, then $\inf_{\partial D} u \leq u \leq \sup_{\partial D} u$ on D.*

The unique continuation property for harmonic functions is very useful.

Lemma 2.5 (i) *Let u be a harmonic function in D and $u = 0$ in a non-empty open subset of D; then $u = 0$ in D.*
(ii) *Let u be a harmonic function in D and $u = \partial u/\partial \nu = 0$ on a non-empty smooth hypersurface; then $u = 0$ in D. Here $\partial/\partial \nu$ denotes the outward normal derivative at points of the hypersurface.*

We recall the following Runge approximation by harmonic functions in $\mathbb{R}^d$.

Lemma 2.6 *Let D be a Lipschitz bounded domain in $\mathbb{R}^d$ such that $\mathbb{R}^d \setminus \overline{D}$ is connected. Then, for any function u, which is harmonic in an open set containing $\overline{D}$ and any positive number δ, there is a harmonic polynomial v such that $|u - v| < \delta$ in D.*

The following result is also of interest to us. As it is not completely standard, we give its proof.

Lemma 2.7 *For a multi-index $i = (i_1, \ldots, i_d) \in \mathbb{N}^d$, let $x^i := x_1^{i_1} \cdots x_d^{i_d}$. Let $f(x) = \sum_{|i| \leq n} a_i x^i$ be a harmonic polynomial and D be a bounded Lipschitz domain in $\mathbb{R}^d$. There is a constant C depending only on the Lipschitz character of D and n such that*

$$\|\nabla f\|_{L^2(\partial D)} \leq C \|\nabla f\|_{L^2(D)} . \tag{2.3}$$

Proof. Let us fix a notation first. For $r > 0$, set

$$(\partial D)_r := \{x : \operatorname{dist}(x, \partial D) < r\} ,$$

and let $Z_r(x)$ denote the cylinder whose side length is $2r$, radius is r, and center is x. As D is a Lipschitz domain, there is an $r > 0$ such that for any $z \in \partial D$, $Z_{2r}(z) \cap \partial D$ is a Lipschitz graph that lies in $Z_{2r}(z) \cap (\partial D)_r$. Fix a $z \in \partial D$. By the mean value property of harmonic functions (2.2), for any $x \in Z_r(z) \cap \partial D$,

$$|\nabla f(x)|^2 \le \frac{C}{r^d} \int_{Z_r(0)} |\nabla f(x+y)|^2 \, dy$$

for some C depending only on the space dimension d. Thus we get

$$\int_{Z_r(z)\cap\partial D} |\nabla f(x)|^2 \, d\sigma(x) \le \frac{C}{r^d} \int_{Z_r(z)\cap\partial D} \int_{Z_r(0)} |\nabla f(x+y)|^2 \, dy \, d\sigma(x)$$

$$\le \frac{C}{r^d} \int_{Z_r(0)} \int_{Z_r(z)\cap\partial D} |\nabla f(x+y)|^2 d\sigma(x) \, dy \ . \quad (2.4)$$

After rotation and translation if necessary, we may assume that $z = 0$ and $Z_{2r}(z) \cap (\partial D)$ is given by a Lipschitz graph

$$x_d = \varphi(x'), \quad x = (x', x_d), \ |x'| < 2r \ .$$

It then follows from (2.4) that

$$\int_{Z_r(z)\cap\partial D} |\nabla f(x)|^2 d\sigma(x)$$
$$\le \frac{C}{r^d} \int_{|y'|<r} \int_{-r}^{r} \int_{|x'|<r} |\nabla f(x' + y', \psi(x') + y_d)|^2 \sqrt{1 + |\nabla \varphi(x')|^2} \, dx' \, dy_d \, dy' \ .$$

As $|\nabla \varphi|$ is bounded, we get

$$\int_{Z_r(z)\cap\partial D} |\nabla f(x)|^2 \, d\sigma(x) \le \frac{C}{r} \int_{Z_{2r}(z)\cap(\partial D)_{2r}} |\nabla f(x)|^2 \, dx \ .$$

Using the partition of unity, we then get

$$\int_{\partial D} |\nabla f(x)|^2 \, d\sigma(x) \le C \int_{(\partial D)_{2r}} |\nabla f(x)|^2 \, dx \ , \quad (2.5)$$

where C depends only on r and $\|\nabla \varphi\|_{L^\infty}$ or, in other words, the Lipschitz character of D. Let $D_r := \{x : \mathrm{dist}(x, D) < r\}$. As f is a polynomial of degree at most n, it follows from (2.5) that

$$\int_{\partial D} |\nabla f(x)|^2 d\sigma(x) \le C \int_{D_{2r}} |\nabla f(x)|^2 \, dx \le C' \int_{D} |\nabla f(x)|^2 \, dx \ ,$$

where the positive constant C' depends only on n and the Lipschitz character of D. This finishes the proof. $\qquad\square$

2.1.5 Divergence Theorem and Stokes's and Green's Formulae

We recall the following formulation of the divergence theorem.

Lemma 2.8 *Let D be a bounded Lipschitz domain, and let $\partial/\partial\nu$ denote the outward normal derivative on ∂D.*

(i) *If $u \in W^{1,2}(D)$ satisfies $\Delta u = 0$ in D, then*

$$\int_D |\nabla u|^2(y)\, dy = \int_{\partial D} \frac{\partial u}{\partial \nu}(y) u(y)\, d\sigma(y) .$$

(ii) *If $u \in W^{1,2}_{loc}(D)$ satisfies $\Delta u = 0$ in $\mathbb{R}^d \setminus \overline{D}$ with $|u(x)| = O(|x|^{2-d})$ if $d \geq 3$, and $|u(x)| = O(|x|^{-1})$ if $d = 2$, then*

$$\int_{\mathbb{R}^d \setminus \overline{D}} |\nabla u|^2(y)\, dy = -\int_{\partial D} \frac{\partial u}{\partial \nu}(y) u(y)\, d\sigma(y) .$$

Two other basic results are the Stokes's and Green's formulae. The next lemma states the Stokes' formula.

Lemma 2.9 *Let D be a bounded Lipschitz domain, and let ν_y denote the outward normal to ∂D at y. Then for any $u \in W^{1,2}(D)^d$,*

$$\int_D (\nabla \cdot u)(y)\, dy = \int_{\partial D} u(y) \cdot \nu_y\, d\sigma(y) .$$

We refer to (2.6) as the Green's formula.

Lemma 2.10 *Let D be a bounded Lipschitz domain. Then for any functions $u, v \in W^{2,2}(D)$*

$$\int_D \left(\Delta v u - \Delta u v \right)(y)\, dy = \int_{\partial D} \left(\frac{\partial v}{\partial \nu} u - \frac{\partial u}{\partial \nu} v \right)(y)\, d\sigma(y) , \qquad (2.6)$$

where $\partial/\partial\nu$ denotes the outward normal derivative at points of ∂D.

2.1.6 Variational Solutions

Let us now turn to the concept of variational solutions. Let $(a_{pq})^d_{p,q=1}$ be a real symmetric $d \times d$ matrix-valued bounded function. We assume that $(a_{pq})^d_{p,q=1}$ is strongly elliptic, i.e.,

$$\frac{1}{C}|\xi|^2 \leq \sum_{p,q} a_{pq}(x)\xi_p\xi_q \leq C|\xi|^2$$

for any $\xi = (\xi_p)^d_{p=1} \in \mathbb{R}^d \setminus \{0\}$, where C is a positive constant. Let D be a bounded Lipschitz domain in $\mathbb{R}^d$, and let ν_q denote the q-component of the outward normal to ∂D. Given $g \in W^2_{-\frac{1}{2}}(\partial D)$, with $\langle 1, g \rangle_{\frac{1}{2}, -\frac{1}{2}} = 0$, we say that $u \in W^{1,2}(D)$ is the (variational) solution to the Neumann problem:

$$\begin{cases} \displaystyle\sum_{p,q=1}^d \frac{\partial}{\partial x_p} a_{pq} \frac{\partial}{\partial x_q} u = 0 & \text{in } D , \\[2mm] \displaystyle\frac{\partial u}{\partial \widetilde{\nu}}\bigg|_{\partial \Omega} = g , \end{cases} \qquad (2.7)$$

where the p-component of $\widetilde{\nu}$, $\widetilde{\nu}_p = \sum_q a_{pq}\nu_q$, if given any $\eta \in W^{1,2}(D)$ we have

$$\int_D \sum_{p,q=1}^d a_{pq}\frac{\partial u}{\partial x_p}\frac{\partial \eta}{\partial x_q}\,dx = \langle \eta, g\rangle_{\frac{1}{2},-\frac{1}{2}}\,.$$

The Lax–Milgram lemma [211] shows that a unique (modulo constants) $u \in W^{1,2}(D)$ exists that solves (2.7).

2.2 Layer Potentials on Smooth Domains

Let us first review some well-known properties of the layer potentials for the Laplacian and prove some useful identities. The theory of layer potentials has been developed in relation to boundary value problems in a Lipschitz domain [190]. It also plays a central role in the study of boundary value problems defined over unbounded domains. This is primarily due to the fact that integral equations not only allow one to replace a problem over an unbounded domain by one over a bounded surface but also reduce the dimensionality of the problem [101, 231, 255].

2.2.1 Fundamental Solution

To give a fundamental solution to the Laplacian in the general case of the dimension d, we recall that ω_d denotes the area of the unit sphere in $\mathbb{R}^d$. Even though the following result is elementary, we give its proof for the reader's convenience.

Lemma 2.11 *A fundamental solution to the Laplacian is given by*

$$\Gamma(x) = \begin{cases} \dfrac{1}{2\pi}\ln|x|\,, & d = 2\,, \\[2ex] \dfrac{1}{(2-d)\omega_d}|x|^{2-d}\,, & d \geq 3\,. \end{cases} \tag{2.8}$$

Proof. The Laplacian is radially symmetric, so it is natural to seek Γ in the form $\Gamma(x) = w(r)$ where $r = |x|$. Since

$$\Delta w = \frac{d^2 w}{d^2 r} + \frac{(d-1)}{r}\frac{dw}{dr} = \frac{1}{r^{d-1}}\frac{d}{dr}\Big(r^{d-1}\frac{dw}{dr}\Big)\,,$$

$\Delta\Gamma = 0$ in $\mathbb{R}^d \setminus \{0\}$ forces that w must satisfy

$$\frac{1}{r^{d-1}}\frac{d}{dr}\Big(r^{d-1}\frac{dw}{dr}\Big) = 0 \quad \text{for } r > 0\,,$$

and hence

$$w(r) = \begin{cases} \dfrac{a_d}{(2-d)}\dfrac{1}{r^{d-2}} + b_d & \text{when } d \geq 3\,, \\[2ex] a_2\ln r + b_2 & \text{when } d = 2\,, \end{cases}$$

for some constants a_d and b_d. The choice of b_d is arbitrary, but a_d is fixed by the requirement that $\Delta\Gamma = \delta_0$ in $\mathbb{R}^d$, where δ_0 is the Dirac function at 0, or in other words

$$\int_{\mathbb{R}^d} \Gamma\Delta\phi = \phi(0) \quad \text{for } \phi \in \mathcal{C}_0^\infty(\mathbb{R}^d) . \tag{2.9}$$

Any test function $\phi \in \mathcal{C}_0^\infty(\mathbb{R}^d)$ has compact support, so we can apply Green's formula over the unbounded domain $\{x : |x| > \epsilon\}$ to arrive at

$$\int_{|x|>\epsilon} \Gamma(x)\Delta\phi(x)\,dx = \int_{|x|=\epsilon} \phi(x)\frac{\partial\Gamma}{\partial\nu}(x)\,d\sigma(x) - \int_{|x|=\epsilon} \Gamma(x)\frac{\partial\phi}{\partial\nu}(x)\,d\sigma(x) ,$$
$$\tag{2.10}$$

where $\nu = x/|x|$ on $\{|x| = \epsilon\}$. Since

$$\nabla\Gamma(x) = \frac{dw}{dr}\frac{x}{|x|} = \frac{a_d x}{|x|^d} \quad \text{for } d \geq 2 ,$$

we have

$$\frac{\partial\Gamma}{\partial\nu}(x) = a_d\epsilon^{1-d} \quad \text{for } |x| = \epsilon .$$

Thus by the continuity of ϕ,

$$\int_{|x|=\epsilon} \phi(x)\frac{\partial\Gamma}{\partial\nu}(x)\,d\sigma(x) = \frac{a_d}{\epsilon^{d-1}} \int_{|x|=\epsilon} \phi(x)\,d\sigma(x) \to a_d\omega_d\phi(0)$$

as $\epsilon \to 0$, whereas

$$\int_{|x|=\epsilon} \Gamma(x)\frac{\partial\phi}{\partial\nu}(x)\,d\sigma(x) = \begin{cases} O(\epsilon) & \text{if } d \geq 3 , \\ O(\epsilon|\ln\epsilon|) & \text{if } d = 2 . \end{cases}$$

Thus, if $a_d = 1/\omega_d$, then (2.9) follows from (2.10) after sending $\epsilon \to 0$. $\qquad\square$

Let $p \in \mathbb{R}^d$ and $q \in \mathbb{R}$. The function $q\Gamma(x-z)$ is called the potential due to charges q at the source point z. The function $p\cdot\nabla_z\Gamma(x-z)$ is called the dipole of moment $|p|$ and direction $p/|p|$. It is known that using point charges one can realize a dipole only approximately (two large charges a small distance apart). See [267].

Now we prove Green's identity.

Lemma 2.12 *Assume that D is a bounded Lipschitz domain in $\mathbb{R}^d, d \geq 2$, and let $u \in W^{1,2}(D)$ be a harmonic function. Then for any $x \in D$,*

$$u(x) = \int_{\partial D} \left(u(y)\frac{\partial\Gamma}{\partial\nu_y}(x-y) - \frac{\partial u}{\partial\nu_y}(y)\Gamma(x-y) \right) d\sigma(y) . \tag{2.11}$$

Proof. For $x \in D$ let $B_\epsilon(x)$ be the ball of center x and radius ϵ. We apply Green's formula to u and $\Gamma(x-\cdot)$ in the domain $D \setminus \overline{B_\epsilon}$ for small ϵ and get

$$\int_{D\setminus B_\epsilon(x)} \left(\Gamma\Delta u - u\Delta\Gamma\right) dy = \int_{\partial D} \left(\Gamma\frac{\partial u}{\partial \nu} - u\frac{\partial \Gamma}{\partial \nu}\right) d\sigma(y)$$
$$- \int_{\partial B_\epsilon(x)} \left(\Gamma\frac{\partial u}{\partial \nu} - u\frac{\partial \Gamma}{\partial \nu}\right) d\sigma(y) \, .$$

Since $\Delta\Gamma = 0$ in $D \setminus B_\epsilon(x)$, we have

$$\int_{\partial D} \left(\Gamma\frac{\partial u}{\partial \nu} - u\frac{\partial \Gamma}{\partial \nu}\right) d\sigma(y) = \int_{\partial B_\epsilon(x)} \left(\Gamma\frac{\partial u}{\partial \nu} - u\frac{\partial \Gamma}{\partial \nu}\right) d\sigma(y) \, .$$

For $d \geq 3$, we get by definition of Γ

$$\int_{\partial B_\epsilon(x)} \Gamma\frac{\partial u}{\partial \nu} \, d\sigma(y) = \frac{1}{(2 - d)\omega_d}\epsilon^{2-d} \int_{\partial B_\epsilon(x)} \frac{\partial u}{\partial \nu} \, d\sigma(y) = 0$$

and

$$\int_{\partial B_\epsilon(x)} u\frac{\partial \Gamma}{\partial \nu} \, d\sigma(y) = \frac{1}{\omega_d\epsilon^{d-1}} \int_{\partial B_\epsilon(x)} u \, d\sigma(y) = u(x) \, ,$$

by the mean value property. Proceeding in the same way, we arrive at the same conclusion for $d = 2$. $\qquad\square$

Given a bounded Lipschitz domain D in $\mathbb{R}^d, d \geq 2$, we denote, respectively, the single and double layer potentials of a function $\phi \in L^2(\partial D)$ as $\mathcal{S}_D\phi$ and $\mathcal{D}_D\phi$, where

$$\mathcal{S}_D\phi(x) := \int_{\partial D} \Gamma(x - y)\phi(y) \, d\sigma(y) \, , \quad x \in \mathbb{R}^d, \tag{2.12}$$

$$\mathcal{D}_D\phi(x) := \int_{\partial D} \frac{\partial}{\partial \nu_y}\Gamma(x - y)\phi(y) \, d\sigma(y) \, , \quad x \in \mathbb{R}^d \setminus \partial D \, . \tag{2.13}$$

We begin with the study of their basic properties. We note that, for $x \in \mathbb{R}^d \setminus \partial D$ and $y \in \partial D$, $\partial\Gamma/\partial\nu_y(x - y)$ is an L^∞-function in y and harmonic in x, and it is $O(|x|^{1-d})$ as $|x| \to +\infty$. Therefore we readily see that $\mathcal{D}_D\phi$ and $\mathcal{S}_D\phi$ are well defined and harmonic in $\mathbb{R}^d \setminus \partial D$. Let us list their behavior at $+\infty$.

(i) $\mathcal{D}_D\phi(x) = O(|x|^{1-d})$ as $|x| \to +\infty$.
(ii) $\mathcal{S}_D\phi(x) = O(|x|^{2-d})$ as $|x| \to +\infty$ when $d \geq 3$.
(iii) If $d = 2$, we have

$$\mathcal{S}_D\phi(x) = \frac{1}{2\pi} \int_{\partial D} \phi(y) \, d\sigma(y) \ln|x| + O(|x|^{-1}) \quad \text{as } |x| \to +\infty \, .$$

(iv) If $\int_{\partial D} \phi(y) \, d\sigma = 0$, then $\mathcal{S}_D\phi(x) = O(|x|^{1-d})$ as $|x| \to +\infty$ for $d \geq 2$.

The first three properties are fairly obvious from the definitions. Let us show (iv). If $\int_{\partial D} \phi(y) \, d\sigma = 0$, then

$$\mathcal{S}_D\phi(x) = \int_{\partial D} [\Gamma(x-y) - \Gamma(x-y_0)]\phi(y)d\sigma(y) ,$$

where $y_0 \in D$. Since

$$|\Gamma(x-y) - \Gamma(x-y_0)| \leq C|x|^{1-d} \quad \text{if } |x| \to +\infty \text{ and } y \in \partial D \qquad (2.14)$$

for some constant C, $\mathcal{S}_D\phi(x) = O(|x|^{1-d})$ as $|x| \to +\infty$.

More interesting and more subtle properties are the behaviors of the functions $\mathcal{D}_D\phi(x \pm t\nu_x)$ and $\nabla\mathcal{S}_D\phi(x \pm t\nu_x)$ for $x \in \partial D$ as $t \to 0^+$. A study of these properties for general Lipschitz domains is beyond the scope of this book. Nevertheless, in view of its importance, a detailed discussion of the behavior near the boundary ∂D of $\mathcal{D}_D\phi$ and $\nabla\mathcal{S}_D\phi$ for a smooth domain D and a density $\phi \in L^2(\partial D)$ may be appropriate. For this purpose we shall follow [122, 126].

Assume that D is a bounded $C^{1+\alpha}$-domain for some $\alpha > 0$. Then we have the bound

$$\left| \frac{\langle x-y, \nu_x \rangle}{|x-y|^d} \right| \leq C \frac{1}{|x-y|^{d-1-\alpha}} \quad \text{for } x, y \in \partial D, x \neq y , \qquad (2.15)$$

which shows that a positive constant C exists depending only on α and D such that

$$\int_{\partial D} \left(\frac{|\langle x-y, \nu_x \rangle|}{|x-y|^d} + \frac{|\langle x-y, \nu_y \rangle|}{|x-y|^d} \right) d\sigma(y) \leq C \qquad (2.16)$$

and

$$\int_{|y-x|<\epsilon} \left(\frac{|\langle x-y, \nu_x \rangle|}{|x-y|^d} + \frac{|\langle x-y, \nu_y \rangle|}{|x-y|^d} \right) d\sigma(y) \leq C \int_0^\epsilon \frac{1}{r^{d-1-\alpha}} r^{d-2} \, dr$$
$$\leq C\epsilon^\alpha , \qquad (2.17)$$

for any $x \in \partial D$, by integration in polar coordinates.

Introduce the operator $\mathcal{K}_D : L^2(\partial D) \to L^2(\partial D)$ given by

$$\mathcal{K}_D\phi(x) = \frac{1}{\omega_d} \int_{\partial D} \frac{\langle y-x, \nu_y \rangle}{|x-y|^d} \phi(y) \, d\sigma(y) . \qquad (2.18)$$

The estimate (2.16) proves that this operator is bounded. In fact, for $\phi, \psi \in L^2(\partial D)$, we estimate

$$\left| \int_{\partial D} \int_{\partial D} \frac{\langle y-x, \nu_y \rangle}{|x-y|^d} \phi(y) \, \psi(x) \, d\sigma(y) \, d\sigma(x) \right| \qquad (2.19)$$

via the inequality $2ab \leq a^2 + b^2$. Then, by (2.16), (2.19) is dominated by

$$C \left(||\phi||^2_{L^2(\partial D)} + ||\psi||^2_{L^2(\partial D)} \right) .$$

Replacing ϕ, ψ, by $t\phi, (1/t)\psi$, we see that (2.19) is bounded by

$$C\left(t^2\|\phi\|^2_{L^2(\partial D)} + \frac{1}{t^2}\|\psi\|^2_{L^2(\partial D)}\right) ;$$

minimizing over $t \in]0, +\infty[$, via elementary calculus, we see that (2.19) is dominated by $C\|\phi\|_{L^2(\partial D)}\|\psi\|_{L^2(\partial D)}$, proving that $\mathcal{K}_D$ is a bounded operator on $L^2(\partial D)$.

On the other hand, it is easily checked that the operator defined by

$$\mathcal{K}_D^*\phi(x) = \frac{1}{\omega_d} \int_{\partial D} \frac{\langle x - y, \nu_x \rangle}{|x - y|^d} \phi(y)\, d\sigma(y) \tag{2.20}$$

is the L^2-adjoint of $\mathcal{K}_D$.

It is now natural to ask about the compactness of these operators.

Lemma 2.13 *If D is a bounded $\mathcal{C}^{1+\alpha}$-domain for some $\alpha > 0$, then the operators $\mathcal{K}_D$ and $\mathcal{K}_D^*$ are compact operators in $L^2(\partial D)$.*

Proof. According to Lemma A.3 it suffices to prove that $\mathcal{K}_D$ is compact in $L^2(\partial D)$ to assert that $\mathcal{K}_D^*$ is compact as well.

Given $\epsilon > 0$, set $\Gamma_\epsilon(x) = \Gamma(x)$ if $|x| > \epsilon$, $\Gamma_\epsilon(x) = 0$ otherwise, and define

$$\mathcal{K}_D^\epsilon\phi(x) = \int_{\partial D} \frac{\partial \Gamma_\epsilon}{\partial \nu_y}(x - y)\phi(y)\, d\sigma(y) .$$

Then

$$\int_{\partial D}\int_{\partial D} \left|\frac{\partial \Gamma_\epsilon}{\partial \nu_y}(x - y)\right|^2 d\sigma(x)\, d\sigma(y) < +\infty ;$$

hence, the operator norm of $\mathcal{K}_D^\epsilon$ on $L^2(\partial D)$ satisfies

$$\|\mathcal{K}_D^\epsilon\| \leq \left\|\frac{\partial \Gamma_\epsilon}{\partial \nu}\right\|_{L^2(\partial D \times \partial D)} .$$

Let $\{\phi_p\}_{p=1}^{+\infty}$ be an orthonormal basis for $L^2(\partial D)$. It is an easy consequence of Fubini's theorem that, if $\psi_{pq}(x, y) = \phi_p(x)\phi_q(y)$, then $\{\psi_{pq}\}_{p,q=1}^{+\infty}$ is an orthonormal basis for $L^2(\partial D \times \partial D)$. Hence we can write

$$\frac{\partial \Gamma_\epsilon}{\partial \nu_y}(x - y) = \sum_{p,q=1}^{+\infty} \langle \frac{\partial \Gamma_\epsilon}{\partial \nu}, \psi_{pq} \rangle \psi_{pq}(x, y) .$$

Here $\langle , \rangle$ denotes the L^2-product. For $N \in \mathbb{N}, N \geq 2$, let

$$\mathcal{K}_D^{\epsilon, N}\phi(x) = \sum_{p+q \leq N} \int_{\partial D} \langle \frac{\partial \Gamma_\epsilon}{\partial \nu}, \psi_{pq} \rangle \psi_{pq}(x, y)\phi(y)\, d\sigma(y) .$$

It is clear that the range of $\mathcal{K}_D^{\epsilon,N}$ lies in the span of $\phi_1,\ldots,\phi_N$, so $\mathcal{K}_D^{\epsilon,N}$ is of finite rank. Moreover

$$\left\| \mathcal{K}_D^{\epsilon} - \mathcal{K}_D^{\epsilon,N} \right\| \leq \left\| \frac{\partial \Gamma_\epsilon}{\partial \nu} - \sum_{p+q\leq N} \langle \frac{\partial \Gamma_\epsilon}{\partial \nu}, \psi_{pq}\rangle \psi_{pq} \right\|_{L^2(\partial D\times\partial D)} \longrightarrow 0 \quad \text{as } N \to +\infty ,$$

and then $\mathcal{K}_D^{\epsilon}$ is compact by Lemma A.2. On the other hand,

$$\mathcal{K}_D\phi(x) = \frac{1}{\omega_d} \int_{|y-x|>\epsilon} \frac{\langle y-x, \nu_y\rangle}{|x-y|^d}\phi(y)\,d\sigma(y)$$
$$+\frac{1}{\omega_d} \int_{|y-x|<\epsilon} \frac{\langle y-x, \nu_y\rangle}{|x-y|^d}\phi(y)\,d\sigma(y)$$
$$= \mathcal{K}_D^{\epsilon}\phi(x) + \frac{1}{\omega_d} \int_{|y-x|<\epsilon} \frac{\langle y-x, \nu_y\rangle}{|x-y|^d}\phi(y)\,d\sigma(y) ,$$

and then, by the estimate (2.17) the operator norm of $\mathcal{K}_D - \mathcal{K}_D^{\epsilon}$ tends to zero as $\epsilon \to 0$, so $\mathcal{K}_D$ is compact by Lemma A.1. $\qquad\square$

In the special case of the unit sphere, we may simplify the expressions defining the operators $\mathcal{K}_D$ and $\mathcal{K}_D^*$. Assume that D is a two-dimensional disk with radius r. Then, as was observed in [180],

$$\frac{\langle x-y, \nu_x\rangle}{|x-y|^2} = \frac{1}{2r} \quad \forall\, x,y \in \partial D, x \neq y ,$$

and therefore, for any $\phi \in L^2(\partial D)$,

$$\mathcal{K}_D^*\phi(x) = \mathcal{K}_D\phi(x) = \frac{1}{4\pi r} \int_{\partial D} \phi(y)\,d\sigma(y) , \tag{2.21}$$

for all $x \in \partial D$.

For $d \geq 3$, if D denotes a sphere with radius r, then since

$$\frac{\langle x-y, \nu_x\rangle}{|x-y|^d} = \frac{1}{2r}\frac{1}{|x-y|^{d-2}} \quad \forall\, x,y \in \partial D, x \neq y ,$$

we have, as shown by Lemma 2.3 of [182], that for any $\phi \in L^2(\partial D)$,

$$\mathcal{K}_D^*\phi(x) = \mathcal{K}_D\phi(x) = \frac{(2-d)}{2r}\mathcal{S}_D\phi(x) \tag{2.22}$$

for any $x \in \partial D$.

Another useful formula is the expression of $\mathcal{K}_D(y)(x)$, where D is an ellipse whose semi-axes are on the x_1- and x_2-axes and of length a and b, respectively. Using the parametric representation $X(t) = (a\cos t, b\sin t), 0 \leq t \leq 2\pi$, for the boundary ∂D, we find that

$$\mathcal{K}_D \phi(x) = \frac{ab}{2\pi(a^2 + b^2)} \int_0^{2\pi} \frac{\phi(X(t))}{1 - Q\cos(t + \theta)}\, dt\,,$$

where $x = X(\theta)$ and $Q = (a^2 - b^2)/(a^2 + b^2)$, which, combined with the formulae

$$\int_0^{2\pi} \frac{\cos t}{1 - Q\cos t}\, dt = -\frac{2\pi}{Q} + \frac{2\pi}{Q\sqrt{1 - Q^2}}\,, \qquad \int_0^{2\pi} \frac{\sin t}{1 - Q\cos t}\, dt = 0\,,$$

gives

$$\mathcal{K}_D(y)(x) = \frac{a - b}{2(a + b)} \begin{pmatrix} 1 & 0 \\ 0 & -1 \end{pmatrix} x, \qquad x \in \partial D\,, \tag{2.23}$$

which is a formula obtained in [176].

Turning now to the behavior of the double layer potential at the boundary, we first establish that the double layer potential with constant density has a jump.

Lemma 2.14 *If D is a bounded $\mathcal{C}^{1+\alpha}$-domain for some $\alpha > 0$, then $\mathcal{D}_D(1)(x) = 0$ for $x \in \mathbb{R}^d \setminus \overline{D}$, $\mathcal{D}_D(1)(x) = 1$ for $x \in D$, and $\mathcal{K}_D(1)(x) = 1/2$ for $x \in \partial D$.*

Proof. The first equation follows immediately from Green's formula, because $\Gamma(x - y)$ is in $\mathcal{C}^\infty(\overline{D})$ and harmonic in D as a function of y when $x \in \mathbb{R}^d \setminus \overline{D}$. As for the second equation, given $x \in D$, let $\epsilon > 0$ be small enough so that $\overline{B}_\epsilon \subset D$, where B_ϵ is the ball of center x and radius ϵ. We can apply Green's formula to $\Gamma(x - y)$ on the domain $D \setminus \overline{B}_\epsilon$ to obtain

$$0 = \mathcal{D}_D(1)(x) - \frac{\epsilon^{1-d}}{\omega_d} \int_{\partial B_\epsilon} d\sigma(y)$$
$$= \mathcal{D}_D(1)(x) - 1\,.$$

Now we prove the third equation. Given $x \in \partial D$, again let B_ϵ be the ball of center x and radius ϵ. Set $\partial D_\epsilon = \partial D \setminus (\partial D \cap B_\epsilon)$, $\partial B'_\epsilon = \partial B_\epsilon \cap D$, and $\partial B''_\epsilon = \{y \in \partial B_\epsilon : \nu_x \cdot y < 0\}$. (Thus, $\partial B''_\epsilon$ is the hemisphere of ∂B_ϵ lying on the same side of the tangent plane to ∂D at x.) A further application of Green's formula shows that

$$0 = \frac{1}{\omega_d} \int_{\partial D_\epsilon} \frac{\langle y - x, \nu_y \rangle}{|x - y|^d}\, d\sigma(y) + \int_{\partial B'_\epsilon} \frac{\partial \Gamma}{\partial \nu_y}(x - y)\, d\sigma(y)\,.$$

Thus

$$\frac{1}{\omega_d} \int_{\partial D_\epsilon} \frac{\langle y - x, \nu_y \rangle}{|x - y|^d}\, d\sigma(y) = -\int_{\partial B'_\epsilon} \frac{\partial \Gamma}{\partial \nu_y}(x - y)\, d\sigma(y) = \frac{\epsilon^{1-d}}{\omega_d} \int_{\partial B'_\epsilon} d\sigma(y)\,.$$

But on the one hand, clearly

$$\int_{\partial D} \frac{\langle y - x, \nu_y\rangle}{|x - y|^d}\, d\sigma(y) = \lim_{\epsilon \to 0} \int_{\partial D_\epsilon} \frac{\langle y - x, \nu_y\rangle}{|x - y|^d}\, d\sigma(y)\,.$$

On the other hand, as ∂D is $\mathcal{C}^{1+\alpha}$, the distance between the tangent plane to ∂D at x and the points on ∂D at a distance ϵ from x is $O(\epsilon^{1+\alpha})$, so

$$\int_{\partial B_\epsilon'} d\sigma(y) = \int_{\partial B_\epsilon''} d\sigma(y) + O(\epsilon^{1+\alpha}) \cdot O(\epsilon^{d-1}) = \frac{\omega_d \epsilon^{d-1}}{2} + O(\epsilon^{d+\alpha})\,,$$

and the desired result follows. $\qquad\qquad\qquad\qquad\qquad\qquad\qquad\qquad\square$

Lemma 2.14 can be extended to general densities $\phi \in L^2(\partial D)$. For convenience we introduce the following notation. For a function u defined on $\mathbb{R}^d \setminus \partial D$, we denote

$$u|_\pm(x) := \lim_{t \to 0^+} u(x \pm t\nu_x), \quad x \in \partial D$$

and

$$\left.\frac{\partial}{\partial \nu_x} u\right|_\pm (x) := \lim_{t \to 0^+} \langle \nabla u(x \pm t\nu_x), \nu_x\rangle\,, \quad x \in \partial D\,,$$

if the limits exist. Here ν_x is the outward unit normal to ∂D at x, and $\langle,\rangle$ denotes the scalar product in $\mathbb{R}^d$. For ease of notation we will sometimes use the dot for the scalar product in $\mathbb{R}^d$.

We relate in the next lemma the traces $\mathcal{D}_D|_\pm$ of the double layer potential to the operator $\mathcal{K}_D$ defined by (2.18).

Lemma 2.15 *If D is a bounded $\mathcal{C}^{1+\alpha}$-domain for some $\alpha > 0$, then for $\phi \in L^2(\partial D)$*

$$(\mathcal{D}_D\phi)\big|_\pm(x) = \left(\mp \frac{1}{2}I + \mathcal{K}_D\right)\phi(x) \quad a.e.\ x \in \partial D\,.$$

Proof. First we consider a density $f \in \mathcal{C}^0(\partial D)$. If $x \in \partial D$ and $t < 0$ is sufficiently small, then $x + t\nu_x \in D$, so by Lemma 2.14,

$$\mathcal{D}_D f(x + t\nu_x) = f(x) + \int_{\partial D} \frac{\partial \Gamma}{\partial \nu_y}(x + t\nu_x - y)(f(y) - f(x))\, d\sigma(y)\,. \quad (2.24)$$

To prove that the second integral is continuous as $t \to 0^-$, given $\epsilon > 0$, let $\delta > 0$ be such that $|f(y) - f(x)| < \epsilon$ whenever $|y - x| < \delta$. Then

$$\int_{\partial D} \frac{\partial \Gamma}{\partial \nu_y}(x + t\nu_x - y)(f(y) - f(x))d\sigma(y) - \int_{\partial D} \frac{\partial \Gamma}{\partial \nu_y}(x - y)(f(y) - f(x))d\sigma(y)$$

$$= \int_{\partial D \cap B_\delta} \frac{\partial \Gamma}{\partial \nu_y}(x + t\nu_x - y)(f(y) - f(x))\, d\sigma(y)$$

$$- \int_{\partial D \cap B_\delta} \frac{\partial \Gamma}{\partial \nu_y}(x - y)(f(y) - f(x))\, d\sigma(y)$$

$$+ \int_{\partial D \setminus B_\delta} \left(\frac{\partial \Gamma}{\partial \nu_y}(x + t\nu_x - y) - \frac{\partial \Gamma}{\partial \nu_y}(x - y) \right)(f(y) - f(x))\, d\sigma(y)$$

$$= I_1 + I_2 + I_3 \, .$$

Here B_δ is the ball of center x and radius δ. It easily follows from (2.16) that $|I_2| \leq C\epsilon$. Since

$$\left| \frac{\partial \Gamma}{\partial \nu_y}(x + t\nu_x - y) - \frac{\partial \Gamma}{\partial \nu_y}(x - y) \right| \leq C \frac{|t|}{|x - y|^d} \quad \forall \, y \in \partial D \, ,$$

we get $|I_3| \leq CM|t|$, where M is the maximum of f on ∂D. To estimate I_1, we assume that $x = 0$, and near the origin, D is given by $y = (y', y_d)$ with $y_d > \varphi(y')$, where φ is a $C^{1+\alpha}$-function such that $\varphi(0) = 0$ and $\nabla \varphi(0) = 0$. With the local coordinates, we can show that

$$\left| \frac{\partial \Gamma}{\partial \nu_y}(x + t\nu_x - y) \right| \leq C \frac{|\varphi(y')| + |t|}{(|y'|^2 + |t|^2)^{d/2}} \, ,$$

and hence $|I_1| \leq C\epsilon$. A combination of the above estimates yields

$$\limsup_{t \to 0^-} \left| \int_{\partial D} \frac{\partial \Gamma}{\partial \nu_y}(x + t\nu_x - y)(f(y) - f(x))\, d\sigma(y) \right.$$
$$\left. - \int_{\partial D} \frac{\partial \Gamma}{\partial \nu_y}(x - y)(f(y) - f(x)\, d\sigma(y) \right| \leq C\epsilon \, .$$

Since ϵ is arbitrary, we obtain that

$$(\mathcal{D}_D f)\big|_-(x) = f(x) + \int_{\partial D} \frac{\partial \Gamma}{\partial \nu_y}(x - y)(f(y) - f(x))\, d\sigma(y)$$

$$= \left(\frac{1}{2}I + \mathcal{K}_D \right) f(x) \quad \text{for } x \in \partial D \, .$$

If $t > 0$, the argument is the same except that

$$\int_{\partial D} \frac{\partial \Gamma}{\partial \nu_y}(x + t\nu_x - y)\, d\sigma(y) = 0 \, ,$$

and hence we write

$$\mathcal{D}_D f(x + t\nu_x) = \int_{\partial D} \frac{\partial \Gamma}{\partial \nu_y}(x + t\nu_x - y)(f(y) - f(x))\, d\sigma(y), \quad x \in \partial D \, ,$$

instead of (2.24). We leave the rest of the proof to the reader.

Next, consider $\phi \in L^2(\partial D)$. We first note that by (2.16), $\lim_{t \to 0+} \mathcal{D}_D \phi(x \pm t\nu_x)$ exists and

$$\left\| \limsup_{t \to 0+} \mathcal{D}_D \phi(x \pm t\nu_x) \right\|_{L^2(\partial D)} \leq C \|\phi\|_{L^2(\partial D)} ,$$

for some positive constant C independent of ϕ.

To handle the general case, let ϵ be given and choose a function $f \in C^0(\partial D)$ satisfying $\|\phi - f\|_{L^2(\partial D)} < \epsilon$. Then

$$\left| \mathcal{D}_D \phi(x \pm t\nu_x) - \left(\mp \frac{1}{2} I + \mathcal{K}_D \right) \phi(x) \right|$$

$$\leq \left| \mathcal{D}_D f(x \pm t\nu_x) - \left(\mp \frac{1}{2} I + \mathcal{K}_D \right) f(x) \right| + \left| \mathcal{D}_D (\phi - f)(x \pm t\nu_x) \right|$$

$$+ \left| \left(\mp \frac{1}{2} I + \mathcal{K}_D \right) (\phi - f)(x) \right| .$$

For $\lambda > 0$, let

$$A_\lambda = \left\{ x \in \partial D : \limsup_{t \to 0+} \left| \mathcal{D}_D \phi(x \pm t\nu_x) - (\mp \frac{1}{2} I + \mathcal{K}_D) \phi(x) \right| > \lambda \right\} .$$

For a set E, let $|E|$ denote its Lebesgue measure. Then

$$|A_\lambda| \leq \left| \left\{ |\mathcal{D}_D(\phi - f)| > \frac{\lambda}{3} \right\} \right| + \left| \left\{ |\phi - f| > \frac{2\lambda}{3} \right\} \right| + \left| \left\{ |\mathcal{K}_D(\phi - f)| > \frac{\lambda}{3} \right\} \right|$$

$$\leq (\frac{3}{\lambda})^2 \left(\|\phi - f\|^2_{L^2(\partial D)} + \frac{1}{4} \|\phi - f\|^2_{L^2(\partial D)} + \|\mathcal{K}_D(\phi - f)\|^2_{L^2(\partial D)} \right)$$

$$\leq C(\frac{3}{\lambda})^2 \epsilon^2 .$$

Here we have used the L^2-boundedness of $\mathcal{K}_D$, which is an obvious consequence of Lemma 2.13. Since ϵ is arbitrary, $|A_\lambda| = 0$ for all $\lambda > 0$. This implies that

$$\lim_{t \to 0+} \mathcal{D}_D \phi(x \pm t\nu_x) = (\mp \frac{1}{2} I + \mathcal{K}_D) \phi(x) \qquad \text{a.e. } x \in \partial D$$

and completes the proof. $\qquad\qquad\qquad\qquad\qquad\qquad\qquad\qquad\qquad\qquad\qquad\square$

In a similar way, we can describe the behavior of the gradient of the single layer potential at the boundary. The following lemma reveals the connection between the traces $\partial \mathcal{S}_D / \partial \nu |_\pm$ and the operator $\mathcal{K}_D^*$ defined by (2.20).

Lemma 2.16 *If D is a bounded $C^{1+\alpha}$-domain for some $\alpha > 0$, then for $\phi \in L^2(\partial D)$:*

$$\frac{\partial}{\partial T} \mathcal{S}_D \phi \bigg|_+ (x) = \frac{\partial}{\partial T} \mathcal{S}_D \phi \bigg|_- (x) \qquad a.e. \ x \in \partial D$$

and

$$\frac{\partial}{\partial \nu} \mathcal{S}_D \phi \bigg|_\pm (x) = \left(\pm \frac{1}{2} I + \mathcal{K}_D^* \right) \phi(x) \qquad a.e. \ x \in \partial D .$$

2.3 Layer Potentials on Lipschitz Domains

2.3.1 Jump Relations

The next theorem gives the jump relations obeyed by the double layer potential and by the normal derivative of the single layer potential on general Lipschitz domains. The boundedness of these operators is not clear because of the critical singularity of the kernels [which is of order $O(|x - y|^{1-d})$] and the fact that we are dealing with non-convolution type operators. The following results can be proved using the deep theorem of Coifman–McIntosh–Meyer [98] on the boundedness of the Cauchy integral on Lipschitz curves (see Appendix A.2), which together with the method of rotations of Calderón [77] allows one to produce patterns of arguments like those found in [109] for $\mathcal{C}^1$-domains. Complete proofs that are beyond the scope of this book can be found in [298]. The jump relation (2.31), for general Lipschitz domains, is from the paper of Costabel [103].

Theorem 2.17 *Let D be a bounded Lipschitz domain in $\mathbb{R}^d$. For $\phi \in L^2(\partial D)$*

$$\mathcal{S}_D\phi\big|_+ (x) = \mathcal{S}_D\phi\big|_- (x) \quad a.e.\ x \in \partial D \,, \tag{2.25}$$

$$\frac{\partial}{\partial T}\mathcal{S}_D\phi\bigg|_+ (x) = \frac{\partial}{\partial T}\mathcal{S}_D\phi\bigg|_- (x) \quad a.e.\ x \in \partial D \,, \tag{2.26}$$

$$\frac{\partial}{\partial \nu}\mathcal{S}_D\phi\bigg|_\pm (x) = \left(\pm\frac{1}{2}I + \mathcal{K}_D^*\right)\phi(x) \quad a.e.\ x \in \partial D \,, \tag{2.27}$$

$$\mathcal{D}_D\phi\big|_\pm (x) = \left(\mp\frac{1}{2}I + \mathcal{K}_D\right)\phi(x) \quad a.e.\ x \in \partial D \,, \tag{2.28}$$

where $\mathcal{K}_D$ is defined by

$$\mathcal{K}_D\phi(x) = \frac{1}{\omega_d}p.v.\int_{\partial D} \frac{\langle y - x, \nu_y\rangle}{|x - y|^d}\phi(y)\,d\sigma(y) \tag{2.29}$$

and $\mathcal{K}_D^*$ is the L^2-adjoint of $\mathcal{K}_D$; i.e.,

$$\mathcal{K}_D^*\phi(x) = \frac{1}{\omega_d}p.v.\int_{\partial D} \frac{\langle x - y, \nu_x\rangle}{|x - y|^d}\phi(y)\,d\sigma(y) \,. \tag{2.30}$$

Here p.v. denotes the Cauchy principal value. The operators $\mathcal{K}_D$ and $\mathcal{K}_D^*$ are, for a Lipschitz domain D, singular integral operators and bounded on $L^2(\partial D)$. Moreover, for $\phi \in W_{\frac{1}{2}}^2(\partial D)$,

$$\frac{\partial}{\partial \nu}\mathcal{D}_D\phi\bigg|_- (x) = \frac{\partial}{\partial \nu}\mathcal{D}_D\phi\bigg|_+ (x) \quad in\ W_{-\frac{1}{2}}^2(\partial D) \,. \tag{2.31}$$

Note that (2.27) yields the following jump relation:

$$\frac{\partial}{\partial \nu}\mathcal{S}_D\phi\bigg|_{+} - \frac{\partial}{\partial \nu}\mathcal{S}_D\phi\bigg|_{-} = \phi \quad \text{on } \partial D . \tag{2.32}$$

We point out that the operators $\mathcal{K}_D$ and $\mathcal{K}_D^*$ are defined for a Lipschitz domain D as principal values of the integrals in (2.29) and (2.30) because of the critical singularity of their kernels. If D is a $\mathcal{C}^{1+\alpha}$-domain, then the definitions (2.29) and (2.18) coincide since the kernel has in this case a weak singularity. Similarly, the definitions (2.30) and (2.20) coincide if D is of class $\mathcal{C}^{1+\alpha}$, $\alpha > 0$.

Let D be a bounded Lipschitz domain in $\mathbb{R}^d$. Observe that again from Green's formula it follows that $\mathcal{D}_D(1)(x) = 1$ for any $x \in D$, and therefore, the jump relation (2.28) yields $\mathcal{K}_D(1) = 1/2$. It is worth mentioning recent results on two interesting questions in connection with this result.

On one hand, there is a conjecture that has not been resolved completely. Recall that $\mathcal{K}_D^*(1) = 1/2$ provided that D is a ball. The conjecture is that if $\mathcal{K}_D^*(1) = 1/2$ and D is a Lipschitz domain, then D is a ball. The conjecture has been proved to be true for some important classes of domains: piecewise smooth domains in $\mathbb{R}^2$ by Martensen [226], star-shaped $\mathcal{C}^{2+\alpha}$-domains by Payne and Philippin [264] and Philippin [268], and $\mathcal{C}^{2+\alpha}$-domains by Reichel [272, 273]. Recently Mendez and Reichel proved the conjecture for bounded Lipschitz domains in $\mathbb{R}^2$ and bounded Lipschitz convex domains in $\mathbb{R}^d$, $d \geq 3$. See [234].

On the other hand, according to (2.22), if D is a ball in $\mathbb{R}^d$, $d \geq 2$, then $\mathcal{K}_D$ is a self-adjoint operator on $L^2(\partial D)$. The converse is also true. Let D be a Lipschitz domain. If $\mathcal{K}_D$ is self-adjoint, then D is a ball. This was proved by Lim in [219].

2.3.2 Injectivity of $\lambda I - \mathcal{K}_D^*$

Let now D be a bounded Lipschitz domain, and let

$$L_0^2(\partial D) := \left\{\phi \in L^2(\partial D) : \int_{\partial D} \phi\, d\sigma = 0\right\} .$$

Let $\lambda \neq 0$ be a real number. Of particular interest for solving the transmission problem for the Laplacian would be the invertibility of the operator $\lambda I - \mathcal{K}_D^*$ on $L^2(\partial D)$ or $L_0^2(\partial D)$.

First, it was proved by Kellogg in [189] that the eigenvalues of $\mathcal{K}_D^*$ on $L^2(\partial D)$ lie in $]-1/2, 1/2]$ for smooth domains; but this argument goes through for Lipschitz domains [120]. The following injectivity result holds.

Lemma 2.18 *Let λ be a real number, and let D be a bounded Lipschitz domain. The operator $\lambda I - \mathcal{K}_D^*$ is one to one on $L_0^2(\partial D)$ if $|\lambda| \geq 1/2$, and for $\lambda \in]-\infty, -1/2] \cup]1/2, +\infty[$, $\lambda I - \mathcal{K}_D^*$ is one to one on $L^2(\partial D)$.*

Proof.   The argument is by contradiction. Let $\lambda \in]-\infty, -1/2]\cup]1/2, +\infty[$, and assume that $\phi \in L^2(\partial D)$ satisfies $(\lambda I - \mathcal{K}_D^*)\phi = 0$ and ϕ is not identically zero. Since $\mathcal{K}_D(1) = 1/2$ by Green's formula, we have

$$0 = \int_{\partial D} (\lambda I - \mathcal{K}_D^*)\phi \, d\sigma = \int_{\partial D} \phi(\lambda - \mathcal{K}_D(1)) \, d\sigma$$

and thus $\int_{\partial D} \phi \, d\sigma = 0$. Hence $\mathcal{S}_D\phi(x) = O(|x|^{1-d})$ and $\nabla\mathcal{S}_D\phi(x) = O(|x|^{-d})$ at infinity for $d \geq 2$. Since ϕ is not identically zero, both of the following numbers cannot be zero:

$$A = \int_D |\nabla\mathcal{S}_D\phi|^2 \, dx \text{ and } B = \int_{\mathbb{R}^d\setminus\overline{D}} |\nabla\mathcal{S}_D\phi|^2 \, dx \,.$$

In fact, if both of them are zero, then $\mathcal{S}_D\phi = $ constant in D and in $\mathbb{R}^d \setminus \overline{D}$. Hence $\phi = 0$ by (2.32), which is a contradiction.

On the other hand, using the divergence theorem and (2.27), we have

$$A = \int_{\partial D} (-\frac{1}{2}I + \mathcal{K}_D^*)\phi \, \mathcal{S}_D\phi \, d\sigma \text{ and } B = -\int_{\partial D} (\frac{1}{2}I + \mathcal{K}_D^*)\phi \, \mathcal{S}_D\phi \, d\sigma \,.$$

Since $(\lambda I - \mathcal{K}_D^*)\phi = 0$, it follows that

$$\lambda = \frac{1}{2}\frac{B - A}{B + A} \,.$$

Thus, $|\lambda| < 1/2$, which is a contradiction and so, for $\lambda \in]-\infty, -\frac{1}{2}]\cup]\frac{1}{2}, +\infty[$, $\lambda I - \mathcal{K}_D^*$ is one to one on $L^2(\partial D)$.

If $\lambda = 1/2$, then $A = 0$ and hence $\mathcal{S}_D\phi = $ constant in D. Thus $\mathcal{S}_D\phi$ is harmonic in $\mathbb{R}^d \setminus \partial D$, behaves like $O(|x|^{1-d})$ as $|x| \to +\infty$ [since $\phi \in L_0^2(\partial D)$], and is constant on ∂D. By (2.27), we have $\mathcal{K}_D^*\phi = (1/2)\,\phi$, and hence

$$B = -\int_{\partial D} \phi \, \mathcal{S}_D\phi \, d\sigma = C \int_{\partial D} \phi \, d\sigma = 0 \,,$$

which forces us to conclude that $\phi = 0$. This proves that $(1/2)\,I - \mathcal{K}_D^*$ is one to one on $L_0^2(\partial D)$. $\qquad\square$

2.3.3 Surjectivity of $\lambda I - \mathcal{K}_D^*$

Let us now turn to the surjectivity of the operator $\lambda I - \mathcal{K}_D^*$ on $L^2(\partial D)$ or $L_0^2(\partial D)$. If D is a bounded $\mathcal{C}^{1+\alpha}$-domain for some $\alpha > 0$, then as shown in Lemma 2.13, the operators $\mathcal{K}_D$ and $\mathcal{K}_D^*$ are compact operators in $L^2(\partial D)$. If D is a bounded $\mathcal{C}^1$-domain, the operators $\mathcal{K}_D$ and $\mathcal{K}_D^*$ are still compact operators in $L^2(\partial D)$ [122], but more elaborate arguments are needed for a proof. Hence, by the Fredholm alternative (see Appendix A.1), it follows from Lemma 2.18 that $\lambda I - \mathcal{K}_D^*$ is invertible on $L_0^2(\partial D)$ if $|\lambda| \geq 1/2$, and for $\lambda \in]-\infty, -1/2]\cup]1/2, +\infty[$, $\lambda I - \mathcal{K}_D^*$ is invertible on $L^2(\partial D)$.

From (2.15) we can also deduce that a constant C exists such that the estimate

$$\|\mathcal{K}_D\phi\|_{L^\infty(\partial D)} \leq C\|\phi\|_{L^\infty(\partial D)} \tag{2.33}$$

holds for all $\phi \in L^\infty(\partial D)$. Indeed, for any $\lambda \in]-\infty, -1/2] \cup]1/2, +\infty[$ a constant C_λ exists such that

$$\|\phi\|_{L^\infty(\partial D)} \leq C_\lambda\|(\lambda I - \mathcal{K}_D)\phi\|_{L^\infty(\partial D)}, \quad \forall\, \phi \in L^\infty(\partial D)\,. \tag{2.34}$$

Unlike the $\mathcal{C}^1$-case, the operators $\mathcal{K}_D$ and $\mathcal{K}_D^*$ are not compact on a Lipschitz domain and, thus, the Fredholm theory is not applicable. This difficulty for the invertibility of $\lambda I - \mathcal{K}_D^*$ was overcome by Verchota [298] who made the key observation that the following Rellich identities (see [274, 266, 254, 172]) are appropriate substitutes for compactness in the case of Lipschitz domains. In order to explain the Rellich identity, we need to fix a notation first. For a vector field $\boldsymbol{\alpha}$ and a function u, let

$$\langle \boldsymbol{\alpha}, \frac{\partial u}{\partial T}\rangle = \sum_{p=1}^{d-1}\langle \boldsymbol{\alpha}, T_p\rangle\frac{\partial u}{\partial T_p}\,.$$

Here $T_1, \ldots, T_{d-1}$ is an orthonormal basis for the tangent plane to ∂D at x.

Lemma 2.19 (Rellich's identities) *Let D be a bounded Lipschitz domain in $\mathbb{R}^d, d \geq 2$. Let u be a function such that either*

(i) *u is a Lipschitz function in $\overline{D}$ and $\Delta u = 0$ in D, or*
(ii) *u is a Lipschitz function in $\mathbb{R}^d \setminus D$, $\Delta u = 0$ in $\mathbb{R}^d \setminus \overline{D}$, and $|u(x)| = O(1/|x|^{d-2})$ when $d \geq 3$, and $|u(x)| = O(1/|x|)$ when $d = 2$, as $|x| \to +\infty$.*

Let $\boldsymbol{\alpha}$ be a $\mathcal{C}^1$-vector field in $\mathbb{R}^d$ with compact support. Then

$$\int_{\partial D}\langle \boldsymbol{\alpha}, \nu\rangle\left|\frac{\partial u}{\partial \nu}\right|^2 = \int_{\partial D}\langle \boldsymbol{\alpha}, \nu\rangle\left|\frac{\partial u}{\partial T}\right|^2 - 2\int_{\partial D}\langle \boldsymbol{\alpha}, \frac{\partial u}{\partial T}\rangle\frac{\partial u}{\partial \nu}$$
$$+ \begin{cases} \displaystyle\int_D\left(2\langle \nabla\boldsymbol{\alpha}\nabla u, \nabla u\rangle - (\nabla \cdot \boldsymbol{\alpha})|\nabla u|^2\right) & \text{if } u \text{ satisfies (i)}, \\[2ex] \displaystyle\int_{\mathbb{R}^d\setminus\overline{D}}\left(2\langle \nabla\boldsymbol{\alpha}\nabla u, \nabla u\rangle - (\nabla \cdot \boldsymbol{\alpha})|\nabla u|^2\right) & \text{if } u \text{ satisfies (ii)}. \end{cases} \tag{2.35}$$

Proof. Assume that u satisfies (i). Observe that

$$\nabla \cdot (\boldsymbol{\alpha}|\nabla u|^2) = (\nabla \cdot \boldsymbol{\alpha})|\nabla u|^2 + \langle \boldsymbol{\alpha}, \nabla|\nabla u|^2\rangle$$
$$= (\nabla \cdot \boldsymbol{\alpha})|\nabla u|^2 + 2\langle \partial^2 u\boldsymbol{\alpha}, \nabla u\rangle$$

and

$$\nabla \cdot (\nabla u\langle \boldsymbol{\alpha}, \nabla u\rangle) = \langle \boldsymbol{\alpha}, \nabla u\rangle\Delta u + \langle \nabla\langle \boldsymbol{\alpha}, \nabla u\rangle, \nabla u\rangle$$
$$= \langle \nabla\boldsymbol{\alpha}\nabla u, \nabla u\rangle + \langle \partial^2 u\boldsymbol{\alpha}, \nabla u\rangle\,.$$

Here $\partial^2 u$ is the Hessian of u. Combining these identities, we obtain

$$\nabla \cdot (\boldsymbol{\alpha}|\nabla u|^2) = 2\nabla \cdot (\nabla u \langle \boldsymbol{\alpha}, \nabla u\rangle) + (\nabla \cdot \boldsymbol{\alpha})|\nabla u|^2 - 2\langle \nabla \boldsymbol{\alpha} \nabla u, \nabla u\rangle \ .$$

Stokes's formula shows that

$$\int_{\partial D} \langle \boldsymbol{\alpha}, \nu\rangle |\nabla u|^2 = 2\int_{\partial D} \frac{\partial u}{\partial \nu} \langle \boldsymbol{\alpha}, \nabla u\rangle + \int_D \left((\nabla \cdot \boldsymbol{\alpha})|\nabla u|^2 - 2\langle \nabla \boldsymbol{\alpha} \nabla u, \nabla u\rangle \right) \ .$$

Since

$$\boldsymbol{\alpha} = \langle \boldsymbol{\alpha}, \nu\rangle \nu + \sum_{p=1}^{d-1} \langle \boldsymbol{\alpha}, T_p\rangle \, T_p \ ,$$

we get

$$\langle \boldsymbol{\alpha}, \nabla u\rangle = \langle \boldsymbol{\alpha}, \nu\rangle \frac{\partial u}{\partial \nu} + \langle \boldsymbol{\alpha}, \frac{\partial u}{\partial T}\rangle \ .$$

We also get

$$|\nabla u|^2 = \left| \frac{\partial u}{\partial \nu}\right|^2 + \left|\frac{\partial u}{\partial T}\right|^2 \ .$$

Thus, after rearranging, we find

$$\int_{\partial D} \langle \boldsymbol{\alpha}, \nu\rangle \left(\left|\frac{\partial u}{\partial \nu}\right|^2 + \left|\frac{\partial u}{\partial T}\right|^2 \right) = 2\int_{\partial D} \langle \boldsymbol{\alpha}, \nu\rangle \left|\frac{\partial u}{\partial \nu}\right|^2 + 2\int_{\partial D} \langle \boldsymbol{\alpha}, \frac{\partial u}{\partial T}\rangle \frac{\partial u}{\partial \nu}$$

$$+ \int_D (\nabla \cdot \boldsymbol{\alpha})|\nabla u|^2 - 2\langle \nabla \boldsymbol{\alpha} \nabla u, \nabla u\rangle \ .$$

Hence

$$\int_{\partial D} \langle \boldsymbol{\alpha}, \nu\rangle \left|\frac{\partial u}{\partial \nu}\right|^2 = \int_{\partial D} \langle \boldsymbol{\alpha}, \nu\rangle \left|\frac{\partial u}{\partial T}\right|^2 - 2\int_{\partial D} \langle \boldsymbol{\alpha}, \frac{\partial u}{\partial T}\rangle \frac{\partial u}{\partial \nu}$$

$$+ \int_D 2\langle \nabla \boldsymbol{\alpha} \nabla u, \nabla u\rangle - (\nabla \cdot \boldsymbol{\alpha})|\nabla u|^2 \ ,$$

and the identity (2.35) holds.

In order to establish the Rellich identity (2.35) when u satisfies (ii), we merely replace D by $\mathbb{R}^d \setminus \overline{D}$ in the above proof and use the decay estimate at infinity $|u(x)| = O(|x|^{2-d})$ when $d \geq 3$ and $|u(x)| = O(|x|^{-1})$ when $d = 2$ as $|x| \to +\infty$ to apply the Stokes's formula in all $\mathbb{R}^d \setminus \overline{D}$. $\qquad\square$

As an easy consequence of the Rellich identities (2.35), the following important result holds.

Corollary 2.20 *Let u be as in Lemma 2.19. Then a positive constant C exists depending only on the Lipschitz character of D such that*

$$\frac{1}{C} \left\| \frac{\partial u}{\partial T}\right\|_{L^2(\partial D)} \leq \left\| \frac{\partial u}{\partial \nu}\right\|_{L^2(\partial D)} \leq C \left\| \frac{\partial u}{\partial T}\right\|_{L^2(\partial D)} \ . \qquad (2.36)$$

Proof. Let c_0 be a fixed positive number. Let $\boldsymbol{\alpha}$ be a vector field supported in the set $\text{dist}(x, \partial D) < 2c_0$ such that $\boldsymbol{\alpha} \cdot \nu \geq \delta$ for some $\delta > 0$, $\forall\, x \in \partial D$ (here, δ depends only on the Lipschitz character of D). Applying (2.35) we obtain

$$\int_{\partial D} \langle \boldsymbol{\alpha}, \nu \rangle \left| \frac{\partial u}{\partial \nu} \right|^2 = \int_{\partial D} \langle \boldsymbol{\alpha}, \nu \rangle \left| \frac{\partial u}{\partial T} \right|^2$$
$$+ O\left(\left\| \frac{\partial u}{\partial T} \right\|_{L^2(\partial D)} \left\| \frac{\partial u}{\partial \nu} \right\|_{L^2(\partial D)} + \| \nabla u \|_{L^2(D)} \right).$$

Since

$$\| \nabla u \|_{L^2(D)}^2 = \int_{\partial D} u \frac{\partial u}{\partial \nu}\, d\sigma \leq \| u - u_0 \|_{L^2(\partial D)} \left\| \frac{\partial u}{\partial \nu} \right\|_{L^2(\partial D)}$$

(because $\int_{\partial D} \partial u / \partial \nu = 0$), where $u_0 = (1/|\partial D|) \int_{\partial D} u\, d\sigma$, the Poincaré inequality (2.1) yields

$$\| \nabla u \|_{L^2(D)}^2 \leq C \left\| \frac{\partial u}{\partial T} \right\|_{L^2(\partial D)} \left\| \frac{\partial u}{\partial \nu} \right\|_{L^2(\partial D)},$$

where the constant C depends only on the Lipschitz character of D. Thus

$$\int_{\partial D} \langle \boldsymbol{\alpha}, \nu \rangle \left| \frac{\partial u}{\partial \nu} \right|^2 = \int_{\partial D} \langle \boldsymbol{\alpha}, \nu \rangle \left| \frac{\partial u}{\partial T} \right|^2 + O\left(\left\| \frac{\partial u}{\partial T} \right\|_{L^2(\partial D)} \left\| \frac{\partial u}{\partial \nu} \right\|_{L^2(\partial D)} \right).$$

Employing the small constant–large constant argument:

$$2ab \leq \delta a^2 + \frac{1}{\delta} b^2 \quad \text{for small positive } \delta\,,$$

we conclude that estimates (2.36) hold. $\qquad\square$

The following results are due to Verchota [298] and Escauriaza, Fabes, and Verchota [120].

Theorem 2.21 *The operator $\lambda I - \mathcal{K}_D^*$ is invertible on $L_0^2(\partial D)$ if $|\lambda| \geq 1/2$, and for $\lambda \in\,]-\infty, -1/2] \cup]1/2, +\infty[$, $\lambda I - \mathcal{K}_D^*$ is invertible on $L^2(\partial D)$.*

Proof. Let us first prove that the operators $\pm (1/2)\, I + \mathcal{K}_D^* : L_0^2(\partial D) \to L_0^2(\partial D)$ are invertible. Observe that $\pm (1/2)\, I + \mathcal{K}_D^*$ maps $L_0^2(\partial D)$ into $L_0^2(\partial D)$. In fact, since $\mathcal{K}_D(1) = 1/2$, we have

$$\int_{\partial D} \mathcal{K}_D^* f\, d\sigma = \frac{1}{2} \int_{\partial D} f\, d\sigma$$

for all $f \in L^2(\partial D)$.

Let $u(x) = \mathcal{S}_D f(x)$, where $f \in L_0^2(\partial D)$. Then u satisfies conditions (i) and (ii) in Lemma 2.19. By virtue of the second formula (2.26) in Theorem 2.17,

$\partial u / \partial T$ is continuous across the boundary ∂D. Moreover, by the jump formula (2.27)

$$\frac{\partial u}{\partial \nu}\Big|_{\pm} = \left(\pm \frac{1}{2}I + \mathcal{K}_D^* \right) f \,.$$

We now apply Corollary 2.20 in D and $\mathbb{R}^d \setminus \overline{D}$ to obtain that

$$\left\| \frac{\partial u}{\partial \nu}\Big|_{-} \right\|_{L^2(\partial D)} \simeq \left\| \frac{\partial u}{\partial \nu}\Big|_{+} \right\|_{L^2(\partial D)} \,,$$

or equivalently

$$\frac{1}{C} \left\| (\frac{1}{2}I + \mathcal{K}_D^*)f \right\|_{L^2(\partial D)} \leq \left\| (\frac{1}{2}I - \mathcal{K}_D^*)f \right\|_{L^2(\partial D)} \,,$$
$$\left\| (\frac{1}{2}I - \mathcal{K}_D^*)f \right\|_{L^2(\partial D)} \leq C \left\| (\frac{1}{2}I + \mathcal{K}_D^*)f \right\|_{L^2(\partial D)} \,. \tag{2.37}$$

Here the constant C depends only on the Lipschitz character of D. Since

$$f = (\frac{1}{2}I + \mathcal{K}_D^*)f + (\frac{1}{2}I - \mathcal{K}_D^*)f \,,$$

(2.37) shows that

$$\left\| (\frac{1}{2}I + \mathcal{K}_D^*)f \right\|_{L^2(\partial D)} \geq C \|f\|_{L^2(\partial D)} \,. \tag{2.38}$$

In order to keep the technicalities to a minimum, we deal with the case when ∂D is given by a Lipschitz graph by localizing the situation. Assume

$$\partial D = \left\{ (x', x_d) : x_d = \varphi(x') \right\} \,,$$

where $\varphi : \mathbb{R}^{d-1} \to \mathbb{R}$ is a Lipschitz function. To show that $A = (1/2)\,I + \mathcal{K}_D^*$ is invertible, we consider the Lipschitz graph corresponding to $t\varphi$,

$$\partial D_t = \left\{ (x', x_d) : x_d = t\varphi(x') \right\} \quad \text{for } 0 < t < 1 \,,$$

and the corresponding operators $\mathcal{K}_{D_t}^*$ and A_t. Then $A_0 = (1/2)\,I, A_1 = A$, and A_t are continuous in norm as a function of t. Moreover, by (2.38), $\|A_t f\|_{L^2(\partial D_t)} \geq C\|f\|_{L^2(\partial D_t)}$, with C independent of t in $(0, 1)$ because the constant in (2.38) depends only on the Lipschitz character of D. The invertibility of A now follows from the continuity method; see Appendix A.3. This method establishes the invertibility of $(1/2)I + \mathcal{K}_D^*$ on $L_0^2(\partial D)$. The invertibility of $-(1/2)I + \mathcal{K}_D^*$ on $L_0^2(\partial D)$ can be proved in the same way starting from the inequality

$$\left\| (-\frac{1}{2}I + \mathcal{K}_D^*)f \right\|_{L^2(\partial D)} \geq C \|f\|_{L^2(\partial D)} \,.$$

We now show that $(1/2)\,I + \mathcal{K}_D^*$ is invertible on $L^2(\partial D)$. To do that, it suffices to show that it is onto on $L^2(\partial D)$. Since $\mathcal{K}_D(1) = 1/2$, we get

$$\int_{\partial D} (\frac{1}{2}I + \mathcal{K}_D^*)f\,d\sigma = \int_{\partial D} f\,d\sigma$$

for all $f \in L^2(\partial D)$. Let $h := ((1/2)\,I + \mathcal{K}_D^*)(1)$. For a given $g \in L^2(\partial D)$, let

$$g = g - ch + ch := g_0 + ch\,, \quad c = \frac{1}{|\partial D|}\int_{\partial D} g\,d\sigma\,.$$

Since

$$\int_{\partial D} h\,d\sigma = \int_{\partial D} (\frac{1}{2}I + \mathcal{K}_D^*)h\,d\sigma = |\partial D|\,,$$

one can easily see that $g_0 \in L_0^2(\partial D)$. Let $f_0 \in L_0^2(\partial D)$ be such that

$$((1/2)\,I + \mathcal{K}_D^*)f_0 = g_0\,.$$

Then $f := f_0 + c$ satisfies $((1/2)\,I + \mathcal{K}_D^*)f = g$. Thus $(1/2)\,I + \mathcal{K}_D^*$ is onto on $L^2(\partial D)$.

Assume now that $|\lambda| > 1/2$. Let $f \in L^2(\partial D)$ and set $u(x) = \mathcal{S}_D f(x)$. Let c_0 be a fixed positive number. Let $\boldsymbol{\alpha}$ be a vector field supported in the set $\mathrm{dist}(x, \partial D) < 2c_0$ such that $\boldsymbol{\alpha} \cdot \nu \geq \delta$ for some $\delta > 0$, $\forall\, x \in \partial D$. From the Rellich identity (2.35), we have

$$\int_{\partial D} \langle \boldsymbol{\alpha}, \nu \rangle \left|\frac{\partial u}{\partial \nu}\right|^2 = \int_{\partial D} \langle \boldsymbol{\alpha}, \nu \rangle \left|\frac{\partial u}{\partial T}\right|^2 - 2\int_{\partial D} \langle \boldsymbol{\alpha}, \frac{\partial u}{\partial T} \rangle \frac{\partial u}{\partial \nu} \tag{2.39}$$
$$+ \int_D 2\langle \nabla \boldsymbol{\alpha} \nabla u, \nabla u \rangle - (\nabla \cdot \boldsymbol{\alpha})|\nabla u|^2\,.$$

Observe that on ∂D

$$\left.\frac{\partial u}{\partial \nu}\right|_- = (-\frac{1}{2}I + \mathcal{K}_D^*)f = (\lambda - \frac{1}{2})f - (\lambda I - \mathcal{K}_D^*)f$$

and

$$\langle \nabla u, \boldsymbol{\alpha} \rangle = \frac{\partial u}{\partial \nu}\langle \boldsymbol{\alpha}, \nu \rangle + \langle \boldsymbol{\alpha}, \frac{\partial u}{\partial T} \rangle,$$
$$= -\frac{1}{2}\langle \boldsymbol{\alpha}, \nu \rangle f + \mathcal{K}_{\boldsymbol{\alpha}}f\,,$$

where

$$\mathcal{K}_{\boldsymbol{\alpha}}(f) = \frac{1}{\omega_d}\mathrm{p.v.}\int_{\partial D} \frac{\langle x - y, \boldsymbol{\alpha}(x) \rangle}{|x - y|^d} f(y)\,d\sigma(y)\,.$$

We also have

$$\int_D |\nabla u|^2\,dx = \int_{\partial D} u\left.\frac{\partial u}{\partial \nu}\right|_-\,d\sigma$$
$$= \int_{\partial D} \mathcal{S}_D(f)\left[(\lambda - \frac{1}{2})f - (\lambda I - \mathcal{K}_D^*)f\right]d\sigma\,.$$

By using

$$-2\int_{\partial D}\langle\boldsymbol{\alpha},\frac{\partial u}{\partial T}\rangle\frac{\partial u}{\partial\nu} = 2\int_{\partial D}\langle\boldsymbol{\alpha},\nu\rangle\left|\frac{\partial u}{\partial\nu}\right|^2 - 2\int_{\partial D}\frac{\partial u}{\partial\nu}\left[-\frac{1}{2}\langle\boldsymbol{\alpha},\nu\rangle f + \mathcal{K}_{\boldsymbol{\alpha}}(f)\right],$$

we get from (2.39) that

$$\frac{1}{2}\int_{\partial D}\langle\boldsymbol{\alpha},\nu\rangle\left|\frac{\partial u}{\partial\nu}\right|^2 = -\frac{1}{2}\int_{\partial D}\langle\boldsymbol{\alpha},\nu\rangle\left|\frac{\partial u}{\partial T}\right|^2 + \int_{\partial D}\frac{\partial u}{\partial\nu}\left[-\frac{1}{2}\langle\boldsymbol{\alpha},\nu\rangle f + \mathcal{K}_{\boldsymbol{\alpha}}(f)\right]$$
$$- \int_D\langle\nabla\boldsymbol{\alpha}\nabla u,\nabla u\rangle + \frac{1}{2}(\nabla\cdot\boldsymbol{\alpha})|\nabla u|^2 .$$

Thus we obtain

$$\frac{1}{2}\left(\lambda-\frac{1}{2}\right)^2\int_{\partial D}\langle\boldsymbol{\alpha},\nu\rangle f^2\,d\sigma$$
$$\leq \int_{\partial D}\left[-\frac{1}{2}\langle\boldsymbol{\alpha},\nu\rangle f + \mathcal{K}_{\boldsymbol{\alpha}}(f)\right]\left[(\lambda-\frac{1}{2})f - (\lambda I - \mathcal{K}_D^*)(f)\right]d\sigma$$
$$+C\|f\|_{L^2(\partial D)}\left(\|\mathcal{S}_D f\|_{L^2(\partial D)} + \|(\lambda I - \mathcal{K}_D^*)(f)\|_{L^2(\partial D)}\right)$$
$$+C\|\mathcal{S}_D f\|_{L^2(\partial D)}\|(\lambda I - \mathcal{K}_D^*)(f)\|_{L^2(\partial D)} + C\|(\lambda I - \mathcal{K}_D^*)(f)\|^2_{L^2(\partial D)} ,$$

where C denotes a constant depending on the Lipschitz character of D and λ. Multiplying out the integrand in the second integral above and taking to the left-hand side of the inequality the term involving f^2, we obtain

$$\frac{1}{2}\left(\lambda^2-\frac{1}{4}\right)\int_{\partial D}\langle\boldsymbol{\alpha},\nu\rangle f^2\,d\sigma \leq \left(\lambda-\frac{1}{2}\right)\int_{\partial D}\mathcal{K}_{\boldsymbol{\alpha}}(f)f\,d\sigma$$
$$+C\|f\|_{L^2(\partial D)}\left(\|\mathcal{S}_D f\|_{L^2(\partial D)} + \|(\lambda I - \mathcal{K}_D^*)(f)\|_{L^2(\partial D)}\right)$$
$$+C\|\mathcal{S}_D f\|_{L^2(\partial D)}\|(\lambda I - \mathcal{K}_D^*)(f)\|_{L^2(\partial D)} + C\|(\lambda I - \mathcal{K}_D^*)(f)\|^2_{L^2(\partial D)} .$$

If $\mathcal{K}_{\boldsymbol{\alpha}}^*$ denotes the adjoint operator on $L^2(\partial D)$ of the operator $\mathcal{K}_{\boldsymbol{\alpha}}$, it is easy to see that $\mathcal{K}_{\boldsymbol{\alpha}} + \mathcal{K}_{\boldsymbol{\alpha}}^* = R_{\boldsymbol{\alpha}}$, where the operator $R_{\boldsymbol{\alpha}}$ is defined by

$$R_{\boldsymbol{\alpha}}(f) = \frac{1}{\omega_d}\text{p.v.}\int_{\partial D}\frac{\langle x-y,\boldsymbol{\alpha}(x)-\boldsymbol{\alpha}(y)\rangle}{|x-y|^d}f(y)\,d\sigma(y) .$$

By duality, we have

$$\int_{\partial D}\mathcal{K}_{\boldsymbol{\alpha}}(f)f\,d\sigma = \frac{1}{2}\int_{\partial D}R_{\boldsymbol{\alpha}}(f)f\,d\sigma .$$

Since $|\lambda| > 1/2$ and $\boldsymbol{\alpha}\cdot\nu \geq \delta > 0$, using a small constant–large constant argument, we can get from the above inequality that

$$\|f\|_{L^2(\partial D)} \leq C\Big(\|(\lambda I - \mathcal{K}_D^*)(f)\|_{L^2(\partial D)} + \|\mathcal{S}_D f\|_{L^2(\partial D)}$$
$$+ \|R_{\boldsymbol{\alpha}}(f)\|_{L^2(\partial D)} \Big) . \tag{2.40}$$

Since $\mathcal{S}_D$ and $R_{\boldsymbol{\alpha}}$ are compact on $L^2(\partial D)$, we conclude from the above estimate that $\lambda I - \mathcal{K}_D^*$ has a closed range.

We now prove that $\lambda I - \mathcal{K}_D^*$ is surjective on $L^2(\partial D)$ and hence invertible on $L^2(\partial D)$ by Lemma 2.18.

Suppose on the contrary that for some λ real, $|\lambda| > 1/2$, $\lambda I - \mathcal{K}_D^*$ is not invertible on $L^2(\partial D)$. Then the intersection of the spectrum of $\mathcal{K}_D^*$ and the set $\{\lambda \in \mathbb{R} : |\lambda| > 1/2\}$ is not empty, and so a real number λ_0 exists that belongs to this intersection and is a boundary point of this set. To reach a contradiction it suffices to show that $\lambda_0 I - \mathcal{K}_D^*$ is invertible. By (2.40) we know that $\lambda_0 I - \mathcal{K}_D^*$ is injective and has a closed range. Hence a constant C exists such that for all $f \in L^2(\partial D)$ the following estimate holds:

$$\|f\|_{L^2(\partial D)} \leq C\|(\lambda_0 I - \mathcal{K}_D^*)(f)\|_{L^2(\partial D)} . \tag{2.41}$$

Since λ_0 is a boundary point of the intersection of spectrum of $\mathcal{K}_D^*$ and the real line, a sequence of real numbers λ_p exists with $|\lambda_p| > 1/2$, $\lambda_p \to \lambda_0$, as $p \to +\infty$, and $\lambda_p I - \mathcal{K}_D^*$ is invertible on $L^2(\partial D)$. Therefore, given $g \in L^2(\partial D)$, a unique $f_p \in L^2(\partial D)$ exists such that $(\lambda_p I - \mathcal{K}_D^*)(f_p) = g$. If $\|f_p\|_{L^2(\partial D)}$ has a bounded subsequence, then another subsequence exists that converges weakly to some f_0 in $L^2(\partial D)$ and we have

$$\int_{\partial D} (\lambda_p I - \mathcal{K}_D^*)(f_0) h \, d\sigma = \lim_{p \to +\infty} \int_{\partial D} f_p (\lambda_0 I - \mathcal{K}_D)(h) \, d\sigma$$
$$= \lim_{p \to +\infty} \int_{\partial D} (\lambda_0 I - \mathcal{K}_D^*)(f_p) h \, d\sigma = \int_{\partial D} g h \, d\sigma .$$

Hence $(\lambda_0 I - \mathcal{K}_D^*)(f_0) = g$. In the opposite case we may assume that $\|f_p\|_{L^2(\partial D)} = 1$ and $(\lambda_0 I - \mathcal{K}_D^*)(f_p)$ converges to zero in $L^2(\partial D)$.

However, it follows from (2.41) that

$$1 = \|f_p\|_{L^2(\partial D)} \leq C\|(\lambda_0 I - \mathcal{K}_D^*)(f_p)\|_{L^2(\partial D)}$$
$$\leq C|\lambda_0 - \lambda_p| + C\|(\lambda_p I - \mathcal{K}_D^*)(f_p)\|_{L^2(\partial D)} .$$

Since the final two terms converge to zero as $p \to +\infty$, we arrive at a contradiction. We conclude that for any λ real, $|\lambda| > 1/2$, $\lambda I - \mathcal{K}_D^*$ is invertible. $\qquad\square$

2.3.4 Mapping Properties

Analogously to (2.34) we can deduce from Theorem 2.21 that for any $\lambda \in \,]-\infty, -\frac{1}{2}] \cup]\frac{1}{2}, +\infty[$ a constant C_λ exists such that

$$\|\phi\|_{L^2(\partial D)} \leq C_\lambda \|(\lambda I - \mathcal{K}_D)\phi\|_{L^2(\partial D)}, \quad \forall\, \phi \in L^2(\partial D) . \tag{2.42}$$

Moreover,

$$\|\phi\|_{L^2(\partial D)} \leq C\|(-\frac{1}{2}I + \mathcal{K}_D)\phi\|_{L^2(\partial D)}, \quad \forall\, \phi \in L_0^2(\partial D)\,, \tag{2.43}$$

for some positive constant C.

Suppose $D \subset B_1(0)$ is a star-shaped domain with respect to the origin in two-dimensional space, where $B_1(0)$ is the disk of radius 1 and center 0. We can quantify the constant C. In order to do this, define

$$\delta(D) := \inf_{x \in \partial D} \langle x, \nu_x \rangle\,.$$

Note that, since D is a star-shaped domain with respect to the origin, $\delta(D) > 0$. For $\phi \in L_0^2(\partial D)$, set $u := \mathcal{S}_D\phi$. It follows from the Rellich identity (2.35) with $\boldsymbol{\alpha}(x) = x$ that

$$\int_{\partial D} \langle x, \nu \rangle \left|\frac{\partial u}{\partial T}\right|^2 d\sigma = \int_{\partial D} \langle x, \nu \rangle \left|\frac{\partial u}{\partial \nu}\right|_\pm\right|^2 d\sigma + 2\int_{\partial D} \langle x, \frac{\partial u}{\partial T}\rangle \frac{\partial u}{\partial \nu}\right|_\pm d\sigma\,,$$

which leads to the following estimates:

$$\delta\left\|\frac{\partial u}{\partial T}\right\|_{L^2(\partial D)}^2 \leq \left\|\frac{\partial u}{\partial \nu}\right|_\pm\right\|_{L^2(\partial D)}^2 + 2\left\|\frac{\partial u}{\partial \nu}\right|_\pm\right\|_{L^2(\partial D)}\left\|\frac{\partial u}{\partial T}\right\|_{L^2(\partial D)}\,,$$

$$\delta\left\|\frac{\partial u}{\partial \nu}\right|_\pm\right\|_{L^2(\partial D)}^2 \leq \left\|\frac{\partial u}{\partial T}\right\|_{L^2(\partial D)}^2 + 2\left\|\frac{\partial u}{\partial \nu}\right|_\pm\right\|_{L^2(\partial D)}\left\|\frac{\partial u}{\partial T}\right\|_{L^2(\partial D)}\,.$$

Therefore

$$\left\|\frac{\partial u}{\partial T}\right\|_{L^2(\partial D)}^2 \leq \frac{2\delta + 4}{\delta^2}\left\|\frac{\partial u}{\partial \nu}\right|_\pm\right\|_{L^2(\partial D)}^2\,,$$

$$\left\|\frac{\partial u}{\partial \nu}\right|_\pm\right\|_{L^2(\partial D)}^2 \leq \frac{2\delta + 4}{\delta^2}\left\|\frac{\partial u}{\partial T}\right\|_{L^2(\partial D)}^2\,.$$

Thus, by the jump formula (2.27), we get

$$\left\|(\pm\frac{1}{2}I + \mathcal{K}_D^*)\phi\right\|_{L^2(\partial D)} = \left\|\frac{\partial u}{\partial \nu}\right|_\pm\right\|_{L^2(\partial D)}$$

$$\leq \frac{2\delta + 4}{\delta^2}\left\|\frac{\partial u}{\partial \nu}\right|_\pm\right\|_{L^2(\partial D)}$$

$$= \frac{2\delta + 4}{\delta^2}\|(\mp\frac{1}{2}I + \mathcal{K}_D^*)\phi\|_{L^2(\partial D)}\,,$$

to conclude that

$$\|\phi\|_{L^2(\partial D)} \leq \|(\pm\frac{1}{2}I + \mathcal{K}_D^*)\phi\|_{L^2(\partial D)} + \|(\mp\frac{1}{2}I + \mathcal{K}_D^*)\phi\|_{L^2(\partial D)}$$

$$\leq \frac{(\delta + 2)^2}{\delta^2}\|(\pm\frac{1}{2}I + \mathcal{K}_D^*)\phi\|_{L^2(\partial D)}\,.$$

We have proved the following result from [43].

Lemma 2.22 *Let $D \subset B_1(0)$ be a star-shaped domain with respect to the origin, where $B_1(0)$ is the disk of radius 1 and center 0. Define $\delta(D) := \inf_{x \in \partial D}\langle x, \nu_x \rangle$. Then, for any $\phi \in L_0^2(\partial D)$,*

$$\|\phi\|_{L^2(\partial D)} \leq \frac{\left(\delta(D) + 2\right)^2}{\delta(D)^2}\left\|(\pm\frac{1}{2}I + \mathcal{K}_D^*)\phi\right\|_{L^2(\partial D)}\,.$$

Estimate (2.43) will be useful in Chapter 5. A more refined one will be needed in Chapter 4.

Lemma 2.23 *A constant C exists depending only on the Lipschitz character of D such that*

$$\|\phi\|_{L^2(\partial D)} \leq C\frac{|k - 1|}{k + 1}\left\|\left(\frac{k + 1}{2(k - 1)}I - \mathcal{K}_D^*\right)\phi\right\|_{L^2(\partial D)} \tag{2.44}$$

for all $\phi \in L_0^2(\partial D)$.

Proof. By (2.43), a constant C exists depending only on the Lipschitz character of D such that

$$\|\phi\|_{L^2(\partial D)} \leq C\|\left(\frac{1}{2}I - \mathcal{K}_D^*\right)\phi\|_{L^2(\partial D)}$$

for all $\phi \in L_0^2(\partial D)$. Hence we get

$$\|\phi\|_{L^2(\partial D)} \leq C\left\|\left(\frac{k + 1}{2(k - 1)}I - \mathcal{K}_D^*\right)\phi\right\|_{L^2(\partial D)} + \frac{C}{|k - 1|}\|\phi\|_{L^2(\partial D)}\,.$$

It then follows that for $k > C + 1$

$$\|\phi\|_{L^2(\partial D)} \leq \frac{C}{1 - \frac{C}{k-1}}\left\|\left(\frac{k + 1}{2(k - 1)}I - \mathcal{K}_D^*\right)\phi\right\|_{L^2(\partial D)},$$

and hence, if k is larger than $2C + 1$,

$$\|\phi\|_{L^2(\partial D)} \leq 2C\left\|\left(\frac{k + 1}{2(k - 1)}I - \mathcal{K}_D^*\right)\phi\right\|_{L^2(\partial D)}\,.$$

When k is smaller than $1/(C+1)$, we can proceed in the same way starting from the estimate

$$\|\phi\|_{L^2(\partial D)} \leq C \left\| \left(-\frac{1}{2}I - \mathcal{K}_D^* \right) \phi \right\|_{L^2(\partial D)} .$$

Now assume that $|k - 1|$ is small or, equivalently, λ is large. Then

$$\|\phi\|_{L^2(\partial D)} \leq \frac{1}{\lambda}\|\lambda\phi\|_{L^2(\partial D)} \leq \frac{1}{\lambda}\|(\lambda I - \mathcal{K}_D^*)\phi\|_{L^2(\partial D)} + \frac{1}{\lambda}\|\mathcal{K}_D^*\phi\|_{L^2(\partial D)} .$$

Since $\|\mathcal{K}_D^*\phi\|_{L^2(\partial D)} \leq C\|\phi\|_{L^2(\partial D)}$ for some C then, if $\lambda > 2C$, we get

$$\|\phi\|_{L^2(\partial D)} \leq \frac{2}{\lambda}\|(\lambda I - \mathcal{K}_D^*)\phi\|_{L^2(\partial D)} .$$

Since the norm on the right-hand side of (2.44) depends continuously on k, by a compactness argument, the proof is complete. $\qquad\square$

We will also prove the following theorem due to Verchota [298].

Theorem 2.24 *Let D be a bounded Lipschitz domain in $\mathbb{R}^d$. Then the single layer potential $\mathcal{S}_D$ maps $L^2(\partial D)$ into $W_1^2(\partial D)$ boundedly and $\mathcal{K}_D : W_1^2(\partial D) \to W_1^2(\partial D)$ is a bounded operator.*

Proof. That $\mathcal{S}_D$ maps $L^2(\partial D)$ into $W_1^2(\partial D)$ boundedly is clear. In fact, by Corollary 2.20, (2.27), and Theorem 2.21, we get

$$\left\| \frac{\partial(\mathcal{S}_D f)}{\partial T} \right\|_{L^2(\partial D)} \approx \left\| \frac{\partial(\mathcal{S}_D f)}{\partial \nu} \Big|_{-} \right\|_{L^2(\partial D)}$$

$$\approx \|(-\frac{1}{2}I + \mathcal{K}_D^*)f\|_{L^2(\partial D)} \leq C\|f\|_{L^2(\partial D)} .$$

Thus we have

$$\|\mathcal{S}_D f\|_{W_1^2(\partial D)} \leq C\|f\|_{L^2(\partial D)} .$$

Given $h \in W_1^2(\partial D)$, let v be the solution to the problem $\Delta v = 0$ in D and $v = h$ on ∂D. Then $v \in W^{1,2}(D)$. By Green's formula, we get

$$\mathcal{S}_D \left(\frac{\partial v}{\partial \nu}\Big|_{-} \right)(x) = \mathcal{D}_D(v|_{-})(x), \quad x \in \mathbb{R}^d \setminus \overline{D} .$$

It then follows from (2.28) that

$$(-\frac{1}{2}I + \mathcal{K}_D)h = \mathcal{S}_D \left(\frac{\partial v}{\partial \nu}\Big|_{-} \right) \quad \text{on } \partial D .$$

Therefore we get

$$\|\mathcal{K}_D h\|_{W_1^2(\partial D)} \leq \frac{1}{2}\|h\|_{W_1^2(\partial D)} + \left\|\mathcal{S}_D\left(\frac{\partial v}{\partial \nu}\Big|_-\right)\right\|_{W_1^2(\partial D)}$$

$$\leq \frac{1}{2}\|h\|_{W_1^2(\partial D)} + C\left\|\frac{\partial v}{\partial \nu}\Big|_-\right\|_{L^2(\partial D)} \leq C\|h\|_{W_1^2(\partial D)},$$

where the last inequality follows from Corollary 2.20. Thus we obtain that $\mathcal{K}_D : W_1^2(\partial D) \to W_1^2(\partial D)$ is bounded. $\qquad\square$

Finally, it is worth emphasizing that the integral operator $\lambda I - \mathcal{K}_D^*$ is singular as λ approaches $1/2$ (or $k \to +\infty$). The kernel of the operator $(1/2)I - \mathcal{K}_D^*$, $\mathrm{Ker}((1/2)I - \mathcal{K}_D^*)$, has the dimension equal to the number of connected components of D. Since $\lambda I - \mathcal{K}_D^* = (2\lambda - 1)\mathcal{K}_D^*$ on $\mathrm{Ker}((1/2)I - \mathcal{K}_D^*)$, a straightforward calculation shows that

$$\|(\lambda I - \mathcal{K}_D^*)^{-1}\|_{\mathcal{L}(L^2(\partial D), L^2(\partial D))} \geq \frac{1}{|2\lambda - 1|} \frac{1}{\|\mathcal{K}_D^*\|_{\mathcal{L}(L^2(\partial D), L^2(\partial D))}},$$

where $\mathcal{L}(L^2(\partial D), L^2(\partial D))$ denotes the space of continuous, linear transformations from $L^2(\partial D)$ to $L^2(\partial D)$. In fact, as long as $\lambda > 1/2$, the integral equation

$$(\lambda I - \mathcal{K}_D^*)\phi = g \quad \text{for } g \in L^2(\partial D) \tag{2.45}$$

has a unique solution and one simply discretizes it and solves it. When $\lambda \to (1/2)^+$, however, a systematic loss of accuracy occurs. The problem is that, in the limit $\lambda = 1/2$, the integral equation (2.45) is not invertible. See [287, 288, 141].

To solve (2.45), we decompose the right-hand side into a constant and a zero-mean part: $g = g_0 + (g - g_0), g_0 = (1/|\partial D|) \int_{\partial D} g \, d\sigma$. We also decompose the unknown density ϕ into a constant and a zero-mean part: $\phi = \phi_0 + (\phi - \phi_0), \phi_0 = (1/|\partial D|) \int_{\partial D} \phi \, d\sigma$. Since $\mathcal{K}_D(1) = 1/2$, the constant part of the unknown density ϕ is simply given by $\phi_0 = (1/(\lambda - (1/2))) g_0$. Thus, the integral equation (2.45) can be written as

$$(\lambda I - \mathcal{K}_D^*)(\phi - \phi_0) = g - \frac{1}{\lambda - \frac{1}{2}} g_0(\lambda I - \mathcal{K}_D^*)(1) \in L_0^2(\partial D),$$

which is well behaved.

This idea has been suggested (and numerically implemented) by Greengard and Lee [141] for the calculation of the electrostatic and thermal properties of systems made of piecewise, homogeneous, high-contrast materials.

2.3.5 Concept of Capacity

We conclude this section by investigating the invertibility of the single layer potential and by defining the concept of capacity. We shall see that complications develop when $d = 2$.

Lemma 2.25 *Let D be a bounded Lipschitz domain in $\mathbb{R}^d$. Let $\phi \in L^2(\partial D)$ satisfy $\mathcal{S}_D \phi = 0$ on ∂D.*

(i) *If $d \geq 3$, then $\phi = 0$.*
(ii) *If $d = 2$ and $\int_{\partial D} \phi = 0$, then $\phi = 0$.*

Proof. If $\mathcal{S}_D \phi = 0$ on ∂D, then $u = \mathcal{S}_D \phi$ satisfies $\Delta u = 0$ in $\mathbb{R}^d \setminus \partial D$, $u = 0$ on ∂D, and as $|x| \to +\infty$, we have $u(x) = O(|x|^{2-d})$ when $d \geq 3$. Moreover $u(x) = O(|x|^{1-d})$ as $|x| \to +\infty$ for $d \geq 2$ provided that $\int_{\partial D} \phi = 0$. Therefore, for large R,

$$\int_{B_R(0)\setminus \overline{D}} |\nabla u|^2 = \int_{\partial R(0)} \frac{\partial u}{\partial \nu} u = \begin{cases} O(R^{2-d}) & \text{if } d \geq 3 , \\ O(R^{-2}) & \text{if } d = 2 . \end{cases}$$

Sending $R \to +\infty$, we deduce that $\nabla u = 0$ in $\mathbb{R}^d \setminus \overline{D}$, and thus, u is constant in $\mathbb{R}^d \setminus \overline{D}$. Since $u = 0$ on ∂D, it follows that $u = 0$ in $\mathbb{R}^d \setminus \overline{D}$. But $\mathcal{S}_D \phi = 0$ in D, and hence, $\phi = \partial \mathcal{S}_D \phi / \partial \nu|_+ - \partial \mathcal{S}_D \phi / \partial \nu|_- = 0$ on ∂D. $\qquad \square$

Theorem 2.26 *Let D be a bounded Lipschitz domain in $\mathbb{R}^d$.*

(i) *If $d \geq 3$, then $\mathcal{S}_D : L^2(\partial D) \to W_1^2(\partial D)$ has a bounded inverse.*
(ii) *If $d = 2$, then the operator $A : L^2(\partial D) \times \mathbb{R} \to W_1^2(\partial D) \times \mathbb{R}$ defined by*

$$A(\phi, a) = \left(\mathcal{S}_D \phi + a, \int_{\partial D} \phi \right)$$

    has a bounded inverse.
(iii) *Suppose $d = 2$ and let $(\phi_e, a) \in L^2(\partial D) \times \mathbb{R}$ denote the solution of the system*

$$\begin{cases} \mathcal{S}_D \phi_e + a = 0 , \\ \int_{\partial D} \phi_e = 1 , \end{cases} \tag{2.46}$$

    then $\mathcal{S}_D : L^2(\partial D) \to W_1^2(\partial D)$ has a bounded inverse if and only if $a \neq 0$.

Proof. Since $W_1^2(\partial D) \hookrightarrow L^2(\partial D)$ is compact, it follows from Theorem 2.24 that the operator $\mathcal{S}_D : L^2(\partial D) \to W_1^2(\partial D)$ is Fredholm with zero index (see Appendix A.1). But, by Lemma 2.25, we have $\mathrm{Ker}(\mathcal{S}_D) = \{0\}$ when $d \geq 3$, and therefore, $\mathcal{S}_D$ has a bounded inverse.

We now establish that A has a bounded inverse. Since $\mathcal{S}_D : L^2(\partial D) \to W_1^2(\partial D)$ is Fredholm with zero index, we need only to prove injectivity. In fact, if $\mathcal{S}_D \phi + a = 0$ and $\int_{\partial D} \phi = 0$, then $\int_{\partial D} \mathcal{S}_D \phi \, \phi = 0$. But

$$\int_{\partial D} (\mathcal{S}_D \phi_e) \phi_e \, d\sigma = \int_{\partial D} \mathcal{S}_D \phi_e \left(\frac{\partial}{\partial \nu} \mathcal{S}_D \phi_e \Big|_+ - \frac{\partial}{\partial \nu} \mathcal{S}_D \phi_e \Big|_- \right)$$
$$= - \int_{\mathbb{R}^d} |\nabla \mathcal{S}_D \phi_e|^2 \, dx , \tag{2.47}$$

and consequently, $\mathcal{S}_D\phi = 0$ since $\mathcal{S}_D\phi \to 0$ as $|x| \to +\infty$. According to Lemma 2.25, this implies $\phi = 0$ and in turn $a = 0$.

Turning to part (iii), we note that if $a = 0$, then $\mathcal{S}_D$ cannot be invertible because $\mathcal{S}_D\phi_e = 0$. Thus, suppose that $a \neq 0$ and $\phi \in L^2(\partial D)$ exists such that $\mathcal{S}_D\phi = 0$. Define $\phi_0 = \phi - (\int_{\partial D} \phi)\phi_e$, and observe that

$$\mathcal{S}_D\phi_0 = -(\int_{\partial D} \phi)\mathcal{S}_D\phi_e = a \int_{\partial D} \phi \text{ and } \int_{\partial D} \phi_0 = 0 \,.$$

Hence $\int_{\partial D} \mathcal{S}_D\phi_0 \, \phi_0 = 0$ and therefore $\phi_0 = 0$. In turn, $\int_{\partial D} \phi = 0$ because $a \neq 0$, giving $\phi = 0$ by Lemma 2.25. Thus, the homogeneous equation $\mathcal{S}_D\phi = 0$ has only the trivial solution, and $\mathcal{S}_D$ is invertible. $\square$

Analogously to part (ii) in the above theorem, if $d \geq 3$, a unique $\phi_e \in L^2(\partial D)$ exists such that $\mathcal{S}_D\phi_e$ is constant on ∂D, and $\int_{\partial D} \phi_e = 1$. Moreover, because of (2.47), we get $\mathcal{S}_D\phi_e < 0$. The reciprocal of the positive constant $-\mathcal{S}_D\phi_e$ is called the capacity of ∂D, which is a quantity we denote by $\mathrm{cap}(\partial D)$, so that

$$\frac{1}{\mathrm{cap}(\partial D)} = -\mathcal{S}_D\phi_e \quad \text{when } d \geq 3 \,. \tag{2.48}$$

This terminology has its origins in electrostatics. The capacity of an isolated conductor is defined as the ratio of the charge in equilibrium on it to the value of the potential at its surface. This definition may be restated as follows. We form the solution u of the Dirichlet problem for the domain outside the conductor D, with boundary values 1. The capacity $\mathrm{cap}(\partial D)$ is given by

$$\mathrm{cap}(\partial D) = -\int_{\partial D} \frac{\partial u}{\partial \nu}\Big|_+ (x)\, d\sigma(x) \quad \left(= \int_{\mathbb{R}^d \setminus D} |\nabla u|^2 \, dx\right) \,.$$

The solution u behaves like the point source $-\mathrm{cap}(\partial D)\Gamma(x)$ at infinity.

In the two-dimensional case, we introduce the logarithmic capacity,

$$\mathrm{cap}(\partial D) = e^{2\pi a} \,,$$

where a is defined by (2.46).

In the case of the unit ball $B_1(0)$, it is clear that $\mathrm{cap}(\partial B_1(0)) = 1$ if $d = 2$, and $\mathrm{cap}(\partial B_1(0)) = (d-2)\omega_d$ if $d \geq 3$.

Additional interesting properties of the capacity are given in the books by Hille [151], Landkof [210], and Armitage and Gardiner [47].

2.4 Neumann and Dirichlet Functions

Let Ω be a bounded Lipschitz domain in $\mathbb{R}^d, d \geq 2$. Let $N(x, z)$ be the Neumann function for $-\Delta$ in Ω corresponding to a Dirac mass at z. That is, N is the solution to

$$\begin{cases} -\Delta_x N(x, z) = \delta_z & \text{in } \Omega \, , \\ \dfrac{\partial N}{\partial \nu_x}\Big|_{\partial\Omega} = -\dfrac{1}{|\partial\Omega|} \, , \displaystyle\int_{\partial\Omega} N(x, z)\, d\sigma(x) = 0 & \text{for } z \in \Omega \, . \end{cases} \qquad (2.49)$$

Note that the Neumann function $N(x, z)$ is defined as a function of $x \in \overline{\Omega}$ for each fixed $z \in \Omega$.

The operator defined by $N(x, z)$ is the solution operator for the Neumann problem

$$\begin{cases} \Delta U = 0 & \text{in } \Omega \, , \\ \dfrac{\partial U}{\partial \nu}\Big|_{\partial\Omega} = g \, ; \end{cases} \qquad (2.50)$$

namely, the function U defined by

$$U(x) := \int_{\partial\Omega} N(x, z) g(z) \, d\sigma(z)$$

is the solution to (2.50) satisfying $\int_{\partial\Omega} U \, d\sigma = 0$.

Now we discuss some properties of N as a function of x and z.

Lemma 2.27 *The Neumann function N is symmetric in its arguments; that is, $N(x, z) = N(z, x)$ for $x \neq z \in \Omega$. It furthermore has the form*

$$N(x, z) = \begin{cases} -\dfrac{1}{2\pi} \ln |x - z| + R_2(x, z) & \text{if } d = 2 \, , \\[2ex] \dfrac{1}{(d-2)\omega_d} \dfrac{1}{|x - z|^{d-2}} + R_d(x, z) & \text{if } d \geq 3 \, , \end{cases} \qquad (2.51)$$

where $R_d(\cdot, z)$ belongs to $W^{\frac{3}{2}, 2}(\Omega)$ for any $z \in \Omega, d \geq 2$ and solves

$$\begin{cases} \Delta_x R_d(x, z) = 0 & \text{in } \Omega \, , \\ \dfrac{\partial R_d}{\partial \nu_x}\Big|_{\partial\Omega} = -\dfrac{1}{|\partial\Omega|} + \dfrac{1}{\omega_d} \dfrac{\langle x - z, \nu_x \rangle}{|x - z|^d} & \text{for } x \in \partial\Omega \, . \end{cases}$$

Proof. Pick $z_1, z_2 \in \Omega$ with $z_1 \neq z_2$. Let $B_r(z_p) = \{|x - z_p| < r\}$, $p = 1, 2$. Choose $r > 0$ so small that $B_r(z_1) \cap B_r(z_2) = \emptyset$. Set $N_1(x) = N(x, z_1)$ and $N_2(x) = N(x, z_2)$. We apply Green's formula in $\Omega' = \Omega \setminus B_r(z_1) \cup B_r(z_2)$ to get

$$\int_{\Omega'} \left(N_1 \Delta N_2 - N_2 \Delta N_1 \right) dx = \int_{\partial\Omega} \left(N_1 \frac{\partial N_2}{\partial \nu} - N_2 \frac{\partial N_1}{\partial \nu} \right) d\sigma$$

$$- \int_{\partial B_r(z_1)} \left(N_1 \frac{\partial N_2}{\partial \nu} - N_2 \frac{\partial N_1}{\partial \nu} \right) d\sigma - \int_{\partial B_r(z_2)} \left(N_1 \frac{\partial N_2}{\partial \nu} - N_2 \frac{\partial N_1}{\partial \nu} \right) d\sigma \, ,$$

where all the derivatives are with respect to the x-variable with z fixed. Since N_p, $p = 1, 2$, is harmonic for $x \neq z_p$, $\partial N_1/\partial\nu = \partial N_2/\partial\nu = -1/|\partial\Omega|$, and $\int_{\partial\Omega}(N_1 - N_2) \, d\sigma = 0$, we have

$$\int_{\partial B_r(z_1)} \left(N_1 \frac{\partial N_2}{\partial \nu} - N_2 \frac{\partial N_1}{\partial \nu} \right) d\sigma + \int_{\partial B_r(z_2)} \left(N_1 \frac{\partial N_2}{\partial \nu} - N_2 \frac{\partial N_1}{\partial \nu} \right) d\sigma = 0 \; .$$
$$(2.52)$$

Thanks to (2.51), which will be proved shortly, the left-hand side of (2.52) has the same limit as $r \to 0$ as the left-hand side of the following identity:

$$\int_{\partial B_r(z_1)} \left(\Gamma \frac{\partial N_2}{\partial \nu} - N_2 \frac{\partial \Gamma}{\partial \nu} \right) d\sigma + \int_{\partial B_r(z_2)} \left(N_1 \frac{\partial \Gamma}{\partial \nu} - \Gamma \frac{\partial N_1}{\partial \nu} \right) d\sigma = 0 \; .$$

Since

$$\int_{\partial B_r(z_1)} \Gamma \frac{\partial N_2}{\partial \nu} \, d\sigma \to 0 \; , \quad \int_{\partial B_r(z_2)} \Gamma \frac{\partial N_1}{\partial \nu} \, d\sigma \to 0 \quad \text{as } r \to 0 \; ,$$

and

$$\int_{\partial B_r(z_1)} N_2 \frac{\partial \Gamma}{\partial \nu} \, d\sigma \to N_2(z_1) \; , \quad \int_{\partial B_r(z_2)} N_1 \frac{\partial \Gamma}{\partial \nu} \, d\sigma \to N_1(z_2) \quad \text{as } r \to 0 \; ,$$

we obtain $N_2(z_1) - N_1(z_2) = 0$, or equivalently $N(z_2, z_1) = N(z_1, z_2)$ for any $z_1 \neq z_2 \in \Omega$.

Now let $R_d, d \geq 2$, be defined by

$$R_d(x, z) = \begin{cases} N(x, z) + \dfrac{1}{2\pi} \ln |x - z| & \text{if } d = 2 \; , \\[2mm] N(x, z) + \dfrac{1}{(2 - d)\omega_d} \dfrac{1}{|x - z|^{d-2}} & \text{if } d \geq 3 \; . \end{cases}$$

Since $R_d(\cdot, z)$ is harmonic in Ω and $\partial R_d(\cdot, z)/\partial \nu \in L^2(\partial\Omega)$, it follows from the standard elliptic regularity theory, (see [172] for example) that $R_d(\cdot, z) \in W^{\frac{3}{2}, 2}(\Omega)$ for any $z \in \Omega$. $\qquad\square$

For D, a subset of Ω, let

$$N_D f(x) := \int_{\partial D} N(x, y) f(y) \, d\sigma(y), \quad x \in \Omega \; .$$

The following lemma from [22] relates the fundamental solution Γ to the Neumann function N.

Lemma 2.28 *For $z \in \Omega$ and $x \in \partial\Omega$, let $\Gamma_z(x) := \Gamma(x - z)$ and $N_z(x) := N(x, z)$. Then*

$$\left(-\frac{1}{2} I + \mathcal{K}_\Omega \right)(N_z)(x) = \Gamma_z(x) \quad \text{modulo constants}, \quad x \in \partial\Omega \; , \qquad (2.53)$$

or, to be more precise, for any simply connected Lipschitz domain D compactly contained in Ω and for any $g \in L_0^2(\partial D)$, we have for any $x \in \partial\Omega$

$$\int_{\partial D} \left(-\frac{1}{2} I + \mathcal{K}_\Omega \right)(N_z)(x) g(z) \, d\sigma(z) = \int_{\partial D} \Gamma_z(x) g(z) \, d\sigma(z) \qquad (2.54)$$

or, equivalently,

$$\left(-\frac{1}{2}I + \mathcal{K}_\Omega\right)\left((N_D g)\big|_{\partial\Omega}\right)(x) = \mathcal{S}_D g(x) \ . \tag{2.55}$$

Proof. Let $f \in L_0^2(\partial\Omega)$ and define

$$u(z) := \int_{\partial\Omega} \left(-\frac{1}{2}I + \mathcal{K}_\Omega\right)(N_z)(x) f(x)\, d\sigma(x), \quad z \in \Omega \ .$$

Then

$$u(z) = \int_{\partial\Omega} N(x,z)\left(-\frac{1}{2}I + \mathcal{K}_\Omega^*\right)f(x)\, d\sigma(x) \ .$$

Therefore, $\Delta u = 0$ in Ω and

$$\frac{\partial u}{\partial \nu}\bigg|_{\partial\Omega} = (-\frac{1}{2}I + \mathcal{K}_\Omega^*)f \ .$$

Hence by the uniqueness modulo constants of a solution to the Neumann problem, we have

$$u(z) - \mathcal{S}_\Omega f(z) = \text{constant}, \quad z \in \Omega \ .$$

Thus if $g \in L_0^2(\partial D)$, we obtain

$$\int_{\partial\Omega}\int_{\partial D}\left(-\frac{1}{2}I + \mathcal{K}_\Omega\right)(N_z)(x)g(z)f(x)\, d\sigma(z)\, d\sigma(x)$$
$$= \int_{\partial\Omega}\int_{\partial D} \Gamma_z(x)g(z)f(x)\, d\sigma(z)\, d\sigma(x) \ .$$

Since f is arbitrary, we have (2.53) or, equivalently, (2.54). This completes the proof. $\square$

The following simple observation is useful.

Lemma 2.29 *Let $f \in L^2(\partial\Omega)$ satisfy $\left(\frac{1}{2}I - \mathcal{K}_\Omega\right)f = 0$. Then f is constant.*

Proof. Let $f \in L^2(\partial\Omega)$ be such that $((1/2)I - \mathcal{K}_\Omega)f = 0$. Then for any $g \in L^2(\partial\Omega)$

$$\int_{\partial\Omega} (\frac{1}{2}I - \mathcal{K}_\Omega)f(x)g(x)\, d\sigma(x) = 0$$

or, equivalently,

$$\int_{\partial\Omega} f(x)(\frac{1}{2}I - \mathcal{K}_\Omega^*)g(x)\, d\sigma(x) = 0 \ .$$

But $\text{Range}((1/2)I - \mathcal{K}_\Omega^*) = L_0^2(\partial\Omega)$ and so, f is constant. $\square$

In Chapter 5 we will be dealing with conductivity inclusions of the form $D = \epsilon B + z$ where B is a bounded Lipschitz domain in $\mathbb{R}^d$. For the purpose of use in Chapter 5, we now expand $N(x, \epsilon y + z)$ asymptotically for $x \in \partial\Omega$, $z \in \Omega$, and $y \in \partial B$, and as $\epsilon \to 0$.

Recall that if $j = (j_1, \ldots, j_d)$ is a multi-index (an ordered d-tuple of non-negative integers), then we write $j! = j_1! \ldots j_d!$, $y^j = y_1^{j_1} \ldots y_d^{j_d}$, $|j| = j_1 + \cdots + j_d$, and $\partial^j = \partial^{|j|}/\partial y_1^{j_1} \ldots \partial y_d^{j_d}$.

By (2.53) we have the following relation:

$$\left(-\frac{1}{2}I + \mathcal{K}_\Omega\right)\left[N(\cdot, \epsilon y + z)\right](x) = \Gamma(x - z - \epsilon y) \quad \text{modulo constants,} \quad x \in \partial\Omega .$$

Using the Taylor expansion

$$\Gamma(x - \epsilon y) = \sum_{|j|=0}^{+\infty} \frac{(-1)^{|j|}}{j!} \epsilon^{|j|} \partial^j \Gamma(x) y^j ,$$

we obtain

$$\left(-\frac{1}{2}I + \mathcal{K}_\Omega\right)\left[N(\cdot, \epsilon y + z)\right](x) = \sum_{|j|=0}^{+\infty} \frac{(-1)^{|j|}}{j!} \epsilon^{|j|} \partial^j (\Gamma(x - z)) y^j$$

$$= \sum_{|j|=0}^{+\infty} \frac{(-1)^{|j|}}{j!} \epsilon^{|j|} \partial_x^j \left(\left(-\frac{1}{2}I + \mathcal{K}_\Omega\right) N(\cdot, z)(x)\right) y^j$$

$$= \sum_{|j|=0}^{+\infty} \frac{1}{j!} \epsilon^{|j|} \left(\left(-\frac{1}{2}I + \mathcal{K}_\Omega\right) \partial_z^j N(\cdot, z)(x)\right) y^j$$

$$= \left(-\frac{1}{2}I + \mathcal{K}_\Omega\right)\left[\sum_{|j|=0}^{+\infty} \frac{1}{j!} \epsilon^{|j|} \partial_z^j N(\cdot, z) y^j\right](x) .$$

Since $\int_{\partial\Omega} N(x, w) \, d\sigma(x) = 0$ for all $w \in \Omega$, we have the following asymptotic expansion of the Neumann function.

Lemma 2.30 *For $x \in \partial\Omega$, $z \in \Omega$, and $y \in \partial B$, and as $\epsilon \to 0$,*

$$N(x, \epsilon y + z) = \sum_{|j|=0}^{+\infty} \frac{1}{j!} \epsilon^{|j|} \partial_z^j N(x, z) y^j . \tag{2.56}$$

We mention that the Neumann function for the ball $B_R(0)$ is given, for any $x, z \in B_R(0)$, by

$$N(x, z) = \frac{1}{4\pi |x - z|} + \frac{1}{4\pi |\frac{R}{|x|} x - \frac{|x|}{R} z|}$$

$$+ \frac{1}{4\pi R} \ln \frac{2}{1 - \frac{x \cdot z}{R^2} + \frac{1}{R}|\frac{|x|}{R} z - \frac{R}{|x|} x|} - \frac{1}{2\pi R} \quad \text{for } d = 3 , \tag{2.57}$$

and by

$$N(x,z) = -\frac{1}{2\pi}\left(\ln|x-z| + \ln\left|\frac{R}{|x|}x - \frac{|x|}{R}z\right| \right) + \frac{\ln R}{\pi} \quad \text{for } d = 2 . \quad (2.58)$$

See [212].

Now we turn to the properties of the Dirichlet function. Let $G(x,z)$ be the Green's function for the Dirichlet problem in Ω; that is, the unique solution to

$$\begin{cases} \Delta_x G(x,z) = -\delta_z & \text{in } \Omega , \\ G(x,z) = 0 & \text{on } \partial\Omega , \end{cases}$$

and let $G_z(x) = G(x,z)$. Then for any $x \in \partial\Omega$ and $z \in \Omega$, we can prove in the same way as (2.53) that

$$\left(\frac{1}{2}I + \mathcal{K}_\Omega^*\right)^{-1}\left(\frac{\partial\Gamma_z(y)}{\partial\nu_y}\right)(x) = -\frac{\partial G_z}{\partial\nu_x}(x) . \quad (2.59)$$

Moreover, we would like to mention the following important properties of G (see [143]):

(i) the Green's function G is symmetric in $\Omega \times \Omega$;

(ii) the maximum principle implies that for $x, z \in \Omega$ with $x \neq z$

$$0 > G(x,z) > -\Gamma(x-z) \quad \text{for } d \geq 3 ,$$

$$0 > G(x,z) > -\Gamma(x-z) + \frac{1}{2\pi}\ln \operatorname{diam}(\Omega) \quad \text{for } d = 2 ;$$

(iii) the Green's function for the ball $B_R(0)$ is given by

$$G(x,z) = \frac{1}{(2-d)\omega_d}\left(|x-z|^{2-d} - \left|\frac{R}{|x|}x - \frac{|x|}{R}z\right|^{2-d} \right) \quad \text{for } d \geq 3 ,$$

$$G(x,z) = \frac{1}{2\pi}\left(\ln|x-z| - \ln\left|\frac{R}{|x|}x - \frac{|x|}{R}z\right| \right) \quad \text{for } d = 2 ;$$

(iv) the normal derivative of the Green's function on the sphere $\partial B_R(0)$ is given by

$$\frac{\partial G}{\partial\nu}(x,z) = \frac{R^2 - |z|^2}{\omega_d R|x-z|^d} \quad \text{for any } z \in B_R(0) \text{ and } x \in \partial B_R(0) .$$

We shall also recall, in connection with part (iv), that the function

$$\frac{R^2 - |z|^2}{\omega_d R|x-z|^d} \quad (z \in B_R(0), x \in \partial B_R(0))$$

is the Poisson kernel of the ball $B_R(0)$. On the other hand, if we consider the half-space $\mathbb{R}^d_+ = \{z = (z', z_d) \in \mathbb{R}^d : z_d > 0\}$, then the function

$$\frac{2z_d}{\omega_d |x - z|^d} \quad (z \in \mathbb{R}_+^d, x \in \partial\mathbb{R}_+^d)$$

is the Poisson kernel for $\mathbb{R}_+^d$, and for any $g \in \mathcal{C}^0(\mathbb{R}^{d-1}) \cap L^\infty(\mathbb{R}^{d-1})$, the following formula holds:

$$\lim_{z \to y, z \in \mathbb{R}_+^d} \frac{2z_d}{\omega_d} \int_{\partial\mathbb{R}_+^d} \frac{g(x')}{|(x',0) - z|^d} \, dx' = g(y) \quad \text{for each } y \in \partial\mathbb{R}_+^d . \tag{2.60}$$

2.5 Representation Formula

Let Ω be a bounded domain in $\mathbb{R}^d$ with a connected Lipschitz boundary and conductivity equal to 1. Consider a bounded domain $D \subset\subset \Omega$ with a connected Lipschitz boundary and conductivity $0 < k \neq 1 < +\infty$.

Let $g \in L_0^2(\partial\Omega)$, and let u and U be, respectively, the (variational) solutions of the Neumann problems

$$\begin{cases} \nabla \cdot \left(1 + (k-1)\chi(D)\right)\nabla u = 0 \quad \text{in } \Omega , \\[2mm] \left.\dfrac{\partial u}{\partial \nu}\right|_{\partial\Omega} = g , \\[2mm] \displaystyle\int_{\partial\Omega} u(x)\, d\sigma(x) = 0 , \end{cases} \tag{2.61}$$

and

$$\begin{cases} \Delta U = 0 \quad \text{in } \Omega , \\[2mm] \left.\dfrac{\partial U}{\partial \nu}\right|_{\partial\Omega} = g , \\[2mm] \displaystyle\int_{\partial\Omega} U(x)\, d\sigma(x) = 0 , \end{cases} \tag{2.62}$$

where $\chi(D)$ is the characteristic function of D. Clearly, the Lax–Milgram lemma shows that, given $g \in L_0^2(\partial\Omega)$, unique u and U in $W^{1,2}(\Omega)$ exist, which solve (2.61) and (2.62).

At this point we have all the necessary ingredients to state and prove a decomposition formula of the steady-state voltage potential u into a harmonic part and a refraction part, which will be the main tool for both deriving the asymptotic expansion in Chapter 5 and providing efficient reconstruction algorithms in Chapter 7. This decomposition formula is unique and seems to inherit geometric properties of the inclusion D, as shown in Chapter 4.

The following theorem was proved in [180, 181, 183].

Theorem 2.31 *Suppose that D is a domain compactly contained in Ω with a connected Lipschitz boundary and conductivity $0 < k \neq 1 < +\infty$. Then the solution u of the Neumann problem (2.61) is represented as*

$$u(x) = H(x) + \mathcal{S}_D\phi(x), \quad x \in \mathbb{R}^d \setminus \partial\Omega , \tag{2.63}$$

where the harmonic function H is given by

$$H(x) = -\mathcal{S}_\Omega(g)(x) + \mathcal{D}_\Omega(f)(x), \quad x \in \Omega , \quad f := u|_{\partial\Omega} \in W_{\frac{1}{2}}^2(\partial\Omega) , \tag{2.64}$$

and $\phi \in L_0^2(\partial D)$ satisfies the integral equation

$$\left(\frac{k+1}{2(k-1)}I - \mathcal{K}_D^*\right)\phi = \left.\frac{\partial H}{\partial\nu}\right|_{\partial D} \quad on \ \partial D . \tag{2.65}$$

The decomposition (2.63) into a harmonic part and a refraction part is unique. Moreover, $\forall \, n \in \mathbb{N}$, a constant $C_n = C(n, \Omega, \mathrm{dist}(D, \partial\Omega))$ exists independent of D and the conductivity k such that

$$\|H\|_{\mathcal{C}^n(\overline{D})} \leq C_n \|g\|_{L^2(\partial\Omega)} . \tag{2.66}$$

Furthermore, the following holds:

$$H(x) + \mathcal{S}_D\phi(x) = 0, \quad \forall \, x \in \mathbb{R}^d \setminus \overline{\Omega} . \tag{2.67}$$

Proof.   Consider the following two-phase transmission problem:

$$\begin{cases} \nabla \cdot \left(1 + (k-1)\chi(D)\right)\nabla v = 0 & \text{in } \mathbb{R}^d \setminus \partial\Omega , \\[2mm] v\big|_- - v\big|_+ = f & \text{on } \partial\Omega , \\[2mm] \dfrac{\partial v}{\partial\nu}\Big|_- - \dfrac{\partial v}{\partial\nu}\Big|_+ = g & \text{on } \partial\Omega , \\[2mm] v(x) = O(|x|^{1-d}) & \text{as } |x| \to +\infty . \end{cases} \tag{2.68}$$

Let $v_1 := -\mathcal{S}_\Omega g + \mathcal{D}_\Omega f + \mathcal{S}_D\phi$ in $\mathbb{R}^d$. Since $\phi \in L_0^2(\partial D)$ and $g \in L_0^2(\partial\Omega)$, $v_1(x) = O(|x|^{1-d})$ and hence v_1 is a solution of (2.68) by the jump formulae (2.27), (2.28), and (2.31). If we put $v_2 = u$ in Ω and $v_2 = 0$ in $\mathbb{R}^d \setminus \overline{\Omega}$, then v_2 is also a solution of (2.68). Therefore, in order to prove (2.63) and (2.67), it suffices to show that the problem (2.68) has a unique solution in $W_{\mathrm{loc}}^{1,2}(\mathbb{R}^d \setminus \partial\Omega)$.

Suppose that $v \in W_{\mathrm{loc}}^{1,2}(\mathbb{R}^d \setminus \partial\Omega)$ is a solution of (2.68) with $f = g = 0$. Then v is a variational solution of $\nabla \cdot (1 + (k-1)\chi(D))\nabla v = 0$ in the entire domain $\mathbb{R}^d$. Therefore, for a large R,

$$\int_{B_R(0)} |\nabla v|^2 \leq \frac{1+k}{k}\int_{B_R(0)} \left(1 + (k-1)\chi(D)\right)|\nabla v|^2$$

$$\leq \frac{1+k}{k}\int_{\partial B_R(0)} v\frac{\partial v}{\partial\nu}$$

$$\leq -\frac{1+k}{k}\int_{\mathbb{R}^d \setminus \overline{B_R(0)}} |\nabla v|^2 \leq 0 ,$$

where $B_R(0) = \{|x| < R\}$. This inequality holds for all R and hence v is constant. Since $v(x) \to 0$ at infinity, we conclude that $v \equiv 0$.

To prove the uniqueness of the representation, suppose that H' is harmonic in Ω and

$$H + S_D\phi = H' + S_D\phi' \quad \text{in } \Omega .$$

Then $S_D(\phi - \phi')$ is harmonic in Ω and hence

$$\left.\frac{\partial}{\partial\nu}S_D(\phi - \phi')\right|_{-} = \left.\frac{\partial}{\partial\nu}S_D(\phi - \phi')\right|_{+} \quad \text{on } \partial D .$$

It then follows from (2.27) that $\phi - \phi' = 0$ on ∂D and $H = H'$.

We finally prove estimate (2.66). Suppose that $\text{dist}(D, \partial\Omega) > c_0$ for some constant $c_0 > 0$. From the definition of H in (2.64), it is easy to see that

$$\|H\|_{C^n(\overline{D})} \le C_n \left(\|g\|_{L^2(\partial\Omega)} + \|u|_{\partial\Omega}\|_{L^2(\partial\Omega)} \right) , \tag{2.69}$$

where C_n depends only on n, $\partial\Omega$, and c_0.

It suffices then to show as in Corollary 2.20 that

$$\|u|_{\partial\Omega}\|_{L^2(\partial\Omega)} \le C \|g\|_{L^2(\partial\Omega)} . \tag{2.70}$$

To do so, we use the Rellich identity. Let $\boldsymbol{\alpha}$ be a vector field supported in the set $\text{dist}(x, \partial\Omega) < c_0$ such that $\boldsymbol{\alpha} \cdot \nu_x \ge \delta$ for some $\delta > 0$, $\forall x \in \partial\Omega$. Using the Rellich identity (2.35) with this $\boldsymbol{\alpha}$, we can show that

$$\left\|\frac{\partial u}{\partial T}\right\|_{L^2(\partial\Omega)} \le C\left(\|g\|_{L^2(\partial\Omega)} + \|\nabla u\|_{L^2(\Omega\setminus\overline{D})}\right) ,$$

where C depends only on $\partial\Omega$ and c_0. Observe that

$$\begin{aligned}
\|\nabla u\|^2_{L^2(\Omega\setminus\overline{D})} &\le \int_\Omega \left(1 + (k-1)\chi(D)\right)\nabla u \cdot \nabla u \, dx \\
&\le \int_{\partial\Omega} gu \, d\sigma \\
&\le \|g\|_{L^2(\partial\Omega)} \|u|_{\partial\Omega}\|_{L^2(\partial\Omega)} .
\end{aligned}$$

Since $\int_{\partial\Omega} u \, d\sigma = 0$, it follows from the Poincaré inequality (2.1) that

$$\|u|_{\partial\Omega}\|_{L^2(\partial\Omega)} \le C\left\|\frac{\partial u}{\partial T}\right\|_{L^2(\partial\Omega)} .$$

Thus we obtain

$$\|u|_{\partial\Omega}\|^2_{L^2(\partial\Omega)} \le C\left(\|g\|^2_{L^2(\partial\Omega)} + \|g\|_{L^2(\partial\Omega)} \|u|_{\partial\Omega}\|_{L^2(\partial\Omega)} \right) ,$$

and hence (2.70). From (2.69) we finally obtain (2.66). $\qquad\square$

It is important to note that, based on this representation formula, Kang and Seo proved global uniqueness results for the inverse conductivity problem with one measurement when the conductivity inclusion D is a disk or a ball in three-dimensional space [180, 182]; see Sect. 3.2.

Another useful expression of the harmonic part H of u is given in the following lemma.

Lemma 2.32 *We have*

$$
H(x) = \begin{cases} u(x) - (k-1)\displaystyle\int_D \nabla_y \Gamma(x-y) \cdot \nabla u(y)\, dy, & x \in \Omega\,, \\[2em] -(k-1)\displaystyle\int_D \nabla_y \Gamma(x-y) \cdot \nabla u(y)\, dy, & x \in \mathbb{R}^d \setminus \overline{\Omega}\,. \end{cases} \tag{2.71}
$$

Proof. We claim that

$$
\phi = (k-1)\frac{\partial u}{\partial \nu}\bigg|_- \,. \tag{2.72}
$$

In fact, it follows from the jump formula (2.27) and (2.63) and (2.65) that

$$
\frac{\partial u}{\partial \nu}\bigg|_- = \frac{\partial H}{\partial \nu} + \frac{\partial}{\partial \nu}\mathcal{S}_D\phi\bigg|_- = \frac{\partial H}{\partial \nu} + (-\frac{1}{2}I + \mathcal{K}_D^*)\phi = \frac{1}{k-1}\phi \quad \text{on } \partial D\,.
$$

Then (2.71) follows from (2.67) and (2.72) by Green's formula. $\qquad\square$

Let $g \in L_0^2(\partial\Omega)$ and

$$
U(y) := \int_{\partial\Omega} N(x,y)g(x)\, d\sigma(x)\,.
$$

Then U is the solution to the Neumann problem (2.62) and the following representation holds.

Theorem 2.33 *The solution u of (2.61) can be represented as*

$$
u(x) = U(x) - N_D\phi(x), \quad x \in \partial\Omega\,, \tag{2.73}
$$

where ϕ is defined in (2.65).

Proof. By substituting (2.63) into (2.64), we obtain

$$
H(x) = -\mathcal{S}_\Omega(g)(x) + \mathcal{D}_\Omega\Big(H|_{\partial\Omega} + (\mathcal{S}_D\phi)|_{\partial\Omega} \Big)(x), \quad x \in \Omega\,.
$$

It then follows from (2.28) that

$$
\left(\frac{1}{2}I - \mathcal{K}_\Omega\right)(H|_{\partial\Omega}) = -(\mathcal{S}_\Omega g)|_{\partial\Omega} + \left(\frac{1}{2}I + \mathcal{K}_\Omega\right)((\mathcal{S}_D\phi)|_{\partial\Omega}) \quad \text{on } \partial\Omega\,. \tag{2.74}
$$

Since $U = -\mathcal{S}_\Omega(g) + \mathcal{D}_\Omega(U|_{\partial\Omega})$ in Ω by Green's formula, we have

$$\left(\frac{1}{2}I - \mathcal{K}_\Omega\right)(U|_{\partial\Omega}) = -(\mathcal{S}_\Omega g)|_{\partial\Omega} . \tag{2.75}$$

Since $\phi \in L_0^2(\partial D)$, it follows from (2.53) that

$$-\left(\frac{1}{2}I - \mathcal{K}_\Omega\right)((N_D\phi)|_{\partial\Omega}) = (\mathcal{S}_D\phi)|_{\partial\Omega} . \tag{2.76}$$

Then, from (2.74), (2.75), and (2.76), we conclude that

$$\left(\frac{1}{2}I - \mathcal{K}_\Omega\right)\left(H|_{\partial\Omega} - U|_{\partial\Omega} + \left(\frac{1}{2}I + \mathcal{K}_\Omega\right)((N_D\phi)|_{\partial\Omega})\right) = 0 .$$

Therefore, we have from Lemma 2.29

$$H|_{\partial\Omega} - U|_{\partial\Omega} + \left(\frac{1}{2}I + \mathcal{K}_\Omega\right)((N_D\phi)|_{\partial\Omega}) = C \text{ (constant)}. \tag{2.77}$$

Note from (2.55) that

$$(\frac{1}{2}I + \mathcal{K}_\Omega)((N_D\phi)|_{\partial\Omega}) = (N_D\phi)|_{\partial\Omega} + (\mathcal{S}_D\phi)|_{\partial\Omega} .$$

Thus we get from (2.63) and (2.77) that

$$u|_{\partial\Omega} = U|_{\partial\Omega} - (N_D\phi)|_{\partial\Omega} + C . \tag{2.78}$$

Since all the functions entering in (2.78) belong to $L_0^2(\partial\Omega)$, we conclude that $C = 0$, and the theorem is proved. $\qquad\square$

We have a similar representation for solutions of the Dirichlet problem. Let $f \in W_{\frac{1}{2}}^2(\partial\Omega)$, and let v and V be the (variational) solutions of the Dirichlet problems:

$$\begin{cases} \nabla \cdot \left(1 + (k-1)\chi(D)\right)\nabla v = 0 & \text{in } \Omega , \\ v = f & \text{on } \partial\Omega , \end{cases} \tag{2.79}$$

and

$$\begin{cases} \Delta V = 0 & \text{in } \Omega , \\ V = f & \text{on } \partial\Omega . \end{cases} \tag{2.80}$$

The following representation theorem holds.

Theorem 2.34 *Let v and V be the solutions of the Dirichlet problems (2.79) and (2.80). Then $\partial v/\partial\nu$ on ∂D can be represented as*

$$\frac{\partial v}{\partial\nu}(x) = \frac{\partial V}{\partial\nu}(x) - \frac{\partial}{\partial\nu}\mathcal{G}_D\phi(x), \quad x \in \partial\Omega , \tag{2.81}$$

where ϕ is defined in (2.65) with H given by (2.64) and $g = \partial v/\partial \nu$ on $\partial \Omega$, and

$$G_D \phi(x) := \int_{\partial D} G(x,y)\phi(y)\, d\sigma(y)\ .$$

Theorem 2.34 can be proved in the same way as Theorem 2.33. In fact, it is simpler because of the solvability of the Dirichlet problem or, equivalently, the invertibility of $(1/2)\, I + \mathcal{K}_\Omega^*$. So we omit the proof.

2.6 Energy Identities

For later use, we shall establish the following energy identities, which are from [184, 10].

Lemma 2.35 *The solutions u and U of (2.61) and (2.62) satisfy*

$$\int_\Omega |\nabla(u-U)|^2\, dx + (k-1)\int_D |\nabla u|^2\, dx = \int_{\partial\Omega}(U-u)g\, d\sigma\ , \quad (2.82)$$

$$\int_\Omega \left(1 + (k-1)\chi(D)\right)|\nabla(u-U)|^2\, dx - (k-1)\int_D |\nabla U|^2\, dx \quad (2.83)$$
$$= -\int_{\partial\Omega}(U-u)g\, d\sigma\ .$$

Proof. From the variational formulations of the Neumann problems (2.61) and (2.62), it follows that

$$\int_\Omega \nabla(u-U)\cdot\nabla\eta\, dx + (k-1)\int_D \nabla u\cdot\nabla\eta\, dx = 0\ , \quad (2.84)$$

for every test function $\eta \in W^{1,2}(\Omega)$. Substituting $\eta = u$ in (2.84) and integrating by parts, we have

$$\int_\Omega |\nabla(u-U)|^2\, dx + (k-1)\int_D |\nabla u|^2\, dx = \int_{\partial\Omega}(U-u)g\, d\sigma\ ,$$

whereas substituting $\eta = u - U$ yields

$$\int_\Omega (1+(k-1)\chi(D))|\nabla(u-U)|^2\, dx - (k-1)\int_D |\nabla U|^2\, dx = -\int_{\partial\Omega}(U-u)g\, d\sigma\ .$$

Then Lemma 2.35 immediately follows from the above two identities. $\square$

2.7 Anisotropic Transmission Problem

Let D be a bounded Lipschitz domain in $\mathbb{R}^d$, $d = 2, 3$. Let A be a positive-definite symmetric matrix and A_* be the positive-definite symmetric matrix such that $A^{-1} = A_*^2$. Let $\Gamma^A(x)$ be a fundamental solution of the operator $\nabla \cdot A\nabla$:

$$\Gamma^A(x) := \begin{cases} \dfrac{1}{2\pi\sqrt{\det(A)}} \ln\|A_*x\|, & d = 2, \\[2ex] -\dfrac{1}{4\pi\sqrt{\det(A)}\|A_*x\|}, & d = 3, \end{cases}$$

where $\det(A)$ is the determinant of A and $\|\cdot\|$ is the usual norm of the vector in $\mathbb{R}^d$.

The single and double layer potentials associated with A of the density function $\phi \in L^2(\partial D)$ are, respectively, defined by

$$\mathcal{S}_D^A\phi(x) := \int_{\partial D} \Gamma^A(x - y)\phi(y)\, d\sigma(y)\,, \quad x \in \mathbb{R}^d,$$

and

$$\mathcal{D}_D^A\phi(x) := \int_{\partial D} \nu_y \cdot A\nabla\Gamma^A(x - y)\phi(y)\, d\sigma(y), \quad x \in \mathbb{R}^d \setminus \partial D\,.$$

Corresponding to Theorem 2.17 for the single and double layer potentials for the Laplacian, we have the following jump formulae:

$$\begin{cases} \nu_x \cdot A\nabla\mathcal{S}_D^A\phi(x)|_+ - \nu_x \cdot A\nabla\mathcal{S}_D^A\phi(x)|_- = \phi(x) & \text{a.e. } x \in \partial D\,, \\ \mathcal{D}_D^A\phi(x)|_+ - \mathcal{D}_D^A\phi(x)|_- = -\phi(x) & \text{a.e. } x \in \partial D\,. \end{cases} \tag{2.85}$$

Now consider $\widetilde{A}$ to be a constant $d \times d$ positive-definite symmetric matrix with $\widetilde{A} \neq A$. Throughout the remainder of the book, we will always assume that $\widetilde{A} - A$ is either positive-definite or negative-definite and use $\mathcal{S}_D^{\widetilde{A}}$ as a notation for the single layer potential associated with the domain D and the matrix $\widetilde{A}$.

The following result of Escauriaza and Seo [121] will help us give a representation formula for the solution to the anisotropic transmission problem.

Theorem 2.36 *For each* $(F, G) \in W_1^2(\partial D) \times L^2(\partial D)$, *a unique solution* $(f, g) \in L^2(\partial D) \times L^2(\partial D)$ *of the integral equation exists*

$$\begin{cases} \mathcal{S}_D^{\widetilde{A}}f - \mathcal{S}_D^A g = F \\ \nu \cdot \widetilde{A}\nabla\mathcal{S}_D^{\widetilde{A}}f|_- - \nu \cdot A\nabla\mathcal{S}_D^A g|_+ = G \end{cases} \quad \text{on } \partial D\,. \tag{2.86}$$

Moreover, a constant C exists depending only on the largest and smallest eigenvalues of $\widetilde{A}$, A, and $\widetilde{A} - A$, and the Lipschitz character of D such that

$$\|f\|_{L^2(\partial D)} + \|g\|_{L^2(\partial D)} \leq C(\|F\|_{W_1^2(\partial D)} + \|G\|_{L^2(\partial D)})\,.$$

We can easily see that, if $G \in L^2_0(\partial D)$, then the solution g of (2.86) lies in $L^2_0(\partial D)$. Moreover, if $G = 0$ and $F = \text{constant}$, then $g = 0$. We summarize these facts in the following lemma.

Lemma 2.37 *Let (f, g) be the solution to (2.86). If $G \in L^2_0(\partial D)$, then $g \in L^2_0(\partial D)$. Moreover, if F is constant and $G = 0$, then $g = 0$.*

Let Ω be a bounded Lipschitz domain in $\mathbb{R}^d$, $d = 2, 3$, containing an inclusion D. Assume that the conductivity of the background $\Omega \setminus \overline{D}$ is A and that of D is $\widetilde{A}$. The conductivity profile of the body Ω is then given by $\chi(\Omega \setminus \overline{D})A + \chi(D)\widetilde{A}$.

For a given $g \in L^2_0(\partial\Omega)$, let u denote the steady-state voltage in the presence of the anisotropic conductivity inclusion D, i.e., the solution to

$$
\begin{cases}
\nabla \cdot \left(\chi(\Omega \setminus \overline{D})A + \chi(D)\widetilde{A} \right) \nabla u = 0 \quad \text{in } \Omega \,, \\[2ex]
\nu \cdot A\nabla u \Big|_{\partial\Omega} = g \,, \\[2ex]
\displaystyle\int_{\partial\Omega} u(x)\, d\sigma(x) = 0 \,.
\end{cases}
\tag{2.87}
$$

Introduce

$$
H^A(x) := -\mathcal{S}^A_\Omega(g)(x) + \mathcal{D}^A_\Omega(f)(x), \quad x \in \Omega, \quad f := u|_{\partial\Omega} \in W^2_{\frac{1}{2}}(\partial\Omega) \,. \tag{2.88}
$$

The following representation formula is an immediate consequence of (2.86).

Theorem 2.38 *Let H^A be defined by (2.88). Then the solution u to (2.87) can be represented as*

$$
u(x) = \begin{cases}
H^A(x) + \mathcal{S}^A_D\phi(x) \,, & x \in \Omega \setminus \overline{D} \,, \\[2ex]
\mathcal{S}^{\widetilde{A}}_D\psi(x) \,, & x \in D \,,
\end{cases}
\tag{2.89}
$$

where the pair (ϕ, ψ) is the unique solution in $L^2_0(\partial D) \times L^2(\partial D)$ to the system of integral equations

$$
\begin{cases}
\mathcal{S}^{\widetilde{A}}_D\psi - \mathcal{S}^A_D\phi = H^A \\[2ex]
\nu \cdot \widetilde{A}\nabla\mathcal{S}^{\widetilde{A}}_D\psi|_- - \nu \cdot A\nabla\mathcal{S}^A_D\phi|_+ = \nu \cdot A\nabla H^A
\end{cases}
\quad \text{on } \partial D \,.
$$

2.8 Periodic Isotropic Transmission Problem

We shall now investigate the periodic isotropic transmission problem used in calculating effective properties of dilute composite materials. The results in this section are from [38]. Some of the techniques described in this section can be applied to the mathematical theory of photonic crystals [205, 37].

Let $Y =]-1/2, 1/2[^d$ denote the unit cell and $\overline{D} \subset Y$. Consider the periodic transmission problem:

$$\begin{cases} \nabla \cdot \left(1 + (k-1)\chi(D) \right) \nabla u_p = 0 \quad \text{in } Y \, , \\[2mm] u_p - x_p \text{ periodic (in each direction) with period } 1 \, , \\[2mm] \displaystyle \int_Y u_p \, dx = 0 \, , \end{cases} \tag{2.90}$$

for $p = 1, \ldots, d$.

In order to derive a representation formula for the solution to the periodic transmission problem (2.90), we need to introduce a periodic Green's function. Let

$$G_\sharp(x) = - \sum_{n \in \mathbb{Z}^d \setminus \{0\}} \frac{e^{i2\pi n \cdot x}}{4\pi^2 |n|^2} \, . \tag{2.91}$$

Then we get, in the sense of distributions,

$$\Delta G_\sharp(x) = \sum_{n \in \mathbb{Z}^d \setminus \{0\}} e^{i2\pi n \cdot x} = \sum_{n \in \mathbb{Z}^d} e^{i2\pi n \cdot x} - 1 \, ,$$

and $G_\sharp$ has mean zero. It then follows from the Poisson summation formula:

$$\sum_{n \in \mathbb{Z}^d} e^{i2\pi n \cdot x} = \sum_{n \in \mathbb{Z}^d} \delta(x + n) \, , \tag{2.92}$$

that

$$\Delta G_\sharp(x) = \sum_{n \in \mathbb{Z}^d} \delta(x + n) - 1 \, . \tag{2.93}$$

The appearance of the constant 1 in (2.93) may be somewhat peculiar. It is the volume of Y, and an integration by parts shows that it should be there. In fact,

$$\int_Y \Delta G_\sharp(x) dx = \int_{\partial Y} \frac{\partial G_\sharp}{\partial \nu} \, d\sigma \, ,$$

and the right-hand side is zero because of the periodicity.

The expression (2.91) for $G_\sharp$ is called a lattice sum, and its asymptotic behavior has been studied extensively in many contexts in solid-state physics, e.g., [308].

We state the next lemma for the general case but give in some detail a proof only for $d = 2$, leaving the proof in higher dimensions to the reader. Formulae (2.94) and (2.95) will be applied later in our study of the effective properties of composite materials.

Lemma 2.39 *A smooth function $R_d(x)$ exists in the unit cell Y such that*

$$G_\sharp(x) = \begin{cases} \dfrac{1}{2\pi}\ln|x| + R_2(x), & d = 2\,, \\[2ex] \dfrac{1}{(2-d)\omega_d}\dfrac{1}{|x|^{d-2}} + R_d(x), & d \geq 3\,. \end{cases} \tag{2.94}$$

Moreover, the Taylor expansion of $R_d(x)$ at 0 for $d \geq 2$ is given by

$$R_d(x) = R_d(0) - \frac{1}{2d}(x_1^2 + \ldots + x_d^2) + O(|x|^4)\,. \tag{2.95}$$

Proof.   As mentioned above, we assume that $d = 2$. The proof we give here is not the simplest one but has the advantage that it can be extended to other more complicated periodic Green's functions. Note that the behavior $G_\sharp(x) \sim \Gamma(x)$ as $|x| \to 0$ is to be expected since the effect of the periodic boundary conditions is negligible when x is near the origin.

We begin by writing

$$\begin{aligned} G_\sharp(x) &= -\sum_{n\in\mathbb{Z}^2\setminus\{0\}} \frac{e^{i2\pi n\cdot x}}{4\pi^2|n|^2} = -\frac{1}{4\pi^2}\sum_{n\in\mathbb{Z}^2\setminus\{0\}} \frac{\cos 2\pi n_1 x_1 \cos 2\pi n_2 x_2}{n_1^2 + n_2^2} \\[1ex] &= -\frac{1}{2\pi^2}\sum_{n_1=0}^{+\infty}\cos 2\pi n_1 x_1 \sum_{n_2=1}^{+\infty}\frac{\cos 2\pi n_2 x_2}{n_1^2 + n_2^2} \\[1ex] &\quad -\frac{1}{2\pi^2}\sum_{n_2=0}^{+\infty}\cos 2\pi n_2 x_2 \sum_{n_1=1}^{+\infty}\frac{\cos 2\pi n_1 x_1}{n_1^2 + n_2^2} \\[1ex] &:= G_1 + G_2\,. \end{aligned}$$

After that, let us invoke three summation identities (see for instance [99, pp. 813–814]):

$$\sum_{n_2=1}^{+\infty}\frac{\cos 2\pi n_2 x_2}{n_1^2 + n_2^2} = \begin{cases} -\dfrac{1}{2n_1^2} + \dfrac{\pi}{2n_1}\dfrac{\cosh\pi(2x_2 - 1)n_1}{\sinh\pi n_1} & \text{if } n_1 \neq 0\,, \\[2ex] \dfrac{\pi^2}{6} - \pi^2 x_2 + \pi^2 x_2^2 & \text{if } n_1 = 0\,, \end{cases} \tag{2.96}$$

$$\sum_{n_1=1}^{+\infty}\frac{\cos 2\pi n_1 x_1}{n_1}e^{-2\pi n_1 x_2} = \pi x_2 - \ln 2 - \frac{1}{2}\ln\left(\sinh^2\pi x_2 + \sin^2\pi x_1\right)\,. \tag{2.97}$$

We then compute

$$G_1 = -\frac{1}{2\pi^2}\sum_{n_2=1}^{+\infty}\frac{\cos 2\pi n_2 x_2}{n_2^2}$$

$$- \frac{1}{2\pi^2} \sum_{n_1=1}^{+\infty} \cos 2\pi n_1 x_1 \left(- \frac{1}{2n_1^2} + \frac{\pi}{2n_1} \frac{\cosh \pi (2x_2 - 1)n_1}{\sinh \pi n_1} \right)$$

$$= - \frac{1}{2\pi^2} \sum_{n_2=1}^{+\infty} \frac{\cos 2\pi n_2 x_2}{n_2^2} + \frac{1}{4\pi^2} \sum_{n_1=1}^{+\infty} \frac{\cos 2\pi n_1 x_1}{n_1^2}$$

$$- \frac{1}{4\pi} \sum_{n_1=1}^{+\infty} \frac{\cos 2\pi n_1 x_1}{n_1} \frac{\cosh \pi (2x_2 - 1)n_1}{\sinh \pi n_1}$$

$$= - \frac{1}{12} + \frac{1}{2} x_2 - \frac{1}{2} x_2^2 + \frac{1}{24} - \frac{1}{4} x_1 + \frac{1}{4} x_1^2 - \frac{1}{4\pi} \sum_{n_1=1}^{+\infty} \frac{\cos 2\pi n_1 x_1}{n_1} e^{-2\pi n_1 x_2}$$

$$- \frac{1}{4\pi} \sum_{n_1=1}^{+\infty} \frac{\cos 2\pi n_1 x_1}{n_1} \left(\frac{\cosh \pi (2x_2 - 1)n_1}{\sinh \pi n_1} - e^{-2\pi n_1 x_2} \right)$$

to arrive at

$$G_1 = - \frac{1}{24} + \frac{\ln 2}{4\pi} + \frac{1}{4}(x_2 - x_1) - \frac{1}{4}(2x_2^2 - x_1^2) + \frac{1}{8\pi} \ln \left(\sinh^2 \pi x_2 + \sin^2 \pi x_1 \right) + r_1(x) \, ,$$

where the function $r_1(x)$ is given by

$$r_1(x) = - \frac{1}{4\pi} \sum_{n_1=1}^{+\infty} \frac{\cos 2\pi n_1 x_1}{n_1} \left(\frac{\cosh \pi (2x_2 - 1)n_1}{\sinh \pi n_1} - e^{-2\pi n_1 x_2} \right)$$

$$= - \frac{1}{4\pi} \sum_{n_1=1}^{+\infty} \frac{\cos 2\pi n_1 x_1}{n_1} \frac{e^{2\pi n_1 x_2} + e^{-2\pi n_1 x_2}}{e^{2\pi n_1} - 1} \, .$$

Because of the term $e^{-\pi n_1}$, we can easily see that r_1 is a C^∞-function.

In the same way we can derive

$$G_2 = - \frac{1}{24} + \frac{\ln 2}{4\pi} + \frac{1}{4}(x_1 - x_2) - \frac{1}{4}(2x_1^2 - x_2^2) + \frac{1}{8\pi} \ln \left(\sinh^2 \pi x_1 + \sin^2 \pi x_2 \right) + r_2(x) \, ,$$

where

$$r_2(x) = - \frac{1}{4\pi} \sum_{n_1=1}^{+\infty} \frac{\cos 2\pi n_1 x_2}{n_1} \frac{e^{2\pi n_1 x_1} + e^{-2\pi n_1 x_1}}{e^{2\pi n_1} - 1} \, .$$

By a Taylor expansion, we readily see that

$$\ln \left(\sinh^2 \pi x_2 + \sin^2 \pi x_1 \right) + \ln \left(\sinh^2 \pi x_1 + \sin^2 \pi x_2 \right)$$

$$= 4 \ln \pi + 2 \ln(x_1^2 + x_2^2) + r_3(x) \, ,$$

where $r_3(x)$ is a C^∞-function with $r_3(x) = O(|x|^4)$ as $|x| \to 0$. In short, we obtain

$$G_\sharp(x) = \frac{1}{2\pi} \ln |x| + R_2(x) \, ,$$

where

$$R_2(x) = C - \frac{1}{4}(x_1^2 + x_2^2) + r_1(x) + r_2(x) + r_3(x)$$

for some constant C. By a Taylor expansion again, one can see that

$$r_1(x) + r_2(x) = C + O(|x|^4) \quad \text{as } |x| \to 0 \, ,$$

for some constant C. That R_2 is harmonic follows from (2.93). This concludes the proof. $\qquad\square$

Note that in the two-dimensional case we can expand $R_2(x)$ even further to get

$$R_2(x) = R_2(0) - \frac{1}{4}(x_1^2 + x_2^2) + \sum_{s=3}^{m} R_2^{(s)}(x) + O(|x|^{m+1}) \quad \text{as } |x| \to 0 \, ,$$

where the harmonic polynomial $R_2^{(s)}$ is homogeneous of degree s; i.e., $R_2^{(s)}(tx) = t^s R_2^{(s)}(x)$ for all $t \in \mathbb{R}$ and all $x \in \mathbb{R}^2$. Since

$$R_2(-x_1, x_2) = R_2(x_1, x_2) \quad \text{and } R_2(x_1, -x_2) = R_2(x_1, x_2) \, ,$$

$R_2^{(s)} \equiv 0$ if s is odd, and hence

$$R_2(x) = R_2(0) - \frac{1}{4}(x_1^2 + x_2^2) + \sum_{s=2}^{m} R_2^{(2s)}(x) + O(|x|^{m+2}) \quad \text{as } |x| \to 0 \, . \quad (2.98)$$

We conclude this section by establishing a representation formula for the solution of the periodic transmission problem (2.90).

Let the periodic single layer potential of the density function $\phi \in L_0^2(\partial D)$ be defined by

$$\mathcal{G}_D\phi(x) := \int_{\partial D} G_\sharp(x - y)\phi(y) \, d\sigma(y), \quad x \in \mathbb{R}^2 \, .$$

Lemma 2.39 shows that

$$\mathcal{G}_D\phi(x) = \mathcal{S}_D\phi(x) + \mathcal{R}_D\phi(x) \, , \qquad (2.99)$$

where $\mathcal{R}_D$ is a smoothing operator defined by

$$\mathcal{R}_D\phi(x) := \int_{\partial D} R_d(x - y)\phi(y) \, d\sigma(y) \, .$$

Thanks to (2.99), we have

$$\frac{\partial}{\partial \nu}\mathcal{G}_D\phi\bigg|_{\pm}(x) = \frac{\partial}{\partial \nu}\mathcal{S}_D\phi\bigg|_{\pm}(x) + \frac{\partial}{\partial \nu}\mathcal{R}_D\phi(x), \quad x \in \partial D .$$

Thus we can understand, with the help of Lemma 2.39, $\partial \mathcal{G}_D\phi/\partial \nu|_{\pm}$ as a compact perturbation of $\partial \mathcal{S}_D\phi/\partial \nu|_{\pm}$. Based on this natural idea, we obtain the following results.

Lemma 2.40 (i) *Let $\phi \in L_0^2(\partial D)$. The following behaviors at the boundary hold:*

$$\frac{\partial}{\partial \nu}\mathcal{G}_D\phi\bigg|_{\pm}(x) = (\pm\frac{1}{2}I + \mathcal{B}_D^*)\phi(x) \ on \ \partial D , \tag{2.100}$$

where $\mathcal{B}_D^* : L_0^2(\partial D) \to L_0^2(\partial D)$ is given by

$$\mathcal{B}_D^*\phi(x) = p.v. \int_{\partial D} \frac{\partial}{\partial \nu_x}G_\sharp(x - y)\phi(y)\,d\sigma(y), \quad x \in \partial D . \tag{2.101}$$

(ii) *If $\phi \in L_0^2(\partial D)$, then $\mathcal{G}_D\phi$ is harmonic in D and $Y \setminus \overline{D}$.*
(iii) *If $|\lambda| \geq \frac{1}{2}$, then the operator $\lambda I - \mathcal{B}_D^*$ is invertible on $L_0^2(\partial D)$.*

Proof. Since $\mathcal{B}_D^* = \mathcal{K}_D^* + \nabla_D$ where ∇_D is a smoothing operator, part (i) immediately follows from (2.27). Part (ii) follows from (2.93) and the fact that $\phi \in L_0^2(\partial D)$. As a consequence of parts (i) and (ii), it follows that $\lambda I - \mathcal{B}_D^*$ maps $L_0^2(\partial D)$ into $L_0^2(\partial D)$. To prove part (iii), we observe that ∇_D maps $L^2(\partial D)$ into $W_1^2(\partial D)$, and hence it is a compact operator on $L^2(\partial D)$. Since, by Theorem 2.21, $\lambda I - \mathcal{K}_D^*$ is invertible on $L_0^2(\partial D)$, it suffices, by applying the Fredholm alternative, to show that $\lambda I - \mathcal{B}_D^*$ is one-to-one on $L_0^2(\partial D)$. We shall prove this fact, using the same argument as the one introduced in Lemma 2.18. Let $|\lambda| \geq 1/2$, and suppose that $\phi \in L_0^2(\partial D)$ satisfies $(\lambda I - \mathcal{B}_D^*)\phi = 0$ and $\phi \neq 0$. Let

$$A := \int_D |\nabla\mathcal{G}_D\phi|^2\,dx, \quad B := \int_{Y\setminus\overline{D}} |\nabla\mathcal{G}_D\phi|^2\,dx .$$

Then $A \neq 0$. In fact, if $A = 0$, then $\mathcal{G}_D\phi$ is constant in D. Therefore $\mathcal{G}_D\phi$ in $Y \setminus \overline{D}$ is periodic and satisfies $\mathcal{G}_D\phi|_{\partial D} = $ constant. Hence $\mathcal{G}_D\phi = $ constant in $Y \setminus \overline{D}$. Therefore, by part (i), we get

$$\phi = \frac{\partial}{\partial \nu}\mathcal{G}_D\phi\bigg|_{+} - \frac{\partial}{\partial \nu}\mathcal{G}_D\phi\bigg|_{-} = 0 ,$$

which contradicts our assumption. In a similar way, we can show that $B \neq 0$. On the other hand, using Green's formula and periodicity, we have

$$A = \int_{\partial D}(-\frac{1}{2}I + \mathcal{B}_D^*)\phi\,\mathcal{G}_D\phi\,d\sigma, \quad B = -\int_{\partial D}(\frac{1}{2}I + \mathcal{B}_D^*)\phi\,\mathcal{G}_D\phi\,d\sigma .$$

Since $(\lambda I - \mathcal{B}_D^*)\phi = 0$, it follows that

$$\lambda = \frac{1}{2}\frac{B - A}{B + A} \, .$$

Thus, $|\lambda| < 1/2$, which is a contradiction. This completes the proof. $\square$

Analogously to Theorem 2.31 the following result holds, giving a decomposition formula of the solution of (2.90) into a harmonic part and a refraction part.

Theorem 2.41 *Let u_p be the unique solution to the transmission problem (2.90). Then u_p, $p = 1, \ldots, d$, can be expressed as follows:*

$$u_p(x) = x_p + C_p + \mathcal{G}_D\big(\frac{k+1}{2(k-1)}I - \mathcal{B}_D^*\big)^{-1}(\nu_p)(x) \quad \text{in } Y \, , \tag{2.102}$$

where C_p is a constant and ν_p is the p-component of the outward unit normal ν to ∂D.

Proof.   Observe that $u_p, p = 1, \ldots, d$, satisfies

$$\begin{cases} \Delta u_p = 0 \quad \text{in } D \cup (Y \setminus \overline{D}) \, , \\ u_p|_+ - u_p|_- = 0 \quad \text{on } \partial D \, , \\ \dfrac{\partial u_p}{\partial \nu}\Big|_+ - k\dfrac{\partial u_p}{\partial \nu}\Big|_- = 0 \quad \text{on } \partial D \, , \\ u_p - x_p \quad \text{periodic with period 1} \, , \\ \displaystyle\int_Y u_p \, dx = 0 \, . \end{cases}$$

To prove (2.102), define

$$V_p(x) = \mathcal{G}_D\big(\frac{k+1}{2(k-1)}I - \mathcal{B}_D^*\big)^{-1}(\nu_p)(x) \quad \text{in } Y \, .$$

Then routine calculations show that

$$\begin{cases} \Delta V_p = 0 \quad \text{in } D \cup (Y \setminus \overline{D}) \, , \\ V_p|_+ - V_p|_- = 0 \quad \text{on } \partial D \, , \\ \dfrac{\partial V_p}{\partial \nu}\Big|_+ - k\dfrac{\partial V_p}{\partial \nu}\Big|_- = (k-1)\nu_p \quad \text{on } \partial D \, , \\ V_p \text{ periodic with period 1} \, . \end{cases} \tag{2.103}$$

Thus by choosing C_p so that $\int_Y u_p \, dx = 0$, we get (2.102), which completes the proof. $\square$

2.9 Periodic Anisotropic Transmission Problem

In this section, we derive a Green's function to the periodic anistropic transmission problem and establish a representation formula for its solution. These results are from [28].

Consider the periodic anisotropic transmission problem:

$$\begin{cases} \nabla \cdot ((\chi(Y \setminus \overline{D})A + \chi(D)\widetilde{A})\nabla u_p) = 0 \quad \text{in } Y , \\ u_p - x_p \quad \text{periodic (in each direction) with period 1 ,} \\ \int_Y u_p = 0 , \end{cases} \tag{2.104}$$

for $p = 1, \ldots, d$. The periodic Green's function $G_\sharp^A(x)$ is given by

$$G_\sharp^A(x) = - \sum_{n \in \mathbb{Z}^d \setminus \{0\}} \frac{e^{2\pi i n \cdot x}}{4\pi^2 An \cdot n} . \tag{2.105}$$

In fact, in the sense of distributions, we have

$$\nabla \cdot (A\nabla G_\sharp^A(x)) = \sum_{n \in \mathbb{Z}^d} e^{2\pi i n \cdot x} - 1 ,$$

and hence by the Poisson summation formula (2.92),

$$\nabla \cdot (A\nabla G_\sharp^A(x)) = \sum_{n \in \mathbb{Z}^d} \delta(x + n) - 1 . \tag{2.106}$$

It follows from the standard elliptic regularity theory that $G_\sharp^A(x) - \Gamma^A(x)$ is smooth in the unit cell Y.

Moreover, we can show that a symmetric matrix K exists such that

$$G_\sharp^A(x) = C + \Gamma^A(x) - x \cdot Kx + O(|x|^4), \quad |x| \to 0 .$$

This matrix K plays an essential role in deriving the effective properties of anisotropic composites. We write down an explicit form of K in the two-dimensional case, leaving the general case to the reader.

Let us first fix a notation. If

$$A = \begin{pmatrix} a & b \\ b & c \end{pmatrix}, \quad a, c > 0 \text{ and } ac - b^2 > 0 ,$$

let

$$\alpha := -\frac{b}{c} + i\frac{\sqrt{\det(A)}}{c} \quad \text{and} \quad \beta := -\frac{b}{a} + i\frac{\sqrt{\det(A)}}{a} . \tag{2.107}$$

We also define real-valued functions θ and η by

$$\theta(z) + i\eta(z) := \sum_{n=1}^{+\infty} \frac{n}{1 - e^{-2\pi i n z}}, \quad \Im z > 0 . \tag{2.108}$$

Observe that $\eta(z) = 0$ if z is purely imaginary.

We have from [28] the following lemma, whose proof turns out to be quite difficult.

Lemma 2.42 *Suppose $d = 2$. A smooth function $R^A(x)$ exists in the unit cell Y such that*

$$G_\sharp^A(x) = \Gamma^A(x) + R^A(x) , \tag{2.109}$$

and $R^A(x)$ takes the form

$$R^A(x) = R^A(0) - x \cdot K\, x + O(|x|^4), \quad |x| \to 0 , \tag{2.110}$$

where K is given by

$$K = \frac{1}{4} \begin{pmatrix} \dfrac{1}{a} & 0 \\ 0 & \dfrac{1}{c} \end{pmatrix} + \frac{\pi}{\sqrt{\det(A)}}\left(\frac{1}{24} + \theta(\alpha)\right) \begin{pmatrix} 1 & -\dfrac{b}{c} \\ -\dfrac{b}{c} & \dfrac{2b^2 - ac}{c^2} \end{pmatrix}$$

$$+ \frac{\pi}{\sqrt{\det(A)}}\left(\frac{1}{24} + \theta(\beta)\right) \begin{pmatrix} \dfrac{2b^2 - ac}{a^2} & -\dfrac{b}{a} \\ -\dfrac{b}{a} & 1 \end{pmatrix}$$

$$+ \frac{\pi\eta(\alpha)}{c} \begin{pmatrix} 0 & -1 \\ -1 & \dfrac{2b}{c} \end{pmatrix} + \frac{\pi\eta(\beta)}{a} \begin{pmatrix} \dfrac{2b}{a} & -1 \\ -1 & 0 \end{pmatrix} . \tag{2.111}$$

In particular, the function $u(x) = -x \cdot K\, x$ satisfies the equation $\nabla \cdot A \nabla u = -1$ in $\mathbb{R}^2$.

Proof. Suppose that

$$A = \begin{pmatrix} a & b \\ b & c \end{pmatrix} , \quad a, c > 0 \text{ and } ac - b^2 > 0 .$$

Then, we have

$$4\pi^2 G_\sharp^A(x) = -\sum_{n \in \mathbb{Z}^2 \backslash \{0\}} \frac{e^{2\pi i n \cdot x}}{an_1^2 + 2bn_1 n_2 + cn_2^2}$$

$$= -\sum_{n_1 \neq 0} \sum_{n_2 = -\infty}^{+\infty} \frac{e^{2\pi i n \cdot x}}{an_1^2 + 2bn_1 n_2 + cn_2^2} - \sum_{n_2 \neq 0} \frac{e^{2\pi i n_2 x_2}}{cn_2^2} . \tag{2.112}$$

Since (2.96) gives

$$\sum_{n=1}^{+\infty} \frac{\cos(nx)}{n^2} = \frac{\pi^2}{6} - \frac{\pi}{2}x + \frac{1}{4}x^2 ,$$

we have

$$\sum_{n_2 \neq 0} \frac{e^{2\pi i n_2 x_2}}{cn_2^2} = \frac{1}{c}\left(\frac{\pi^2}{3} - 2\pi^2 x_2 + 2\pi^2 x_2^2 \right) . \tag{2.113}$$

To compute the first term in (2.112), we use a general formula from [99, p. 815]: If $P(z)$ is a holomorphic polynomial and α is real, then

$$\sum_{n=-\infty}^{+\infty} \frac{e^{i\alpha n}}{P(n)} = -2\pi i \sum_{\xi:\ \text{zeros of } P(z)} \text{Residue}\left(\frac{e^{i\alpha z}}{P(z)(e^{2\pi iz}-1)}, \xi\right) . \tag{2.114}$$

Let $P(z) := cz^2 + 2bn_1 z + an_1^2$. Then the zeros of $P(z)$ are αn_1 and $\overline{\alpha} n_1$, where

$$\alpha := -\frac{b}{c} + i\frac{\sqrt{\det(A)}}{c} .$$

It then follows from (2.114) that

$$\sum_{n_2=-\infty}^{+\infty} \frac{e^{2\pi in_2 x_2}}{an_1^2 + 2bn_1 n_2 + cn_2^2} = \frac{2\pi i}{c(\alpha-\overline{\alpha})} \left[\frac{e^{2\pi i\overline{\alpha}n_1 x_2}}{n_1(e^{2\pi i\overline{\alpha}n_1}-1)} - \frac{e^{2\pi i\alpha n_1 x_2}}{n_1(e^{2\pi i\alpha n_1}-1)}\right] .$$

Since $c(\alpha - \overline{\alpha}) = 2i\sqrt{\det(A)}$, we get

$$\sum_{n_1\neq 0} \sum_{n_2=-\infty}^{+\infty} \frac{e^{2\pi in\cdot x}}{an_1^2 + 2bn_1 n_2 + cn_2^2}$$

$$= \frac{\pi}{\sqrt{\det(A)}} \sum_{n_1\neq 0} \left[\frac{e^{2\pi i(x_1+\overline{\alpha}x_2)n_1}}{n_1(e^{2\pi i\overline{\alpha}n_1}-1)} - \frac{e^{2\pi i(x_1+\alpha x_2)n_1}}{n_1(e^{2\pi i\alpha n_1}-1)}\right]$$

$$= -\frac{2\pi}{\sqrt{\det(A)}}\Re \sum_{n_1\neq 0} \frac{e^{2\pi i(x_1+\alpha x_2)n_1}}{n_1(e^{2\pi i\alpha n_1}-1)} . \tag{2.115}$$

We have

$$\sum_{n_1\neq 0} \frac{e^{2\pi i(x_1+\alpha x_2)n_1}}{n_1(e^{2\pi i\alpha n_1}-1)} = -\sum_{n_1>0} \frac{e^{2\pi i(x_1+\alpha x_2)n_1}}{n_1} + r_1(x) , \tag{2.116}$$

where

$$r_1(x) := \sum_{n_1>0} \frac{e^{2\pi i(x_1+\alpha x_2)n_1}}{n_1} \frac{e^{2\pi i\alpha n_1}}{e^{2\pi i\alpha n_1}-1} + \sum_{n_1<0} \frac{e^{2\pi i(x_1+\alpha x_2)n_1}}{n_1} \frac{1}{e^{2\pi i\alpha n_1}-1}$$

$$= \sum_{n_1=1}^{+\infty} \frac{e^{2\pi i(x_1+\alpha x_2)n_1} + e^{-2\pi i(x_1+\alpha x_2)n_1}}{n_1} \frac{e^{2\pi i\alpha n_1}}{e^{2\pi i\alpha n_1}-1} .$$

Observe that since $\Im \alpha > 0$, the above series converges absolutely and uniformly thanks to the factor $e^{2\pi i\alpha n_1}$ and $r_1(x)$ is a smooth function in the variables x_1 and x_2 for $|x_2| < 1$. Moreover, one can see by the Taylor expansion that

$$r_1(x) = C_1 + 4\pi^2\mu(\alpha)(x_1 + \alpha x_2)^2 + O(|x|^4), \quad |x| \to 0 , \tag{2.117}$$

where

$$\mu(\alpha) = \theta(\alpha) + i\eta(\alpha) := \sum_{n=1}^{+\infty} \frac{n}{1 - e^{-2\pi i \alpha n}} \ .$$

In order to compute the first term in the right-hand side of (2.116), we invoke formula (2.97). Since

$$\ln(\sinh^2 \pi x_2 + \sin^2 \pi x_1) = \ln \pi^2 + \ln(x_1^2 + x_2^2) + \frac{\pi^2}{3}(x_2^2 - x_1^2) + O(|x|^4) \ ,$$

we get

$$\sum_{n_1=1}^{+\infty} \frac{\cos(2\pi n_1 x_1)}{n_1} e^{-2\pi n_1 x_2} = \pi x_2 - \ln 2\pi^2 - \frac{1}{2}\ln(x_1^2 + x_2^2) + \frac{\pi^2}{6}(x_1^2 - x_2^2) + O(|x|^4) \ .$$

Thus we obtain

$$\Re \sum_{n_1 > 0} \frac{e^{2\pi i (x_1 + \alpha x_2) n_1}}{n_1} = \sum_{n_1=1}^{+\infty} \frac{\cos 2\pi(x_1 - \frac{b}{c}x_2)n_1}{n_1} e^{-2\pi \frac{\sqrt{\det(A)}}{c} n_1 x_2}$$

$$= \frac{\sqrt{\det(A)}}{c}\pi x_2 - \ln 2\pi^2 - \frac{1}{2}\ln\left[(x_1 - \frac{b}{c}x_2)^2 + \frac{\det(A)}{c^2}x_2^2\right]$$

$$+ \frac{\pi^2}{6}\left[(x_1 - \frac{b}{c}x_2)^2 - \frac{\det(A)}{c^2}x_2^2\right] + O(|x|^4) \ .$$

Let $A_* = \sqrt{A^{-1}}$ as before. Then one can see that

$$(x_1 - \frac{b}{c}x_2)^2 + \frac{\det(A)}{c^2}x_2^2 = \frac{\det(A)}{c}(x \cdot A^{-1}x) = \frac{\det(A)}{c}\|A_* x\|^2 \ ,$$

and hence

$$\Re \sum_{n_1 > 0} \frac{e^{2\pi i (x_1 + \alpha x_2) n_1}}{n_1} = C + \frac{\sqrt{\det(A)}}{c}\pi x_2 - \ln\|A_* x\|$$

$$+ \frac{\pi^2}{6}\left[(x_1 - \frac{b}{c}x_2)^2 - \frac{\det(A)}{c^2}x_2^2\right] + O(|x|^4) \ , \qquad (2.118)$$

for some constant C. Combining (2.112), (2.113), (2.115), (2.116), and (2.118) yields

$$4\pi^2 G_\sharp^A(x) = C + \frac{2\pi}{\sqrt{\det(A)}}\ln\|A_* x\| - \frac{\pi^3}{3\sqrt{\det(A)}}\left[(x_1 - \frac{b}{c}x_2)^2 - \frac{\det(A)}{c^2}x_2^2\right]$$

$$- \frac{2\pi^2}{c}x_2^2 + \frac{8\pi^3}{\sqrt{\det(A)}}\Re(\mu(\alpha)(x_1 + \alpha x_2)^2) + O(|x|^4) \ , \qquad (2.119)$$

for some constant C.

In order to obtain a formula for $G_\sharp^A(x)$ in a symmetric form, we now use

$$4\pi^2 G_\sharp^A(x) = -\sum_{n_2\neq 0}\sum_{n_1=-\infty}^{+\infty} \frac{e^{2\pi in\cdot x}}{an_1^2 + 2bn_1n_2 + cn_2^2} - \sum_{n_1\neq 0}\frac{e^{2\pi in_1 x_1}}{an_1^2}\,,$$

and interchange the role of x_1 and x_2 to get

$$4\pi^2 G_\sharp^A(x) = C + \frac{2\pi}{\sqrt{\det(A)}}\ln\|A_*x\| - \frac{\pi^3}{3\sqrt{\det(A)}}\left[(x_2 - \frac{b}{a}x_1)^2 - \frac{\det(A)}{a^2}x_1^2\right]$$

$$-\frac{2\pi^2}{a}x_1^2 + \frac{8\pi^3}{\sqrt{\det(A)}}\Re(\mu(\beta)(x_2 + \beta x_1)^2) + O(|x|^4)\,, \tag{2.120}$$

for some constant C where

$$\beta := -\frac{b}{a} + i\frac{\sqrt{\det(A)}}{a}\,.$$

By taking the average of the formulae in (2.119) and (2.120), we finally arrive at

$$G_\sharp^A(x) = C + \Gamma^A(x) - x\cdot Kx + O(|x|^4), \quad |x|\to 0\,, \tag{2.121}$$

where C is a constant and K is the symmetric matrix given by

$$x\cdot Kx = \frac{\pi}{12\sqrt{\det(A)}}\left[\frac{a^2 + b^2 - \det(A)}{2a^2}x_1^2 - \left(\frac{b}{a} + \frac{b}{c}\right)x_1x_2\right.$$

$$\left. + \frac{c^2 + b^2 - \det(A)}{2c^2}x_2^2\right] + \frac{1}{4}\left(\frac{x_1^2}{a} + \frac{x_2^2}{c}\right)$$

$$-\frac{\pi}{\sqrt{\det(A)}}\Re(\mu(\alpha)(x_1 + \alpha x_2)^2 + \mu(\beta)(x_2 + \beta x_1)^2)\,. \tag{2.122}$$

The formula (2.111) now follows from (2.122) through elementary but tedious computation. $\qquad\square$

Let $\mathrm{Tr}(M)$ denote the trace of the matrix M. Since

$$\nabla\cdot A\nabla(x\cdot Bx) = 2\mathrm{Tr}(AB)$$

for any symmetric matrix B, we infer that the quadratic polynomial u defined by the first matrix in the right-hand side of (2.111) satisfies $\nabla\cdot(A\nabla u(x)) = 1$, whereas those defined by the other matrices satisfy

$$\nabla\cdot(A\nabla u(x)) = 0\,.$$

If A is diagonal, then the formula is particularly simple. If $b = 0$, then $\alpha = i\sqrt{a/c}$ and $\beta = i\sqrt{c/a}$, and hence $\eta(\alpha) = \eta(\beta) = 0$ and K takes the form

$$K = \frac{1}{4}A^{-1}(I + c(A)E) ,\qquad(2.123)$$

where $E = \begin{pmatrix} 1 & 0 \\ 0 & -1 \end{pmatrix}$ and

$$c(A) := \frac{4\pi}{\sqrt{\det(A)}}\left(\frac{a}{24} + a\theta\left(i\sqrt{\frac{a}{c}}\right) - \frac{c}{24} - c\theta\left(i\sqrt{\frac{c}{a}}\right)\right) .\qquad(2.124)$$

Observe that $c(A) = 0$ when $a = c$, i.e., A is isotropic. In fact, $c(A) = 0$ only when A is isotropic. To see this, write $c(A)$ as

$$c(A) = g(\sqrt{\frac{a}{c}}) - g(\sqrt{\frac{c}{a}}) ,$$

where

$$g(x) = 4\pi x \left[\frac{1}{24} + \sum_{n=1}^{+\infty}\frac{n}{1 - e^{2\pi n x}}\right] ,\qquad x > 0 .$$

We can easily see that g is monotonically increasing. Thus $c(A) = 0$ if and only if $a = c$.

Definition 2.43 *A function H is called A-harmonic in an open set D if H is the solution to*

$$\nabla \cdot (A\nabla H) = 0 \quad in\ D .\qquad(2.125)$$

In our later study of composites of anisotropic materials, we will need to extend the representation formula (2.102) to the anisotropic transmission problem (2.104). To this end we introduce the periodic single layer potential for a domain D compactly contained in Y as follows:

$$\mathcal{G}_D^A\phi(x) = \int_{\partial D} G_\sharp^A(x - y)\phi(y)\,d\sigma(y) \qquad \text{for } x \in \mathbb{R}^d, \quad \forall\, \phi \in L_0^2(\partial D) .$$

Observe that $\mathcal{G}_D^A\phi$ is A-harmonic in D and $Y \setminus \overline{D}$ provided that ϕ belongs to $L_0^2(\partial D)$ and is periodic. In fact, by (2.106), we get for $x \in D \cup (Y \setminus \overline{D})$

$$\nabla \cdot (A\nabla \mathcal{G}_D^A\phi)(x) = -\int_{\partial D}\phi\,d\sigma = 0 ,$$

provided that $\phi \in L_0^2(\partial D)$.

Let $\mathcal{S}_D^A$ and $\mathcal{S}_D^{\widetilde{A}}$ be the (non-periodic) single layer potentials corresponding to the conductivities A and $\widetilde{A}$, respectively. By Lemma 2.42, we have

$$\mathcal{G}_D^A\phi(x) = \mathcal{S}_D^A\phi(x) + \mathcal{R}_D^A\phi(x), \quad x \in Y ,\qquad(2.126)$$

where $\mathcal{R}_D^A$ is defined by

$$\mathcal{R}_D^A\phi(x) = \int_{\partial D} R^A(x - y)\phi(y)\,d\sigma(y) .\qquad(2.127)$$

We note that since $R^A(x)$ is a smooth function in Y, $\mathcal{R}_D^A\phi$ is smooth in Y for any $\phi \in L^2(\partial D)$. Therefore, we get, in particular,

$$\nu \cdot A\nabla\mathcal{G}_D^A\phi(x)|_+ - \nu \cdot A\nabla\mathcal{G}_D^A\phi(x)|_- = \phi(x), \quad \text{a.e. } x \in \partial D .\qquad(2.128)$$

Lemma 2.44 *Let D be a bounded Lipschitz domain compactly contained in Y. Then the map $T_\sharp : L^2(\partial D) \times L^2(\partial D) \to W_1^2(\partial D) \times L^2(\partial D)$, defined by*

$$T_\sharp(f,g) = \left(\mathcal{S}_D^{\widetilde{A}}f - \mathcal{G}_D^A g, \nu \cdot \widetilde{A}\nabla \mathcal{S}_D^{\widetilde{A}}f|_- - \nu \cdot A\nabla \mathcal{G}_D^A g|_+ \right), \qquad (2.129)$$

is invertible, and a positive constant C exists such that

$$\|(f,g)\|_{L^2(\partial D) \times L^2(\partial D)} \le C\|T_\sharp(f,g)\|_{W_1^2(\partial D) \times L^2(\partial D)}, \qquad (2.130)$$

for all $(f,g) \in L^2(\partial D) \times L^2(\partial D)$.

Proof. Because of (2.109), $T_\sharp(f,g) = T(f,g) - T_R(g)$, where

$$T(f,g) = \left(\mathcal{S}_D^{\widetilde{A}}f - \mathcal{S}_D^A g, \nu \cdot \widetilde{A}\nabla \mathcal{S}_D^{\widetilde{A}}f|_- - \nu \cdot A\nabla \mathcal{S}_D^A g|_+ \right) \qquad (2.131)$$

and

$$T_R(g) = \left(\mathcal{R}_D^A g, \nu \cdot A\nabla \mathcal{R}_D^A g \right). \qquad (2.132)$$

Observe that

$$\nu \cdot A\nabla \mathcal{R}_D^A g \in X := \left\{ \nu \cdot F \mid F \in W_1^2(\partial D) \right\}$$

and X is compact in $L^2(\partial D)$. Therefore T_R is a compact operator on $L^2(\partial D) \times L^2(\partial D)$. Since T is invertible by (2.86), it suffices to show that $T_\sharp$ is injective on $L^2(\partial D) \times L^2(\partial D)$ by the Fredholm alternative.

Suppose that $T_\sharp(f,g) = (0,0)$. Then

$$\int_{\partial D} \nu \cdot A\nabla \mathcal{G}_D^A g|_+ \, d\sigma = \int_{\partial D} \nu \cdot \widetilde{A}\nabla \mathcal{S}_D^{\widetilde{A}}f|_- \, d\sigma = 0 ,$$

and hence we get from (2.128) that $\int_{\partial D} g \, d\sigma = 0$.

Now, let

$$u = \mathcal{S}_D^{\widetilde{A}}f\chi(D) + \mathcal{G}_D^A g\chi(Y \setminus \overline{D}) .$$

Then u is periodic and satisfies $\nabla \cdot (\chi(Y \setminus \overline{D})A + \chi(D)\widetilde{A})\nabla u = 0$ in Y. So $u = C$, where C is a constant. In particular, $\mathcal{G}_D^A g = C$ in $Y \setminus \overline{D}$ and so $\mathcal{G}_D^A g = C$ on ∂D. Since $\mathcal{G}_D^A g$ is A-harmonic in D, $\mathcal{G}_D^A g = C$ in D and hence $g = 0$ on ∂D by (2.128). Observe that if $g = 0$, then $T_\sharp(f,g) = T(f,g)$ and hence $T(f,g) = 0$. By the invertibility of T, we get $(f,g) = (0,0)$. This completes the proof. $\qquad\square$

Lemma 2.44 gives us a representation of the solution to (2.104).

Theorem 2.45 *Suppose $d = 2$. Let $(f_p, g_p) \in L^2(\partial D) \times L^2(\partial D)$, $p = 1,2$, be the solution to*

$$T_\sharp(f_p, g_p) = (x_p, \nu \cdot A\nabla x_p) , \qquad (2.133)$$

where $T_\sharp$ is defined in (2.129). Then the solution u_p to (2.104) can be represented as

$$u_p(x) = C_p + \begin{cases} x_p + \mathcal{G}_D^A g_p(x) \,, \\ \mathcal{S}_D^{\tilde{A}} f_p(x) \,, \end{cases} \tag{2.134}$$

where the constant C_p is chosen so that $\int_Y u_p\, dx = 0$.

Proof. It is enough to show that $g_p \in L_0^2(\partial D)$ so that $\mathcal{G}_D^A g_p$ is A-harmonic in $Y \setminus \overline{D}$. But since $\nu \cdot A\nabla x_p \in L_0^2(\partial D)$, we get $\nu \cdot A\nabla \mathcal{G}_D^A g_p|_+ \in L_0^2(\partial D)$. By the jump relation (2.128), we get $g_p \in L_0^2(\partial D)$, as before. $\square$

2.10 Further Results and Open Problems

The representation formulae (2.63), (2.73), and (2.102) can be extended for the solution to the transmission problem for the Helmholtz equation; see [25] and [26]. Based on the work of Mitrea, Mitrea and Pipher[238], similar results for the time-harmonic Maxwell's equations could be established.

The numerical solutions of the periodic transmission problems (2.90) and (2.104) require evaluations of the periodic Green's functions (2.91) and (2.105), and so the feasibility of our layer potential technique for solving periodic transmission problems is strongly influenced by how efficiently these functions can be computed. The standard representations (2.91) and (2.105) contain series that converge slowly and so are unsuitable for numerical work. Nevertheless, many analytic techniques can be used for efficient and accurate numerical constructions of the periodic Green's functions. These methods include those based on Ewald's summation, Kummer's transformation, and fast evaluations of lattice sums through alternative formulations of the periodic Green's functions. See [269, 221, 68, 140, 111].

3

Uniqueness for Inverse Conductivity Problems

Introduction

Let Ω be a simply connected Lipschitz domain in $\mathbb{R}^d, d \geq 2$, and let D be a subdomain of Ω such that $\overline{D} \subset \Omega$. Let $g \in L_0^2(\partial\Omega)$. Fix $0 < k \neq 1 < +\infty$, and let u be the solution to

$$
\begin{cases}
\nabla \cdot \left(1 + (k-1)\chi(D)\right)\nabla u = 0 & \text{in } \Omega , \\[2mm]
\dfrac{\partial u}{\partial \nu}\bigg|_{\partial\Omega} = g , \\[2mm]
\displaystyle\int_{\partial\Omega} u(x)\, d\sigma(x) = 0 .
\end{cases}
\tag{3.1}
$$

The inverse conductivity problem is to find the inclusion D (and its conductivity k) given $f = u|_{\partial\Omega}$ for one or finitely many g (one measurement problem) or for all g (many measurements problem). In some applied situations, it is f that is prescribed on $\partial\Omega$ and g that is measured on $\partial\Omega$. This makes some difference (not significant theoretically and computationally) in the case of single boundary measurements but makes no difference in the case of many boundary measurements, since actually it is the set of Cauchy data (f, g) that is given.

This problem lays a mathematical foundation to electrical impedance tomography, which is a method of imaging the interior of a body by measurements of current flows and voltages on its surface. On the surface one prescribes current sources (such as electrodes) and measures voltage (or vice versa) for some or all positions of these sources. The same mathematical model works in a variety of applications, such as breast cancer imaging [40, 282, 209] and mine detection [129].

For the many measurements problem there is a well-established theory. We refer the reader to the survey papers of Sylvester and Uhlmann [286], and of Uhlmann [295, 296], as well as to the book by Isakov [167]. When

$d \geq 2$, many boundary measurements provide much more information about the conductivity profile of Ω than a finite number of measurements. Thus, the inverse conductivity problem with finite measurements is more difficult than the one with many boundary measurements and not much was known about it until recently. Fortunately, there has been over the last few years a considerable amount of interesting work and new techniques dedicated to both theoretical and numerical aspects of this problem. In this chapter, we restrict ourselves to uniqueness results. Later, we shall describe some of the numerical techniques, in particular, those later on for the reconstruction of diametrically small conductivity inclusions.

This chapter begins with a proof of the uniqueness with many measurements, which will be applied later in our study of the generalized polarization tensors. After that, we consider the monotone case for which global uniqueness holds for general domains and prove the unique determination of disk-shaped inclusions with one boundary measurement.

3.1 Uniqueness With Many Measurements

Our purpose here is to state and prove a special case of the general uniqueness result due to Isakov [165]; see also Druskin [116]. Let U be the solution to

$$
\begin{cases}
\Delta U = 0 & \text{in } \Omega , \\
\dfrac{\partial U}{\partial \nu}\bigg|_{\partial \Omega} = g , \\
\displaystyle\int_{\partial \Omega} U(x)\, d\sigma(x) = 0 .
\end{cases}
\tag{3.2}
$$

We will need the following lemma, which was first obtained in [184].

Lemma 3.1 *Let u and U be, respectively, the solutions of* (3.1) *and* (3.2). *Then there are positive constants C_1 and C_2 depending only on k such that*

$$
C_1 \left| \int_{\partial \Omega} (U - u) g \, d\sigma \right| \leq \int_D |\nabla U|^2 \, dx \leq C_2 \left| \int_{\partial \Omega} (U - u) g \, d\sigma \right| .
\tag{3.3}
$$

Moreover, if $k > 1$, then

$$
C_1 = \frac{1}{k-1}, \quad C_2 = \frac{(\sqrt{k-1}+1)^2}{k-1} ,
$$

and if $0 < k < 1$, then

$$
C_1 = \frac{(1 - \sqrt{1-k})^2}{1-k}, \quad C_2 = \frac{1}{1-k} .
$$

Proof. This lemma is a direct consequence of Lemma 2.35. Suppose first that $k > 1$. It follows from (2.82) that

$$\int_{\partial\Omega} (U - u)g\, d\sigma > 0 \, ,$$

and hence by (2.83)

$$\int_{\partial\Omega} (U - u)g\, d\sigma \leq (k - 1) \int_{D} |\nabla U|^2\, dx \, .$$

On the other hand, using (2.82), we have for any positive τ,

$$\int_{D} |\nabla U|^2\, dx \leq \left(1 + \frac{1}{\tau}\right) \int_{D} |\nabla u|^2\, dx + (1 + \tau) \int_{D} |\nabla (u - U)|^2\, dx$$

$$\leq \left(1 + \tau + \frac{1 + \frac{1}{\tau}}{k - 1}\right) \int_{\partial\Omega} (U - u)g\, d\sigma \, .$$

The factor $1 + \tau + (1 + 1/\tau)/(k - 1)$ has its minimum value when $\tau = 1/\sqrt{k - 1}$, and in this case, we arrive at

$$\int_{D} |\nabla U|^2\, dx \leq \frac{(\sqrt{k - 1} + 1)^2}{k - 1} \left| \int_{\partial\Omega} (U - u)g\, d\sigma \right| \, .$$

If $0 < k < 1$, then

$$\int_{\partial\Omega} (U - u)g\, d\sigma < 0 \, ,$$

and, it then follows from (2.83) that

$$\int_{D} |\nabla U|^2\, dx \leq \frac{1}{1 - k} \left| \int_{\partial\Omega} (U - u)g\, d\sigma \right| \, .$$

From (2.82), we see that

$$\left| \int_{\partial\Omega} (U - u)g\, d\sigma \right| \leq (1 - k) \int_{D} |\nabla u|^2\, dx \, ,$$

and obtain that, for any positive τ,

$$\int_{D} |\nabla u|^2\, dx \leq \left(1 + \frac{1}{\tau}\right) \int_{D} |\nabla U|^2\, dx + (1 + \tau) \int_{D} |\nabla (u - U)|^2\, dx \, ,$$

which implies that

$$\int_{D} |\nabla u|^2\, dx \leq \frac{1 + \frac{1}{\tau}}{1 + (k - 1)(1 + \tau)} \int_{D} |\nabla U|^2\, dx \, .$$

The minimum of $(1 + 1/\tau)/(1 + (k - 1)(1 + \tau))$ with the function value being positive occurs when $\tau + 1 = 1/\sqrt{1 - k}$, and in this case, we obtain

$$\left| \int_{\partial\Omega} (U - u)g\, d\sigma \right| \leq \frac{1 - k}{(1 - \sqrt{1 - k})^2} \int_D |\nabla U|^2\, dx \,,$$

which completes the proof. $\qquad\qquad\qquad\qquad\qquad\qquad\qquad\qquad\qquad$ $\square$

We define the set of Cauchy data

$$\mathcal{C}_{D,k} = \left\{ (u|_{\partial\Omega}, \frac{\partial u}{\partial \nu}\Big|_{\partial\Omega}) \ : \ u \in W^{1,2}(\Omega), \Delta u = 0 \text{ in } (\Omega\backslash\overline{D})\cup D, \frac{\partial u}{\partial \nu}\Big|_+ = k\frac{\partial u}{\partial \nu}\Big|_- \right\} .$$

In fact, $\mathcal{C}_{D,k}$ is a graph, namely

$$\mathcal{C}_{D,k} = \left\{ (f, \Lambda(f)) \in W^2_{\frac{1}{2}}(\partial\Omega) \times W^2_{-\frac{1}{2}}(\partial\Omega) \right\} ,$$

where $\Lambda(f) = \partial u/\partial\nu|_{\partial\Omega}$ with $u \in W^{1,2}(\Omega)$ the solution of

$$\begin{cases} \nabla \cdot \left(1 + (k - 1)\chi(D) \right)\nabla u = 0 & \text{in } \Omega \,, \\ u|_{\partial\Omega} = f \,. \end{cases}$$

The operator Λ is called the Dirichlet-to-Neumann (DtN) map.

The following theorem is a special case of the general uniqueness theorem due to Isakov [165]. Later, in Chapter 4, we shall use this result for our study of the generalized polarization tensors.

Theorem 3.2 *Let Ω be a Lipschitz bounded domain in $\mathbb{R}^d, d \geq 2$. Suppose that D_1 and D_2 are bounded Lipschitz domains such that, for $p = 1, 2, \overline{D_p} \subset \Omega$ and $\Omega \setminus \overline{D_p}$ are connected. Suppose that the conductivity of D_p is $0 < k_p \neq 1 < +\infty$, $p = 1, 2$. If $\mathcal{C}_{D_1,k_1} = \mathcal{C}_{D_2,k_2}$, then $D_1 = D_2$ and $k_1 = k_2$.*

Proof.   For a fixed but arbitrary $g \in L^2_0(\partial\Omega)$, let u_p, $p = 1, 2$, be the solution to

$$\begin{cases} \nabla \cdot \left(1 + (k_p - 1)\chi(D_p) \right)\nabla u_p = 0 & \text{in } \Omega \,, \\ \dfrac{\partial u_p}{\partial \nu}\Big|_{\partial\Omega} = g \in L^2_0(\partial\Omega), \quad \displaystyle\int_{\partial\Omega} u_p = 0 \,, \end{cases}$$

and U be the solution to (3.2). If $\mathcal{C}_{D_1,k_1} = \mathcal{C}_{D_2,k_2}$, then $u_1 = u_2$ on $\partial\Omega$, and hence

$$\int_{\partial\Omega} (U - u_1)g\, d\sigma = \int_{\partial\Omega} (U - u_2)g\, d\sigma \,.$$

It then follows from Lemma 3.1 that

$$\int_{D_1} |\nabla U|^2\, dx \approx \int_{D_2} |\nabla U|^2\, dx \,. \qquad\qquad\qquad (3.4)$$

Observe that (3.4) holds for all $U \in W^{1,2}(\Omega)$ harmonic in Ω.

Suppose that $D_1 \neq D_2$. Then there is z_0 in ∂D_1 (or ∂D_2) such that z_0 is further away from $\overline{D_2}$ (or $\overline{D_1}$). For $z \notin \overline{D_1 \cup D_2}$ let $\Gamma_z(x) := \Gamma(x - z)$ where Γ is the fundamental solution for Δ. Then, Γ_z is harmonic in a neighborhood of $\overline{D_1 \cup D_2}$. Therefore, by the Runge approximation (see Lemma 2.6), there is a sequence of entire harmonic functions that converges uniformly on $\overline{D_1 \cup D_2}$ to $\Gamma_z(x)$. It then follows from (3.4) that

$$\int_{D_1} |\nabla \Gamma_z|^2 \, dx \approx \int_{D_2} |\nabla \Gamma_z|^2 \, dx \, , \tag{3.5}$$

regardless of z.

Since $|\nabla \Gamma_z(x)| \approx |x - z|^{1-d}$ for x in a vicinity of z, as $z \to z_0$, the left-hand side of (3.5) goes to $+\infty$, whereas the right-hand side stays bounded since z_0 is away from $\overline{D_2}$. This contradiction forces us to conclude that $D_1 = D_2$.

Let $g \in L_0^2(\partial\Omega)$ be non-trivial. Let $f = u_1 = u_2$ on $\partial\Omega$ and

$$\lambda_p = (k_p + 1)/(2(k_p - 1)) \quad \text{for } p = 1, 2 \, .$$

Let $H = -\mathcal{S}_\Omega g + \mathcal{D}_\Omega f$ in $\mathbb{R}^d \setminus \partial\Omega$. By the representation formula (2.63), it follows that for $p = 1, 2$,

$$u_p = H + \mathcal{S}_{D_p}(\lambda_p I - \mathcal{K}_{D_p}^*)^{-1}\left(\frac{\partial H}{\partial \nu}\bigg|_{\partial D_p}\right) \quad \text{in } \Omega \, .$$

Then

$$\mathcal{S}_{D_1}(\lambda_1 I - \mathcal{K}_{D_1}^*)^{-1}\left(\frac{\partial H}{\partial \nu}\bigg|_{\partial D_1}\right) = \mathcal{S}_{D_1}(\lambda_2 I - \mathcal{K}_{D_1}^*)^{-1}\left(\frac{\partial H}{\partial \nu}\bigg|_{\partial D_1}\right) \quad \text{in } \Omega \setminus \overline{D_1} \, ,$$

and hence in Ω by the maximum principle (see Lemma 2.4). Thus by the jump formula, we have

$$(\lambda_1 I - \mathcal{K}_{D_1}^*)^{-1}\left(\frac{\partial H}{\partial \nu}\bigg|_{\partial D_1}\right) = (\lambda_2 I - \mathcal{K}_{D_1}^*)^{-1}\left(\frac{\partial H}{\partial \nu}\bigg|_{\partial D_1}\right) \, ,$$

which gives

$$(\lambda_1 - \lambda_2)(\lambda_2 I - \mathcal{K}_{D_1}^*)^{-1}\left(\frac{\partial H}{\partial \nu}\bigg|_{\partial D_1}\right) = 0 \, .$$

Since $\partial H/\partial \nu \not\equiv 0$ on ∂D_1, we get $\lambda_1 = \lambda_2$, which completes the proof. $\square$

It is worth mentioning that if $D_1 = D_2$, then a single measurement is sufficient to have $k_1 = k_2$.

3.2 Uniqueness With One Measurement

Let Ω be a simply connected Lipschitz domain in $\mathbb{R}^d$, and let $D_p, p = 1, 2$, be compact subdomains of Ω. Fix $0 < k \neq 1 < +\infty$, and let u_p, $p = 1, 2$, be the solutions of

$$\begin{cases} \nabla \cdot \Big(1 + (k-1)\chi(D_p)\Big)\nabla u_p = 0 \quad \text{in } \Omega \,, \\[2mm] \dfrac{\partial u_p}{\partial \nu}\Big|_{\partial\Omega} = g \in L_0^2(\partial\Omega), \quad \int_{\partial\Omega} u_p = 0 \,. \end{cases} \tag{3.6}$$

The question of uniqueness here is whether from $u_1 = u_2$ on $\partial\Omega$ for a certain g, it follows that $D_1 = D_2$. This question has been studied extensively recently. However, it is still wide open. The global uniqueness results thus far are obtained only when D is restricted to convex polyhedrons (with very restricted g) and balls in three-dimensional space and polygons and disks in the plane (see [58, 55, 131, 168, 281, 181, 182]). Even the uniqueness within the classes of ellipses and ellipsoids is not known. The uniqueness for multiple disks and multiple balls is also a challenging problem with practical implications.

3.2.1 Uniqueness in the Monotone Case

In the following monotone case, global uniqueness holds for general domains [57, 2].

Theorem 3.3 *Let Ω be a simply connected Lipschitz domain in $\mathbb{R}^d$, and let D_1 and D_2 be two Lipschitz bounded domains compactly contained within Ω. Suppose that $D_1 \subset D_2$; then for any non-zero $g \in L_0^2(\partial\Omega)$, if $u_1 = u_2$ on $\partial\Omega$ then $D_1 = D_2$.*

Proof. Assume that $D_1 \subset D_2$. Then $\partial u_1/\partial\nu = \partial u_2/\partial\nu$ on $\partial\Omega$ implies

$$\int_\Omega (1 + (k-1)\chi(D_1))\nabla u_1 \cdot \nabla\eta = \int_\Omega (1 + (k-1)\chi(D_2))\nabla u_2 \cdot \nabla\eta \,,$$

for all $\eta \in W^{1,2}(\Omega)$ and hence,

$$\int_\Omega (1 + (k-1)\chi(D_1))\nabla(u_1 - u_2) \cdot \nabla\eta = (k-1)\int_{D_2\backslash D_1} \nabla u_2 \cdot \nabla\eta \,. \tag{3.7}$$

Since $u_1 = u_2$ on $\partial\Omega$, we have

$$\int_\Omega (1 + (k-1)\chi(D_1))\nabla u_1 \cdot \nabla(u_1 - u_2) = 0 \,.$$

Consequently, substituting $\eta = u_1$ and $\eta = u_1 - u_2$ in (3.7), we obtain

$$\int_\Omega (1 + (k-1)\chi(D_1))|\nabla(u_1 - u_2)|^2 + (k-1)\int_{D_2\backslash D_1} |\nabla u_2|^2 = 0 \,.$$

So, if $k > 1$, then $u_1 = u_2$ in Ω, and therefore by the transmission condition, we conclude that $D_1 = D_2$ since otherwise $u_1 = u_2 \equiv 0$ in Ω. If $0 < k < 1$, we interchange the roles of D_1 and D_2 to arrive at

$$\int_\Omega (1 + (k-1)\chi(D_2))|\nabla(u_1 - u_2)|^2 + (1-k)\int_{D_2\backslash D_1} |\nabla u_1|^2 = 0 \,,$$

which yields the same conclusion. $\qquad\square$

3.2.2 Uniqueness of Disks With One Measurement

We give here a proof due to Kang and Seo [180] for the unique determination of disks with one measurement.

Theorem 3.4 *Let Ω be a simply connected Lipschitz domain in $\mathbb{R}^2$, and let D_1 and D_2 be two disk-shaped conductivity inclusions compactly contained in Ω, having the same conductivity k. For any non-zero $g \in L_0^2(\partial\Omega)$, if $u_1 = u_2$ on $\partial\Omega$, then $D_1 = D_2$.*

Proof. Let $f = u_1 = u_2$ on $\partial\Omega$ and $\lambda = (k+1)/(2(k-1))$. Let $H = -\mathcal{S}_\Omega g + \mathcal{D}_\Omega f$ in $\mathbb{R}^2 \setminus \partial\Omega$. Recall from (2.21) that $\mathcal{K}_{D_p}^* \equiv 0$ on $L_0^2(\partial D_p)$. By the representation formula (2.63), it follows that for $p = 1, 2$,

$$u_p = H + \frac{1}{\lambda}\mathcal{S}_{D_p}\Big(\frac{\partial H}{\partial\nu}\Big|_{\partial D_p}\Big) \quad \text{in } \Omega .$$

(i) The monotone case. Assume that $D_1 \subset D_2$. Then, by Theorem 3.3, $u_1 = u_2$ on $\partial\Omega$ implies that $D_1 = D_2$.

(ii) The disjoint case. If D_1 and D_2 are disjoint, then

$$\mathcal{S}_{D_1}\Big(\frac{\partial H}{\partial\nu}\Big|_{\partial D_1}\Big) = \mathcal{S}_{D_2}\Big(\frac{\partial H}{\partial\nu}\Big|_{\partial D_2}\Big) \quad \text{in } \mathbb{R}^2 \setminus D_1 \cup D_2$$

implies that $\mathcal{S}_{D_1}(\partial H/\partial\nu|_{\partial D_1})$ is harmonic on $\mathbb{R}^2$ and hence $\partial H/\partial\nu = 0$ on ∂D_1 by (2.32), and hence H is a constant function, which is a contradiction.

(iii) The non-monotone case. From $u_1 = u_2$ on $\partial\Omega$, it follows by using the representation formula (2.63) that

$$\mathcal{S}_{D_1}\Big(\frac{\partial H}{\partial\nu}\Big|_{\partial D_1}\Big) = \mathcal{S}_{D_2}\Big(\frac{\partial H}{\partial\nu}\Big|_{\partial D_2}\Big) \quad \text{in } \mathbb{R}^2 \setminus D_1 \cup D_2 .$$

Assume that D_1 and D_2 are two disks with a non-empty intersection. Since

$$\frac{\partial}{\partial\nu}\mathcal{S}_{D_p}\Big(\frac{\partial H}{\partial\nu}\Big|_{\partial D_p}\Big)\Big|_{-} = -\frac{1}{2}\frac{\partial H}{\partial\nu}\Big|_{\partial D_p} \quad \text{on } \partial D_p , \ p = 1, 2$$

by (2.21) and (2.27), it follows from the uniqueness of a solution to the Neumann boundary value problem for the Laplacian that

$$\mathcal{S}_{D_p}\Big(\frac{\partial H}{\partial\nu}\Big|_{\partial D_p}\Big) = -\frac{1}{2}H + c_p \quad \text{in } D_p$$

for some constant c_p. Hence

$$\mathcal{S}_{D_1}\Big(\frac{\partial H}{\partial \nu}\Big|_{\partial D_1}\Big) = \mathcal{S}_{D_2}\Big(\frac{\partial H}{\partial \nu}\Big|_{\partial D_2}\Big) + \text{ constant} \quad \text{in } D_1 \cap D_2 \ .$$

Since

$$\mathcal{S}_{D_1}\Big(\frac{\partial H}{\partial \nu}\Big|_{\partial D_1}\Big) = \mathcal{S}_{D_2}\Big(\frac{\partial H}{\partial \nu}\Big|_{\partial D_2}\Big) \quad \text{in } \mathbb{R}^2 \setminus \overline{D_1 \cup D_2} \ ,$$

we get by the continuity of the single layer potential that

$$\mathcal{S}_{D_1}\Big(\frac{\partial H}{\partial \nu}\Big|_{\partial D_1}\Big) = \mathcal{S}_{D_2}\Big(\frac{\partial H}{\partial \nu}\Big|_{\partial D_2}\Big) \quad \text{in } D_1 \cap D_2 \ .$$

Hence

$$\mathcal{S}_{D_1}\Big(\frac{\partial H}{\partial \nu}\Big|_{\partial D_1}\Big) = \mathcal{S}_{D_2}\Big(\frac{\partial H}{\partial \nu}\Big|_{\partial D_2}\Big) \quad \text{on } \partial(D_1 \setminus D_2) \cup \partial(D_2 \setminus D_1) \ ,$$

and by the maximum principle,

$$\mathcal{S}_{D_1}\Big(\frac{\partial H}{\partial \nu}\Big|_{\partial D_1}\Big) = \mathcal{S}_{D_2}\Big(\frac{\partial H}{\partial \nu}\Big|_{\partial D_2}\Big) \quad \text{in } \mathbb{R}^2 \ .$$

It implies that $\mathcal{S}_{D_1}(\partial H/\partial \nu|_{\partial D_1})$ is a harmonic function in the entire domain $\mathbb{R}^2$, and so $\partial H/\partial \nu = 0$ on ∂D_1 and H is a constant function, which is a contradiction. $\qquad \square$

3.3 Further Results and Open Problems

Given $g \in L_0^2(\partial\Omega)$, by comparing $u|_{\partial\Omega}$ with $U|_{\partial\Omega}$, where u and U are the solutions of (3.1) and (3.2), upper and lower bounds of the size of the inclusion D can be obtained; see [10, 184]. A Hölder stability estimate for disks can also be derived under some condition on the Neumann data g; see [123]. Based on the representation formula (2.63), a numerical algorithm for identifying disk-shaped conductivity inclusions from one boundary measurement is proposed and implemented in [185].

One interesting problem is to establish global uniqueness for the inverse isotropic conductivity problem with one measurement within the classes of ellipses, ellipsoids, and multiple disks and balls. Another open question concerns uniqueness or non-uniqueness for the inverse anisotropic conductivity problem with a finite number of measurements.

4

Generalized Isotropic and Anisotropic Polarization Tensors

Introduction

In this chapter we introduce the notion of generalized polarization tensors (GPTs) associated with a bounded Lipschitz domain and an isotropic or an anisotropic conductivity and study their basic properties. The GPTs generalize the concepts of classic Pólya–Szegö polarization tensors, which have been extensively studied by many authors for various purposes [83, 38, 84, 115, 225, 222, 132, 195, 202, 266, 271, 280, 106]. The notion of Pólya–Szegö polarization tensors, appeared in problems of potential theory related to certain questions arising in hydrodynamics and in electrostatics. If the conductivity of the inclusion is zero, namely, if the inclusion is insulated, the polarization tensor of Pólya–Szegö is called the virtual mass.

As it will be shown later, in Chapter 5, the GPTs are the basic building blocks for the full asymptotic expansions of the boundary voltage perturbations due to the presence of a small conductivity inclusion inside a conductor. The use of these GPTs leads to stable and accurate algorithms for the numerical computations of the steady-state voltage in the presence of small conductivity inclusions. It is known that small size features cause difficulties in the numerical solution of the conductivity problem by the finite element or finite difference methods, because such features require refined meshes in their neighborhoods, with their attendant problems [187].

On the other hand, it is important from an imaging point of view to precisely characterize these GPTs and derive some of their properties, such as symmetry, positivity, and optimal bounds on their elements, in order to develop efficient algorithms for reconstructing conductivity inclusions of small volume. The GPTs seem to contain significant information about the inclusion and its conductivity, which is yet to be investigated.

The concept of polarization tensors also occurs in several other interesting contexts, in particular in asymptotic models of dilute electrical composites [245, 38, 81, 114]. The determination of the effective or macroscopic property of a two-phase medium consisting of inclusions of one material of known shape embedded homogeneously in another one, having physical properties different from the former one's, has been one of the classic problems in physics. Later in this book, we shall present a general unified layer potential technique for rigorously deriving very accurate asymptotic expansions of electrical effective properties of dilute media for general inclusions in terms of the volume fraction. Our approach is valid for high contrast mixtures and inclusions with Lipschitz boundaries. These asymptotic expansions are expressed via the GPTs of the inclusions.

This chapter lays down the main concept, which forms the unifying thread throughout the whole book. We begin by giving two slightly different but equivalent definitions of the GPTs. We then prove that the knowledge of the set of all GPTs allows for uniquely determining the domain and the constitutive parameter. Furthermore, we show important properties of symmetry and positivity of the GPTs and derive isoperimetric inequalities satisfied by the tensor elements of the GPTs. We also establish relations that can be used to provide bounds on the weighted volume. We understand an isoperimetric inequality to be any inequality that relates two or more geometric and/or physical quantities associated with the same domain. The inequality must be optimal in the sense that the equality sign holds for some domain or in the limit as the domain degenerates [263]. The classic isoperimetric inequality — the one after which all such inequalities are named — states that of all plane curves of given perimeter the circle encloses the largest area. This inequality was known already to the ancient Greeks. The reader is referred to [271, 53, 263, 265] for a variety of important isoperimetric inequalities. After that, we consider the polarization tensors associated with multiple inclusions. We prove their symmetry and positivity. We then estimate their eigenvalues in terms of the total volume of the inclusions. We also give explicit formulae for the GPTs in the multi-disk case. We conclude the chapter by establishing similar results for the (generalized) anisotropic polarization tensors (APTs). These tensors are defined in the same way as the GPTs. However, they occur due to not only the presence of discontinuity but also the difference of the anisotropy.

The properties of the GPTs and APTs investigated here will be used in Chapter 7 to obtain accurate reconstructions of small conductivity inclusions from a small number of boundary measurements. They also play an essential role in deriving the effective properties of dilute electrical composites; see Chapter 8.

4.1 Definition

Let B be a Lipschitz bounded domain in $\mathbb{R}^d$, and let the conductivity of B be k, $0 < k \neq 1 < +\infty$. Denote $\lambda := (k+1)/(2(k-1))$.

To motivate the definition of the GPTs, we begin with deriving the far-field expansion of the solution to the transmission problem in free space.

Suppose that the origin $O \in B$. Let H be a harmonic function in $\mathbb{R}^d$, and let u be the solution to the following problem:

$$\begin{cases} \nabla \cdot ((1 + (k-1)\chi(B))\nabla u) = 0 & \text{in } \mathbb{R}^d , \\ u(x) - H(x) = O(|x|^{1-d}) & \text{as } |x| \to +\infty . \end{cases} \tag{4.1}$$

For a multi-index $i = (i_1, \ldots, i_d) \in \mathbb{N}^d$, let $\partial^i f = \partial_1^{i_1} \cdots \partial_d^{i_d} f$ and $x^i := x_1^{i_1} \cdots x_d^{i_d}$. Following the same lines as in the derivation of (2.63), we can easily prove that we have

$$u(x) = H(x) + \mathcal{S}_B(\lambda I - \mathcal{K}_B^*)^{-1}\left(\frac{\partial H}{\partial \nu}\big|_{\partial B}\right)(x) \quad \text{for } x \in \mathbb{R}^d , \tag{4.2}$$

which together with the Taylor expansion

$$\Gamma(x-y) = \sum_{i,|i|=0}^{+\infty} \frac{(-1)^{|i|}}{i!}\partial_x^i \Gamma(x)y^i, \quad y \text{ in a compact set}, \quad |x| \to +\infty ,$$

yields the far-field expansion

$$(u-H)(x) = \sum_{|i|,|j|=1}^{+\infty} \frac{(-1)^{|i|}}{i!j!}\partial_x^i \Gamma(x)\partial^j H(0) \int_{\partial B} (\lambda I - \mathcal{K}_B^*)^{-1}\left(\nu_x \cdot \nabla x^i\right)(y)y^j \, do(y) \tag{4.3}$$

as $|x| \to +\infty$.

Definition 4.1 *For $i, j \in \mathbb{N}^d$, we define the generalized polarization tensor M_{ij} by*

$$M_{ij} := \int_{\partial B} y^j \phi_i(y) \, d\sigma(y) , \tag{4.4}$$

where ϕ_i is given by

$$\phi_i(y) := (\lambda I - \mathcal{K}_B^*)^{-1}\left(\nu_x \cdot \nabla x^i\right)(y), \quad y \in \partial B . \tag{4.5}$$

Here $\mathcal{K}_B^*$ is the singular integral operator defined by (2.30). If $|i| = |j| = 1$, we denote M_{ij} by $(m_{pq})_{p,q=1}^d$ and call $M = (m_{pq})_{p,q=1}^d$ the polarization tensor of Pólya–Szegö.

Formula (4.3) shows that through the GPTs we have complete information about the far-field expansion of u:

$$(u - H)(x) = \sum_{|i|,|j|=1}^{+\infty} \frac{(-1)^{|i|}}{i!j!}\partial_x^i \Gamma(x)M_{ij}\partial^j H(0)$$

as $|x| \to +\infty$.

We can also represent the GPTs in terms of solutions to transmission problems. As a first step, we prove the following existence and uniqueness result.

Lemma 4.2 *For any multi-index* $i = (i_1, \ldots, i_d) \in \mathbb{N}^d$, *there is a unique solution* ψ_i *to the following transmission problem:*

$$
\begin{cases}
\Delta\psi_i(x) = 0, \quad x \in B \cup (\mathbb{R}^d \setminus \overline{B}) , \\[2mm]
\psi_i\big|_+(x) - \psi_i\big|_-(x) = 0, \quad x \in \partial B , \\[2mm]
\dfrac{\partial\psi_i}{\partial\nu}\bigg|_+(x) - k\dfrac{\partial\psi_i}{\partial\nu}\bigg|_-(x) = \nu \cdot \nabla x^i, \quad x \in \partial B , \\[2mm]
\psi_i(x) \to 0 \;\; as \;\; |x| \to +\infty \quad if\; d = 3 , \\[2mm]
\psi_i(x) - \dfrac{1}{2\pi}\ln|x| \displaystyle\int_{\partial B} \nu \cdot \nabla y^i \, d\sigma(y) \to 0 \;\; as \;\; |x| \to +\infty \quad if\; d = 2 .
\end{cases}
\tag{4.6}
$$

Moreover, ψ_i *satisfies the following decay estimate at infinity:*

$$
\psi_i(x) - \Gamma(x)\int_{\partial B} \nu \cdot \nabla y^i \, d\sigma(y) = O\left(\frac{1}{|x|^{d-1}}\right) \quad as \;\; |x| \to +\infty .
\tag{4.7}
$$

Proof.   The existence and uniqueness of ψ_i can be established using single layer potentials with suitably chosen densities. Fairly simple manipulations show that $\partial\psi_i/\partial\nu|_-$ satisfies the integral equation

$$
(\lambda I - \mathcal{K}_B^*)\left(\frac{\partial\psi_i}{\partial\nu}\bigg|_-\right)(x) = \frac{1}{k-1}\left(-\frac{1}{2}I + \mathcal{K}_B^*\right)(\nu \cdot \nabla y^i)(x) , \quad x \in \partial B .
\tag{4.8}
$$

Since $\mathcal{K}_B(1) = 1/2$, we have

$$
\int_{\partial B}\left(-\frac{1}{2}I + \mathcal{K}_B^*\right)(\nu \cdot \nabla y^i)(x)\, d\sigma(x) = \int_{\partial B}(\nu \cdot \nabla x^i)\left(-\frac{1}{2}I + \mathcal{K}_B\right)(1)\, d\sigma(x) = 0 ,
$$

and consequently, according to Theorem 2.21, a unique solution exists $\partial\psi_i/\partial\nu|_- \in L_0^2(\partial B)$ to the integral equation (4.8). Furthermore, we can express $\psi_i(x)$ for all $x \in \mathbb{R}^d$ as follows:

$$
\psi_i(x) = \frac{1}{k-1}\mathcal{S}_B(\lambda I - \mathcal{K}_B^*)^{-1}(\nu \cdot \nabla y^i)(x) , \quad x \in \mathbb{R}^d .
\tag{4.9}
$$

To obtain the behavior at infinity of ψ_i we write

$$
\psi_i(x) = \frac{1}{k-1}\int_{\partial B}\left(\Gamma(x-y) - \Gamma(x)\right)(\lambda I - \mathcal{K}_B^*)^{-1}(\nu \cdot \nabla z^i)(y)\, d\sigma(y)
$$
$$
+ \Gamma(x)\frac{1}{k-1}\int_{\partial B}(\lambda I - \mathcal{K}_B^*)^{-1}(\nu \cdot \nabla z^i)(y)\, d\sigma(y) .
$$

Note that since $\mathcal{K}_B(1) = 1/2$, $(\lambda I - \mathcal{K}_B^*)^{-1}(1) = k - 1$, and hence

$$
\int_{\partial B}(\lambda I - \mathcal{K}_B^*)^{-1}(\nu \cdot \nabla y^i)(z)\, d\sigma(z) = \int_{\partial B}(\nu \cdot \nabla y^i)(\lambda I - \mathcal{K}_B^*)^{-1}(1)\, d\sigma(y)
$$
$$
= (k-1)\int_{\partial B}\nu \cdot \nabla y^i \, d\sigma(y) .
$$

Thus we obtain

$$\psi_i(x) - \Gamma(x) \int_{\partial B} \nu \cdot \nabla y^i \, d\sigma(y)$$
$$= \frac{1}{k-1} \int_{\partial B} \Big(\Gamma(x-y) - \Gamma(x) \Big) (\lambda I - \mathcal{K}_B^*)^{-1} (\nu \cdot \nabla z^i)(y) \, d\sigma(y) \ .$$

Now the desired decay estimate (4.7) follows from (2.14).

Observe that the uniqueness of a solution ψ_i to (4.6) can be proved in a straightforward way from the decay estimate (4.7). Let θ be the difference of two solutions, so that

$$\begin{cases} \nabla \cdot \Big(1 + (k-1)\chi(B) \Big) \nabla \theta = 0 \quad \text{in } \mathbb{R}^d, \\ \theta(x) = O(|x|^{1-d}) \quad \text{as } |x| \to +\infty \ . \end{cases}$$

Integrating by parts yields the energy identity

$$\int_{|y|<R} (1 + (k-1)\chi(B)) |\nabla \theta|^2 = \int_{|y|=R} \frac{\partial \theta}{\partial \nu}(y) \, \theta(y) \, d\sigma(y) \ .$$

Now let $R \to +\infty$; we have

$$\frac{\partial \theta}{\partial \nu}(y)\theta(y) = O(R^{-2d+1}) \quad \text{for } |y| = R \ ,$$

so that

$$\int_{\mathbb{R}^d} (1 + (k-1)\chi(B)) |\nabla \theta|^2 = 0 \ .$$

This implies that θ is constant in $\mathbb{R}^d$, and in fact $\theta \equiv 0$ in $\mathbb{R}^d$ because $\theta(y)$ goes to 0 as $|y| \to +\infty$. $\qquad \square$

We are now able to prove the following.

Lemma 4.3 *For all $i, j \in \mathbb{N}^d$, $M_{ij}(k, B)$ can be rewritten in the following form:*

$$M_{ij}(k, B) = (k-1) \int_{\partial B} x^j \frac{\partial x^i}{\partial \nu} \, d\sigma(x) + (k-1)^2 \int_{\partial B} x^j \frac{\partial \psi_i}{\partial \nu}\Big|_{-} (x) \, d\sigma(x) \ , \quad (4.10)$$

where ψ_i is the unique solution to the transmission problem (4.6).

Proof. From the expression (4.9) of ψ_i and the identity

$$-\frac{1}{2}I + \mathcal{K}_B^* = -(\lambda I - \mathcal{K}_B^*) + (\lambda - \frac{1}{2})I \ ,$$

we compute by using the jump relation (2.27)

$$\int_{\partial B} x^j \frac{\partial \psi_i}{\partial \nu}\bigg|_-(x) = \frac{1}{k-1}\int_{\partial B} x^j \left[(\lambda I - \mathcal{K}_B^*)^{-1}(-\frac{1}{2}I + \mathcal{K}_B^*)(\nu\cdot\nabla y^i)(x)\right]d\sigma(x)$$

$$= \frac{1}{k-1}\int_{\partial B} x^j \left[(\lambda - \frac{1}{2})(\lambda I - \mathcal{K}_B^*)^{-1}(\nu\cdot\nabla y^i)(x) - \nu\cdot\nabla x^i\right]d\sigma(x) ,$$

which immediately leads to (4.10). $\square$

One significant advantage of using boundary integrals for defining the GPTs is that all the computation can be carried out on ∂B without having to deal with unbounded spaces.

The following observation is from [46] and simply follows from a change of variables.

Lemma 4.4 *If $|i| + |j|$ is odd and B is symmetric about the origin, then $M_{ij}(k, B)$ is zero.*

Proof.   Set $\theta_i(x) = \psi_i(-x)$. Then the function θ_i satisfies

$$\begin{cases} \Delta\theta_i(x) = 0, \quad x \in B \cup (\mathbb{R}^d \setminus \overline{B}) , \\[4pt] \theta_i\bigg|_+(x) - \theta_i\bigg|_-(x) = 0 \quad x \in \partial B , \\[4pt] \dfrac{\partial\theta_i}{\partial\nu}\bigg|_+(x) - k\dfrac{\partial\theta_i}{\partial\nu}\bigg|_-(x) = (-1)^{|i|}\nu\cdot\nabla x^i \quad x \in \partial B , \\[4pt] \theta_i(x) \to 0 \text{ as } |x| \to +\infty \quad \text{if } d \geq 3 , \\[4pt] \theta_i(x) + (-1)^{|i|+1}\dfrac{1}{2\pi}\ln|x|\displaystyle\int_{\partial B}\nu\cdot\nabla y^i \, d\sigma(y) \to 0 \text{ as } |x| \to +\infty \quad \text{if } d = 2 , \end{cases}$$

which implies that $\theta_i(x) = (-1)^{|i|}\psi_i(x)$. With the change of variables $y = -x$

$$\int_{\partial B} x^j \frac{\partial x^i}{\partial\nu}\, d\sigma(x) = (-1)^{|i|+|j|}\int_{\partial B} y^j \frac{\partial y^i}{\partial\nu}\, d\sigma(y)$$

and

$$\int_{\partial B} x^j \frac{\partial\psi_i}{\partial\nu}\bigg|_-(x)\, d\sigma(x) = (-1)^{|j|+1}\int_{\partial B} y^j \frac{\partial\psi_i}{\partial\nu}\bigg|_-(-y)\, d\sigma(y)$$

$$= (-1)^{|i|+|j|}\int_{\partial B} y^j \frac{\partial\psi_i}{\partial\nu}\bigg|_-(y)\, d\sigma(y) .$$

Hence $M_{ij}(k, B)$ is zero provided that $|i| + |j|$ is odd. $\square$

The following lemma, which can be proved by simple changes of variables, is also of importance to us.

Lemma 4.5 *Let $0 < k \neq 1 < +\infty$. Let B' be a domain and $B = \mathcal{R}B'$ where $\mathcal{R}$ is a unitary transformation, and let $M(k, B)$ and $M(k, B')$ be the first-order polarization tensors associated with B and B', respectively. Then*

$$M(k, B) = \mathcal{R}M(k, B')\mathcal{R}^T .$$

4.2 Explicit Formulae

The polarization tensor M of Pólya–Szegö can be explicitly computed for disks and ellipses in the plane and balls and ellipsoids in three-dimensional space [195]. The following analytical expression has been derived by Brühl, Hanke, and Vogelius [73].

Proposition 4.6 *If B is an ellipse whose semi-axes are on the x_1- and x_2-axes and of length a and b, respectively, then its polarization tensor of Pólya–Szegö M takes the form*

$$M(k, B) = (k - 1)|B| \begin{pmatrix} \dfrac{a+b}{a+kb} & 0 \\ 0 & \dfrac{a+b}{b+ka} \end{pmatrix}, \tag{4.11}$$

where $|B|$ denotes the volume of B.

Proof. To fix notation, let B be the ellipse with focal interval $[-R, R]$ on the x_1-axis and eccentricity $1/\cosh\rho$, or in other words, the ellipse whose major axis is of length $a = R\cosh\rho$ and lies on the x_1-axis, and whose semi-minor axis is of length $b = R\sinh\rho$ and lies on the x_2-axis. In order to determine the solutions ψ_i, for $i = (1, 0)$ and $i = (0, 1)$ to (4.6), we introduce elliptic coordinates (r, ω), as follows:

$$x_1 = R\cos\omega\cosh r, \quad x_2 = R\sin\omega\sinh r, \quad r \geq 0, 0 \leq \omega \leq 2\pi,$$

in which the ellipse B is given by $B = \{(r, \omega) : r < \rho\}$. Separation of variables yields a general solution to the Laplace equation of the form

$$\psi(r, \omega) = A_0 + \sum_{m=1}^{+\infty} \Big(A_m \cos m\omega\, e^{-mr} + B_m \sin m\omega\, e^{-mr} + C_m \cos m\omega\, e^{mr}$$
$$+ D_m \sin m\omega\, e^{mr} \Big)$$

in $B \setminus [-R, R]$ and in the exterior of B, with different sets of coefficients. For the solution in $B \setminus [-R, R]$ to extend to a harmonic function in B, we must furthermore require that

$$\psi(0, \omega) = \psi(0, -\omega) \text{ and } \frac{\partial\psi}{\partial r}(0, \omega) = -\frac{\partial\psi}{\partial r}(0, -\omega). \tag{4.12}$$

The coefficients of the specific solutions ψ_i, for $i = (1, 0)$ and $i = (0, 1)$, are now determined by the condition (4.12), together with the transmission conditions $\psi_i|_+ = \psi_i|_-, \partial\psi_i/\partial\nu|_+ - k\partial\psi_i/\partial\nu|_- = \nu \cdot \nabla x^i$ on ∂B, and the behavior at infinity $\psi_i(x) \to 0$ as $|x| \to +\infty$. The result is

$$\psi_{(1,0)} = -\frac{ab}{a+kb}R_1(r)\cos\omega \quad \text{and} \quad \psi_{(0,1)} = -\frac{ab}{b+ka}R_2(r)\sin\omega$$

with

$$R_1(r) = \begin{cases} \dfrac{\cosh r}{\cosh \rho} & \text{for } r < \rho, \\[2ex] \dfrac{e^{-r}}{e^{-\rho}} & \text{for } r > \rho, \end{cases} \quad \text{and} \quad R_2(r) = \begin{cases} \dfrac{\sinh r}{\sinh \rho} & \text{for } r < \rho, \\[2ex] \dfrac{e^{-r}}{e^{-\rho}} & \text{for } r > \rho. \end{cases}$$

Using this it turns out by Lemma 4.3 that the polarization tensor M takes the diagonal form (4.11), where $|B| = \pi ab$ is the area of the ellipse. $\qquad\square$

For an arbitrary ellipse whose semi-axes are not aligned with the coordinate axes, one can use Lemma 4.5 to compute its Pólya–Szegö polarization tensor.

Kang and Kim [176] used (2.23) to derive (4.11) by a boundary integral method. Following [176], we first observe that

$$M_{ij}(k, B) = \int_{\partial B} y^j \phi_i(y)\, d\sigma(y)$$
$$= \int_{\partial B} y^j \left(\frac{\partial}{\partial \nu} \mathcal{S}_B \phi_i \bigg|_+ - \frac{\partial}{\partial \nu} \mathcal{S}_B \phi_i \bigg|_- \right)(y)\, d\sigma(y) \,.$$

Next, using the definition (4.4), we see from (4.9) that $\mathcal{S}_B \phi_i = (k-1)\psi_i$, where ψ_i is the solution to (4.6), and we have

$$\frac{\partial}{\partial \nu} \mathcal{S}_B \phi_i \bigg|_+ (y) = (k-1)\frac{\partial \psi_i}{\partial \nu} \bigg|_+ (y)$$
$$= (k-1)\left(\frac{\partial \psi_i}{\partial \nu} \bigg|_- (y) + \nu \cdot \nabla y^i \right)$$
$$= k\frac{\partial}{\partial \nu} \mathcal{S}_B \phi_i \bigg|_- (y) + (k-1)\nu \cdot \nabla y^i \,.$$

Hence,

$$M_{ij}(k, B) = (k-1)\int_{\partial B} y^j \frac{\partial}{\partial \nu} \mathcal{S}_B \phi_i \bigg|_- (y)\, d\sigma(y) + (k-1)\int_{\partial B} y^j \frac{\partial y^i}{\partial \nu}\, d\sigma(y)$$
$$= (k-1)\int_{\partial B} y^j \left(-\frac{1}{2}I + \mathcal{K}_B^* \right)\phi_i(y)\, d\sigma(y) + (k-1)\int_{\partial B} y^j \frac{\partial y^i}{\partial \nu}\, d\sigma(y)\,,$$

giving

$$M_{ij}(k, B) = (k-1)\int_{\partial B} \left(-\frac{1}{2}I + \mathcal{K}_B \right)(y^j)\phi_i(y)\, d\sigma(y)$$
$$+ (k-1)\int_{\partial B} y^j \frac{\partial y^i}{\partial \nu}\, d\sigma(y) \,. \tag{4.13}$$

When $|i| = |j| = 1$, (2.23) gives

$$\begin{pmatrix} \dfrac{a+kb}{a+b} & 0 \\ 0 & \dfrac{b+ka}{a+b} \end{pmatrix} M(k,B) = (k-1)|B|I \, ,$$

and hence, (4.11) holds, as desired. This method has been applied to derive the polarization tensors for an anisotropic conductivity inclusion as well [176].

In the three-dimensional case, a domain for which analogous analytical expressions for the elements of its polarization tensor M are available is the ellipsoid. If the coordinate axes are chosen to coincide with the principal axes of the ellipsoid B whose equation then becomes

$$\frac{x_1^2}{a^2} + \frac{x_2^2}{b^2} + \frac{x_3^2}{c^2} = 1, \quad 0 < c \le b \le a \, ,$$

then M takes the form

$$M(k,B) = (k-1)|B| \begin{pmatrix} \dfrac{1}{(1-A)+kA} & 0 & 0 \\ 0 & \dfrac{1}{(1-B)+kB} & 0 \\ 0 & 0 & \dfrac{1}{(1-C)+kC} \end{pmatrix} \, ,$$

$$(4.14)$$

where the constants A, B, and C are defined by

$$A = \frac{bc}{a^2} \int_1^{+\infty} \frac{1}{t^2\sqrt{t^2 - 1 + (\frac{b}{a})^2}\sqrt{t^2 - 1 + (\frac{c}{a})^2}} \, dt \, ,$$

$$B = \frac{bc}{a^2} \int_1^{+\infty} \frac{1}{(t^2 - 1 + (\frac{b}{a})^2)^{\frac{3}{2}}\sqrt{t^2 - 1 + (\frac{c}{a})^2}} \, dt \, ,$$

$$C = \frac{bc}{a^2} \int_1^{+\infty} \frac{1}{\sqrt{t^2 - 1 + (\frac{b}{a})^2}(t^2 - 1 + (\frac{c}{a})^2)^{\frac{3}{2}}} \, dt \, .$$

In the special case, $a = b = c$, the ellipsoid B becomes a sphere and $A = B = C = 1/3$. Hence the polarization tensor of Pólya–Szegö associated with the sphere B is given by

$$M(k,B) = (k-1)|B| \begin{pmatrix} \dfrac{3}{2+k} & 0 & 0 \\ 0 & \dfrac{3}{2+k} & 0 \\ 0 & 0 & \dfrac{3}{2+k} \end{pmatrix} \, .$$

Derivation of the above formulae can be found in [236].

The higher order GPTs can be explicitly computed for disks and ellipses in the plane and balls in three-dimensional space. Recall that a polynomial is homogeneous of degree n if it is a finite linear combination of monomials x^i where $|i| = n$. From [220] the following results hold.

Proposition 4.7(i) *Let B be the disk of radius R and center 0. Suppose that a_i and b_j are constants such that $f = \sum a_i y^i, g = \sum b_j y^j$ are harmonic polynomials of homogeneous degrees n and m, respectively. Then*

$$\sum a_i b_j M_{ij}(k, B) = \begin{cases} \dfrac{n\pi R^{2n}}{\lambda} & \text{if } f = g\,, \\ 0 & \text{otherwise}\,, \end{cases}$$

up to a multiplicative constant that is independent of k and B.

(ii) *Let B be the ellipse with focal interval $[-R, R]$ on the x_1-axis and eccentricity $1/\cosh\rho$. Suppose that a_i and b_j are constants such that $f = \sum a_i y^i$ and $g = \sum b_j y^j$ are harmonic polynomials of homogeneous degrees n and m, respectively. Then, up to a multiplicative constant that is independent of k and B,*

$$\sum a_i b_j M_{ij}(k, B) = (k - 1)\frac{m\pi R^{m+n}}{2^{m+n-1}} \times$$

$$\begin{cases} \displaystyle\sum_{p=1}^{\min(\frac{n}{2}, \frac{m-2}{2})} \frac{4p}{m + 2p} \binom{m-1}{\frac{m}{2} - p} \binom{n}{\frac{n}{2} - p} c_{2p} \sinh 4p\rho \\ \qquad + \mathcal{H}(n - m + 2) \binom{n}{\frac{n-m}{2}} c_m \sinh 2m\rho \\ \quad \text{if } n \text{ and } m \text{ are even,} \\[2ex] \displaystyle\sum_{p=0}^{\min(\frac{n-1}{2}, \frac{m-3}{2})} \frac{4p + 2}{m + 2p + 1} \binom{m-1}{\frac{m-1}{2} - p} \binom{n}{\frac{n-1}{2} - p} c_{2p+1} \sinh(4p + 2)\rho \\ \qquad + \mathcal{H}(n - m + 2) \binom{n}{\frac{n-m}{2}} c_m \sinh 2m\rho \\ \quad \text{if } n \text{ and } m \text{ are odd,} \\[2ex] 0 \qquad \text{otherwise,} \end{cases}$$

where $\dbinom{n}{p} = n!/((n - p)!p!),$

$$c_n = \frac{\sinh n\rho + \cosh n\rho}{k \sinh n\rho + \cosh n\rho}, \tag{4.15}$$

and $\mathcal{H}$ is the characteristic function of $]0, +\infty[$.

(iii) *Let B be the ball of radius R and center 0. Then*

$$\sum a_i b_j M_{ij}(k, B) = \frac{(k-1)n(2n+1)}{nk+n+1} R^{2n+1} \delta_{nm} \delta_{ll'} \, ,$$

where $\sum a_i y^i = |y|^n Y_{n,l}(y/|y|)$ and $\sum b_j y^j = |y|^m Y_{m,l'}(y/|y|)$. Here $\{Y_{n,1}, \ldots, Y_{n,2n+1}\}$ is a set of orthonormal harmonics of degree n and δ_{nm} denotes the Kronecker symbol.

Proof.   Let $\psi = \sum a_i \psi_i$, where ψ_i is the solution to (4.6). By (4.9) we know that

$$\psi = \frac{1}{k-1} \mathcal{S}_B (\lambda I - \mathcal{K}_B^*)^{-1} \left(\frac{\partial f}{\partial \nu} \right) . \tag{4.16}$$

With this formula, we have that

$$(k-1) \int_{\partial B} g \frac{\partial \psi}{\partial \nu} \bigg|_+ d\sigma = \int_{\partial B} g \left(\frac{1}{2} I + \mathcal{K}_B^* \right) (\lambda I - K_B^*)^{-1} \left(\frac{\partial f}{\partial \nu} \right) d\sigma$$

$$= - \int_{\partial B} g \frac{\partial f}{\partial \nu} d\sigma + \left(\lambda + \frac{1}{2} \right) \int_{\partial B} g (\lambda I - \mathcal{K}_B^*)^{-1} \left(\frac{\partial f}{\partial \nu} \right) d\sigma$$

$$= - \int_{\partial B} g \frac{\partial f}{\partial \nu} d\sigma + \frac{k}{k-1} \sum a_i b_j M_{ij}(k, B) \, ,$$

and therefore

$$\sum a_i b_j M_{ij}(k, B) = \left(1 - \frac{1}{k} \right) \left[\int_{\partial B} g \frac{\partial f}{\partial \nu} d\sigma + (k-1) \int_{\partial B} g \frac{\partial \psi}{\partial \nu} \bigg|_+ d\sigma \right] . \tag{4.17}$$

Define $\phi := (k-1)\psi + f$. Obviously, ϕ is the unique solution to the following transmission problem:

$$\begin{cases} \Delta \phi = 0 & \text{in } B \cup \mathbb{R}^2 \setminus \overline{B} \, , \\ \phi|_+ - \phi|_- = 0 & \text{on } \partial B \, , \\ \dfrac{\partial \phi}{\partial \nu} \bigg|_+ - k \dfrac{\partial \phi}{\partial \nu} \bigg|_- = 0 & \text{on } \partial B \, , \\ (\phi - f)(x) \to 0 & \text{as } |x| \to +\infty \, . \end{cases} \tag{4.18}$$

Formula (4.17) can now be simplified as follows:

$$\sum a_i b_j M_{ij}(k, B) = \left(1 - \frac{1}{k} \right) \int_{\partial B} g \frac{\partial \phi}{\partial \nu} \bigg|_+ d\sigma$$

$$= (k-1) \int_{\partial B} g \frac{\partial \phi}{\partial \nu} \bigg|_- d\sigma \tag{4.19}$$

$$= (k-1) \int_B \nabla g \cdot \nabla \phi \, dx \, .$$

We claim that there are functions U^- and U^+ holomorphic in B and $\mathbb{R}^2\backslash\overline{B}$, respectively, so that

$$\phi = \begin{cases} \Re U^- & \text{in } B \text{ ,} \\ \Re U^+ & \text{in } \mathbb{R}^2 \setminus \overline{B} \text{ .} \end{cases}$$

In fact, the existence of U^- is obvious since B is simply connected. In view of (4.16), we have

$$\psi(z) = \frac{1}{(k-1)2\pi} \int_{\partial B} \ln(z-\zeta)(\lambda I - \mathcal{K}_B^*)^{-1}(\frac{\partial f}{\partial \nu})(\zeta)\,d\sigma(\zeta), \quad z \in \mathbb{R}^2 \setminus \overline{B} \text{ ,}$$

and the integral is well-defined since $\int_{\partial B}(\lambda I - \mathcal{K}_B^*)^{-1}(\frac{\partial f}{\partial \nu})d\sigma = 0$.

The transmission condition in (4.18) implies

$$\frac{k}{k-1}U^- = \frac{k+1}{2(k-1)}U^+ + \frac{1}{2}\overline{U^+} + iC \quad \text{on } \partial B \text{ ,} \tag{4.20}$$

for some real constant C. By using the polynomial expansion of holomorphic functions together with (4.20), it is easy to show that the solution ϕ of (4.18) with $f = \Re z^n$, $z = x_1 + ix_2$, is precisely the real part of the function

$$U^-(z) = \frac{2}{k+1}z^n \text{ .}$$

Thus, with $g = \Re z^m$, (4.19) reads as follows:

$$\begin{aligned} \sum a_i b_j M_{ij}(k, B) &= (k-1)\int_B \nabla(\Re z^m) \cdot \nabla(\Re U^-)\,dx \\ &= \frac{2(k-1)}{(k+1)}\int_B \nabla(\Re z^m) \cdot \nabla(\Re z^n)\,dx \\ &= \frac{mn}{\lambda}\Re\int_B z^{m-1}\overline{z}^{n-1}\,dx \\ &= \frac{n\pi R^{2n}}{\lambda}\delta_{nm} \quad (z = x_1 + ix_2) \text{ .} \end{aligned}$$

In precisely the same fashion, we may show that if $f = \Im z^n$ and $g = \Im z^m$, then $\sum a_i b_j M_{ij}(k, B) = (n\pi R^{2n}/\lambda)\delta_{nm}$, whereas if $f = \Im z^n$ and $g = \Re z^m$ (or vice versa), then $\sum a_i b_j M_{ij}(k, B) = 0$. Since a harmonic polynomial of degree, say n, is either the real or the imaginary part of z^n, up to a multiplicative constant, the proof of (i) is complete.

We now prove (ii). In order to determine the function ϕ, we introduce, as in the proof of Proposition 4.6, the modified-elliptic coordinates on $\mathbb{C}\backslash[-R, R]$

$$z = \Phi(\xi) := R\cosh(r + i\omega) \qquad (r \geq 0,\ 0 \leq \omega < 2\pi) \text{ ,}$$

in which the ellipse B is given by $\{\xi = r+i\omega : r < \rho\}$. Let $u(\xi) = \phi \circ \Phi(\xi)$. Then holomorphic functions U^+ and U^- exist in $\Phi^{-1}(\mathbb{C}) \setminus \{r \leq \rho\}$ and $\{r < \rho\}$, respectively, so that

$$u = \begin{cases} \Re U^+ & \text{in } \mathbb{R}^2 \setminus \overline{B} , \\ \Re U^- & \text{in } B . \end{cases}$$

By the transmission conditions satisfied by ϕ and the conformality of the map Φ, we have

$$\frac{k}{k-1} U^- = \frac{k+1}{2(k-1)} U^+ + \frac{1}{2}\overline{U^+} + iC \qquad \text{on } r = \rho , \tag{4.21}$$

for some real constant C. Next, suppose for a moment that

$$U^+(\xi) - C' \cosh n\xi \to 0 \quad \text{as } |\xi| \to +\infty ,$$

for some constant C', then we have

$$U^-(\xi) = C' \left(\Re \frac{\sinh n\rho + \cosh n\rho}{k \sinh n\rho + \cosh n\rho} + i\Im \frac{\sinh n\rho + \cosh n\rho}{\sinh n\rho + k \cosh n\rho} \right) \cosh n\xi . \tag{4.22}$$

Let us now calculate $\sum a_i b_j M_{ij}(k, B)$ for $f = \Re z^n$ and $g = \Re z^m$. We shall find ϕ satisfying (4.18) and $(\phi - f)(x) \to 0$ as $|x| \to +\infty$. Therefore, by using the fact that

$$U^+(\xi) - f \circ \Phi(\xi) \to 0 \quad \text{as } |\xi| \to +\infty ,$$

we obtain according to (4.22) that, for $f(z) = \Re z^n$,

$$U^-(\xi) = \begin{cases} \displaystyle\sum_{p=1}^{\frac{n}{2}} \frac{R^n}{2^{n-1}} \binom{n}{\frac{n}{2} - p} c_{2p} \cosh 2p\xi + \frac{R^n}{2^n} \binom{n}{\frac{n}{2}} & \text{if } n \text{ is even,} \\[4mm] \displaystyle\sum_{p=0}^{\frac{n-1}{2}} \frac{R^n}{2^{n-1}} \binom{n}{\frac{n-1}{2} - p} c_{2p+1} \cosh(2p + 1)\xi & \text{if } n \text{ is odd,} \end{cases} \tag{4.23}$$

where c_n is given in (4.15). With this result in hand, (4.19) reads as follows:

$$\sum a_i b_j M_{ij}(k, B) = (k - 1) \int_B \nabla(\Re z^m) \cdot \nabla(\Re U^-) \, dx \qquad (z = x_1 + ix_2)$$

$$= (k - 1) \frac{m R^{m+n-1}}{2^{m+n-3}} \times$$

$$\begin{cases} \displaystyle\Re \int_B \sum_{s=0}^{\frac{m-2}{2}} \sum_{p=1}^{\frac{n}{2}} \binom{m-1}{\frac{m-2}{2} - s} \binom{n}{\frac{n}{2} - p} c_{2p} \cosh(2s + 1)\xi \overline{\frac{\partial}{\partial \xi} \cosh 2t\xi} \, dx \\ \qquad\qquad \text{if } n \text{ and } m \text{ are even,} \\[4mm] \displaystyle\Re \int_B \sum_{s=0}^{\frac{m-1}{2}} \sum_{p=0}^{\frac{n-1}{2}} \binom{m-1}{\frac{m-1}{2} - s} \binom{n}{\frac{n-1}{2} - p} \frac{c_{2p+1}}{1 + \delta_{0s}} \cosh 2s\xi \overline{\frac{\partial}{\partial \xi} \cosh(2p + 1)\xi} \, dx \\ \qquad\qquad \text{if } n \text{ and } m \text{ are odd,} \\[4mm] 0 \qquad\qquad\qquad\qquad \text{otherwise.} \end{cases}$$

But, by a change of variables, we can show that

$$\Re \int_B \cosh n\xi \,\overline{\frac{\partial \cosh m\xi}{\partial z}}\, dx = \frac{\pi R}{4} \sinh 2m\rho \Big(\delta_{(n+1)m} - \delta_{(n-1)m} + \delta_{(n-1)(-m)}\Big)$$

for $m \geq 1$, and $\Re \int_B \cosh n\xi \, dx = 0$, which yields the desired formula. Similarly to (i), we compute the other cases to complete the proof of (ii).

To prove (iii) we observe that the function ϕ is given in this case by

$$\phi(y) = \begin{cases} \dfrac{2n+1}{nk+n+1}|y|^n Y_{n,l}(\dfrac{y}{|y|}), & y \in B\,, \\[2ex] \dfrac{-kn+n}{kn+n+1}R^{2n+1}|y|^{-n-1}Y_{n,l}(\dfrac{y}{|y|}) + |y|^n Y_{n,l}(\dfrac{y}{|y|}), & y \in \mathbb{R}^3 \setminus \overline{B}\,, \end{cases}$$

and therefore

$$\sum a_i b_j M_{ij}(k, B) = (k-1)\int_{\partial B}\Big(\sum b_j y^j\Big)\frac{\partial\phi}{\partial\nu}\Big|_{-} d\sigma$$

$$= (k-1)\int_{\partial B}\frac{n(2n+1)}{nk+n+1}R^{n+n'+1}Y_{n',l'}(\theta)Y_{n,l}(\theta)\,d\sigma(\theta)\,,$$

which, by the orthogonality relation $\int_{\partial B} Y_{n',l'}(\theta)Y_{n,l}(\theta)\,d\sigma(\theta) = \delta_{nn'}\delta_{ll'}$, gives the claim. $\qquad\square$

When B is the disk of radius R and center 0, we see from (4.13) and (2.21) that

$$\frac{k+1}{2}M_{ij}(k, B) = \frac{k-1}{4\pi R}\left(\int_{\partial B}y^j\,d\sigma(y)\right) \times \int_{\partial B}\phi_i(y)\,d\sigma(y)$$

$$+ (k-1)\int_{\partial B}y^j\frac{\partial y^i}{\partial\nu}\,d\sigma(y)\,.$$

Since $\int_{\partial B}\phi_i(y)\,d\sigma(y) = (k-1)\int_{\partial B}\partial y^i/\partial\nu\,d\sigma(y)$, it follows that

$$M_{ij}(k, B) = \frac{1}{\lambda}\left[\frac{k-1}{4\pi R}\left(\int_{\partial B}y^j\,d\sigma(y)\right)\times\int_{\partial B}\frac{\partial y^i}{\partial\nu}\,d\sigma(y) + \int_{\partial B}y^j\frac{\partial y^i}{\partial\nu}\,d\sigma(y)\right]\,,$$

giving the formula in (i).

4.3 Extreme Conductivity Cases

We begin by noting that the definition (4.4) of GPTs is valid even for $k = 0$ or $+\infty$. If $k = 0$, namely, if B is insulated, then

$$M_{ij}(0, B) := \int_{\partial B}y^j\left(-\frac{1}{2}I - \mathcal{K}_B^*\right)^{-1}(\nu_y \cdot \nabla y^i)(y)\,d\sigma(y)\,,$$

whereas if $k = +\infty$, namely, if B is perfectly conducting and the constants $a_i, i \in I$, where I is a finite index set, are such that $\sum_i a_i y^i$ is a harmonic polynomial, then

$$\sum_i a_i M_{ij}(+\infty, B) := \int_{\partial B} y^j \left(\frac{1}{2}I - \mathcal{K}_B^*\right)^{-1} (\nu_y \cdot \nabla \sum_i a_i y^i)(y)\, d\sigma(y) \, .$$

When $|i| = |j| = 1$, these definitions exactly match those introduced by Pólya–Szegö [271] and Schiffer and Szegö [280].[1]

The following lemma is easy to prove.

Lemma 4.8 *The following convergences hold:*

(i) *Let $i, j \in \mathbb{N}^d$. Then*

$$M_{ij}(k, B) \to M_{ij}(0, B) \quad \text{as } k \to 0 \, .$$

(ii) *Let the constants $a_i, i \in I$, where I is a finite index set, be such that $\sum_i a_i y^i$ is a harmonic polynomial. Then*

$$\sum_i a_i M_{ij}(k, B) \to \sum_i a_i M_{ij}(+\infty, B) \quad \text{as } k \to +\infty \, .$$

Suppose $d \geq 3$. Denote by

$$\kappa = \frac{1}{|\partial B|} \int_{\partial B} \left(\mathcal{S}_B(-\frac{1}{2}I + \mathcal{K}_B^*)^{-1}(\nu)(y) - y \right) d\sigma(y) \, .$$

If we form the solution $v(x)$ to the Dirichlet problem for the domain outside the conductor B, with boundary values x, then, as $|x| \to +\infty$,

$$v(x) = \kappa\, \text{cap}(\partial B)\left[\Gamma(x) + \partial\Gamma(x) \int_{\partial B} y\phi_e(y)\, d\sigma(y)\right]$$
$$+ M(+\infty, B)\partial\Gamma(x) + O(\frac{1}{|x|^d}) \, ,$$

where $\text{cap}(\partial B)$ is the capacity of B, which is defined by (2.48), ϕ_e is the unique function in $L^2(\partial B)$ such that $\mathcal{S}_B\phi_e$ is constant on ∂B and $\int_{\partial B} \phi_e = 1$, and

$$M(+\infty, B) = \int_{\partial B} (-\frac{1}{2}I + \mathcal{K}_B^*)^{-1}(\nu)(y)y\, d\sigma(y) \, .$$

Alternatively, the solution w of $\Delta w = 0$ in $\mathbb{R}^d \setminus \overline{B}$, $w(x) = x + \lambda$ on ∂B, and $w(x) = O(|x|^{2-d})$ as $|x| \to +\infty$, behaves like the dipole $M(+\infty, B)\partial\Gamma(x)$ at infinity.

The GPTs seem to carry important geometric and potential theoretics properties of the domain B. In the following sections we investigate some of these properties.

---

[1] When $k = 0$, it is called the virtual mass.

4.4 Uniqueness Result

In this section we prove that the knowledge of all GPTs uniquely determines the geometry and the constitutive parameter of the inclusion. To do so, we relate the GPTs to the Dirichlet-to-Neumann (DtN) map. We prove that we can recover the DtN map from the set of all the GPTs, and, hence by the uniqueness result in Theorem 3.2, B and k are uniquely determined from all GPTs.

Let Ω be a bounded Lipschitz domain in $\mathbb{R}^d$ compactly containing B. Recall that the DtN map $\Lambda : W^2_{\frac{1}{2}}(\partial\Omega) \to W^2_{-\frac{1}{2}}(\partial\Omega)$ corresponding to k and B is defined by, for $f \in W^2_{\frac{1}{2}}(\partial\Omega)$,

$$\Lambda(f) := \left.\frac{\partial u}{\partial \nu}\right|_{\partial\Omega},$$

where u is the unique variational solution to

$$\begin{cases} \nabla \cdot \left(1 + (k-1)\chi(B)\right)\nabla u = 0 & \text{in } \Omega, \\ u|_{\partial\Omega} = f. \end{cases}$$

Let $M_{ij}(k, B)$ denote the GPTs associated with the domain B and conductivity k. The following theorem asserts that we can recover the DtN map and hence B and k from all GPTs.

Theorem 4.9 *Let k_1, k_2 be numbers different from 1, and let B_1, B_2 be bounded Lipschitz domains in $\mathbb{R}^d$. Let Ω be a domain compactly containing $\overline{B_1 \cup B_2}$, and let Λ_p be the DtN map corresponding to k_p and B_p, $p = 1, 2$, on $\partial\Omega$. If $M_{ij}(k_1, B_1) = M_{ij}(k_2, B_2)$ for all multi-indices $i, j \in \mathbb{N}^d$, then $\Lambda_1 = \Lambda_2$, and hence $k_1 = k_2$ and $B_1 = B_2$.*

Proof. Let $\lambda_p = (k_p + 1)/(2(k_p - 1))$, $p = 1, 2$. Let H be an entire harmonic function in $\mathbb{R}^d$. Since

$$\Gamma(x - y) = \sum_{|j|=0}^{+\infty} \frac{1}{j!}\partial^j \Gamma(x)y^j, \quad |x| \to +\infty, \tag{4.24}$$

and y in a compact set, we obtain, for all sufficiently large x,

$$\mathcal{S}_{B_p}(\lambda_p I - \mathcal{K}^*_{B_p})^{-1}(\nu \cdot \nabla H|_{\partial B_p})(x)$$

$$= \int_{\partial B_p} \Gamma(x - y)(\lambda_p I - \mathcal{K}^*_{B_p})^{-1}(\nu \cdot \nabla H|_{\partial B_p})(y)\, d\sigma(y)$$

$$= \sum_{|i|=1}^{\infty} \sum_{|j|=1}^{+\infty} \frac{\partial^i H(0)}{i!j!}\partial^j \Gamma(x) \int_{\partial B_p} y^j(\lambda_p I - \mathcal{K}^*_{B_p})^{-1}(\nu \cdot \nabla y^i|_{\partial B_p})(y)\, d\sigma(y)$$

$$= \sum_{|i|=1}^{+\infty} \sum_{|j|=1}^{+\infty} \frac{\partial^i H(0)}{i!j!}\partial^j \Gamma(x) M_{ij}(k_p, B_p).$$

If $M_{ij}(k_1, B_1) = M_{ij}(k_2, B_2)$ for all i and j, then

$$\mathcal{S}_{B_1}(\lambda_1 I - \mathcal{K}_{B_1}^*)^{-1}(\nu \cdot \nabla H|_{\partial B_1})(x) = \mathcal{S}_{B_2}(\lambda_2 I - \mathcal{K}_{B_2}^*)^{-1}(\nu \cdot \nabla H|_{\partial B_2})(x) \quad (4.25)$$

for all large x. By the unique continuation property of harmonic functions, we conclude that (4.25) holds for $x \in \mathbb{R}^d \setminus \overline{B_1 \cup B_2}$ and entire harmonic functions H.

Let $f \in W_{\frac{1}{2}}^2(\partial\Omega)$ and u_1 be the $W^{1,2}(\Omega)$-solution to the boundary value problem $\nabla \cdot ((1 + (k_1 - 1)\chi(B_1))\nabla u) = 0$ in Ω with $u|_{\partial\Omega} = f$. Let $H(x) := -\mathcal{S}_\Omega(\Lambda_1(f))(x) + \mathcal{D}_\Omega(f)(x)$, $x \in \Omega$.

Then by the representation formula in Theorem 2.31, we have

$$u_1(x) = H(x) + \mathcal{S}_{B_1}(\lambda_1 I - \mathcal{K}_{B_1}^*)^{-1}(\nu \cdot \nabla H|_{\partial B_1})(x), \quad x \in \Omega .$$

Define u_2 by

$$u_2(x) = H(x) + \mathcal{S}_{B_2}(\lambda_2 I - \mathcal{K}_{B_2}^*)^{-1}(\nu \cdot \nabla H|_{\partial B_2})(x), \quad x \in \Omega .$$

Then u_2 is a $W^{1,2}(\Omega)$ solution to the equation $\nabla \cdot ((1 + (k_2 - 1)\chi(B_2))\nabla u) = 0$ in Ω. Since H is harmonic in Ω, then, by the Runge approximation, there is a sequence H_n of entire harmonic functions converging to H uniformly on any compact subset of Ω. Since $\overline{B_1 \cup B_2}$ is a compact subset of Ω, it follows from (4.25) that $u_1 = u_2$ in $\Omega' \setminus \overline{B_1 \cup B_2}$, where Ω' is any relatively compact subset of Ω. By the unique continuation property of harmonic functions, we get $u_1 = u_2$ in $\Omega \setminus \overline{B_1 \cup B_2}$. Therefore, we obtain

$$\Lambda_1(f) = \left.\frac{\partial u_1}{\partial \nu}\right|_{\partial\Omega} = \left.\frac{\partial u_2}{\partial \nu}\right|_{\partial\Omega} = \Lambda_2(f) .$$

Since f is arbitrary, we conclude that $\Lambda_1 = \Lambda_2$.

It now follows from Theorem 3.2 that $k_1 = k_2$ and $B_1 = B_2$. This completes the proof. $\qquad\square$

Theorem 4.9 shows that the set of all GPTs completely characterizes the domain and its conductivity. However, it seems difficult to characterize the geometric information about the domain carried by individual M_{ij}. Nevertheless we will see that the first-order tensor carries information about the volume and orientation of the inclusion and that higher order ones carry information about the weighted volume. Other interesting physical properties of GPTs are investigated in the following sections.

4.5 Symmetry and Positivity of GPTs

We now consider the symmetry and positivity of GPT's. When $|i| = |j| = 1$, these properties were first proved in [84]. For symmetry we have the following theorem.

Theorem 4.10 *Suppose that* $a_i, i \in I$, *and* $b_j, j \in J$, *where* I *and* J *are finite index sets, are constants such that* $\sum_i a_i y^i$ *and* $\sum_j b_j y^j$ *are harmonic polynomials. Then*

$$\sum_{i,j} a_i b_j M_{ij} = \sum_{i,j} a_i b_j M_{ji} \,. \tag{4.26}$$

Proof. Note that

$$\sum_{i,j} a_i b_j M_{ij} = \int_{\partial B} \sum_j b_j y^j \sum_i a_i \phi_i(y) \, d\sigma(y) \,,$$

with ϕ_i given by (4.5). Put $f(y) = \sum_i a_i y^i$, $g(y) = \sum_j b_j y^j$, $\phi = \sum_i a_i \phi_i = (\lambda I - \mathcal{K}_B^*)^{-1}(\frac{\partial f}{\partial \nu})$, and $\psi = (\lambda I - \mathcal{K}_B^*)^{-1}(\frac{\partial g}{\partial \nu})$. Then $\mathcal{S}_B \phi$ and $\mathcal{S}_B \psi$ satisfy the transmission conditions

$$\frac{\partial}{\partial \nu} \mathcal{S}_B \phi\big|_+ - k \frac{\partial}{\partial \nu} \mathcal{S}_B \phi\big|_- = (k-1) \frac{\partial f}{\partial \nu}$$

and

$$\frac{\partial}{\partial \nu} \mathcal{S}_B \psi\big|_+ - k \frac{\partial}{\partial \nu} \mathcal{S}_B \psi\big|_- = (k-1) \frac{\partial g}{\partial \nu}$$

on ∂B. Recall that

$$\sum_{i,j} a_i b_j M_{ij} = \int_{\partial B} g\phi \, d\sigma \quad \text{and} \quad \sum_{i,j} a_i b_j M_{ji} = \int_{\partial B} f\psi \, d\sigma \,.$$

By (2.27) and the transmission condition, we have

$$\begin{aligned}
\int_{\partial B} g\phi \, d\sigma &= \int_{\partial B} g \left[\frac{\partial \mathcal{S}_B \phi}{\partial \nu}\bigg|_+ - \frac{\partial \mathcal{S}_B \phi}{\partial \nu}\bigg|_- \right] d\sigma \\
&= (k-1) \int_{\partial B} g \frac{\partial}{\partial \nu} (\mathcal{S}_B \phi + f)\bigg|_- d\sigma \,.
\end{aligned} \tag{4.27}$$

We then immediately obtain

$$\begin{aligned}
\int_{\partial B} g\phi \, d\sigma &= (k-1) \int_{\partial B} (\mathcal{S}_B \psi + g) \frac{\partial}{\partial \nu} (\mathcal{S}_B \phi + f)\bigg|_- d\sigma \\
&\quad - \int_{\partial B} \mathcal{S}_B \psi \frac{\partial}{\partial \nu} \mathcal{S}_B \phi\bigg|_+ d\sigma + \int_{\partial B} \mathcal{S}_B \psi \frac{\partial}{\partial \nu} \mathcal{S}_B \phi\bigg|_- d\sigma \\
&= (k-1) \int_B \nabla(\mathcal{S}_B \psi + g) \cdot \nabla(\mathcal{S}_B \phi + f) \, dx \\
&\quad + \int_{\mathbb{R}^d \setminus \overline{B}} \nabla \mathcal{S}_B \psi \cdot \nabla \mathcal{S}_B \phi \, dx + \int_B \nabla \mathcal{S}_B \psi \cdot \nabla \mathcal{S}_B \phi \, dx \,.
\end{aligned}$$

The symmetry property (4.26) follows from the above identity. $\qquad\square$

Suppose that $f = g$ in the proof of Theorem 4.10. It then follows from (4.27) that

$$\int_{\partial B} f\phi \, d\sigma = (k-1) \int_{\partial B} \frac{\partial f}{\partial \nu}(\mathcal{S}_B \phi + f) \, d\sigma \,. \tag{4.28}$$

On the other hand, it follows from the transmission condition that

$$
\begin{aligned}
\int_{\partial B} f\phi \, d\sigma &= (k-1) \int_{\partial B} (\mathcal{S}_B \phi + f)\frac{\partial}{\partial \nu}(\mathcal{S}_B \phi + f)\Big|_{-} \, d\sigma \\
&\quad - (k-1) \int_{\partial B} \mathcal{S}_B \phi \frac{\partial}{\partial \nu}\mathcal{S}_B \phi\Big|_{-} \, d\sigma - (k-1) \int_{\partial B} \mathcal{S}_B \phi \frac{\partial f}{\partial \nu} \, d\sigma \\
&= (k-1) \int_{\partial B} (\mathcal{S}_B \phi + f)\frac{\partial}{\partial \nu}(\mathcal{S}_B \phi + f)\Big|_{-} \, d\sigma \\
&\quad - \left(1 - \frac{1}{k}\right) \int_{\partial B} \mathcal{S}_B \phi \frac{\partial}{\partial \nu}\mathcal{S}_B \phi\Big|_{+} \, d\sigma - \left(1 - \frac{1}{k}\right) \int_{\partial B} \mathcal{S}_B \phi \frac{\partial f}{\partial \nu} \, d\sigma \,.
\end{aligned}
\tag{4.29}
$$

Define the quadratic form $Q_D(u)$ by

$$Q_D(u) := \int_D |\nabla u|^2 \, dx \,, \tag{4.30}$$

where D is a Lipschitz domain in $\mathbb{R}^d$. Then, by equating (4.28) and (4.29), we obtain

$$\int_{\partial B} \mathcal{S}_B \phi \frac{\partial f}{\partial \nu} \, d\sigma = \frac{k}{k+1} Q_B(\mathcal{S}_B \phi + f) + \frac{1}{k+1} Q_{\mathbb{R}^d \setminus \overline{B}}(\mathcal{S}_B \phi) - \frac{k}{k+1} Q_B(f) \,.$$

Substituting this identity into (4.28), we get

$$
\begin{aligned}
\int_{\partial B} f\phi \, d\sigma &= \frac{k(k-1)}{k+1} Q_B(\mathcal{S}_B \phi + f) + \frac{k-1}{k+1} Q_{\mathbb{R}^d \setminus \overline{B}}(\mathcal{S}_B \phi) \\
&\quad + \frac{k-1}{k+1} Q_B(f) \,.
\end{aligned}
$$

So we obtain the following theorem of positivity.

Theorem 4.11 *Suppose that a_i, $i \in I$, where I is a finite index set, are constants such that $f(y) = \sum_{i \in I} a_i y^i$ is a harmonic polynomial. Let $\phi = (\lambda I - \mathcal{K}_B^*)^{-1}(\partial f / \partial \nu)$. Then*

$$\sum_{i,j \in I} a_i a_j M_{ij} = \frac{k-1}{k+1}\left[k Q_B(\mathcal{S}_B \phi + f) + Q_{\mathbb{R}^d \setminus \overline{B}}(\mathcal{S}_B \phi) + Q_B(f) \right] \,. \tag{4.31}$$

Theorem 4.11 says that, if $k > 1$, then GPTs are positive-definite, and they are negative definite if $0 < k < 1$.

4.6 Estimates of the Harmonic Moments

If $f(x) = \sum a_i x^i$ is a harmonic polynomial, then $Q_B(f) = \int_B |\nabla(\sum a_i x^i)|^2 \, dx$, where Q_B is defined by (4.30). In particular, if $f(x) = x_p$, $p = 1, \ldots, d$, then $Q_B(f) = |B|$. One can observe from (4.31) that, if $\sum_{i \in I} a_i x^i$ is a harmonic polynomial, then

$$\left| \sum_{i,j \in I} a_i a_j M_{ij} \right| \geq \frac{|k-1|}{k+1} \int_B \left| \nabla \left(\sum a_i x^i \right) \right|^2 dx .$$

We now derive an upper bound for $\sum_{i,j \in I} a_i a_j M_{ij}$ in terms of the harmonic moments, defined as the set of $\int_B |\nabla f|^2$ where f is a harmonic polynomial.

Lemma 4.12 *A constant C exists depending only on the Lipschitz character of B such that, if $f(x) = \sum_{i \in I} a_i x^i$ is a harmonic polynomial, then*

$$\int_B |\nabla f|^2 \, dx \leq \frac{k+1}{|k-1|} \left| \sum_{i,j \in I} a_i a_j M_{ij} \right| \leq C \int_B |\nabla f|^2 \, dx . \tag{4.32}$$

Proof.   By the definition of GPTs, we have

$$\sum_{i,j \in I} a_i a_j M_{ij} = \int_{\partial B} f(y)(\lambda I - \mathcal{K}_B^*)^{-1} \left(\left. \frac{\partial f}{\partial \nu} \right|_{\partial B} \right) (y) \, d\sigma(y) .$$

Since $\int_{\partial B}(\lambda I - \mathcal{K}_B^*)^{-1}(\frac{\partial f}{\partial \nu}|_{\partial B}) \, d\sigma = 0$, we get

$$\sum_{i,j \in I} a_i a_j M_{ij} = \int_{\partial B} (f(y) - f_0)(\lambda I - \mathcal{K}_B^*)^{-1} \left(\left. \frac{\partial f}{\partial \nu} \right|_{\partial B} \right) (y) \, d\sigma(y) ,$$

where $f_0 := \frac{1}{|\partial B|} \int_{\partial B} f \, d\sigma$. It thus follows from Lemma 2.23 that

$$\left| \sum_{i,j \in I} a_i a_j M_{ij} \right| \leq C \frac{|k-1|}{k+1} \| f - f_0 \|_{L^2(\partial B)} \left\| \frac{\partial f}{\partial \nu} \right\|_{L^2(\partial B)} .$$

By the Poincaré inequality,

$$\| f - f_0 \|_{L^2(\partial B)} \leq C \| \nabla f \|_{L^2(\partial B)} .$$

Thus the proof is complete by Lemma 2.7. $\square$

We now set up the variational characterization of (4.31), which will help us to improve estimates (4.32) for $\sum_{i,j \in I} a_i a_j M_{ij}$. To this end, we first introduce the functional spaces

$$W_3 := \left\{ w \in W_{\mathrm{loc}}^{1,2}(\mathbb{R}^3) : \frac{w}{r} \in L^2(\mathbb{R}^3), \nabla w \in L^2(\mathbb{R}^3) \right\} \tag{4.33}$$

and

$$W_2 := \left\{ w \in W_{\mathrm{loc}}^{1,2}(\mathbb{R}^2) : \frac{w}{\sqrt{1 + r^2}\,\ln(2 + r^2)} \in L^2(\mathbb{R}^2), \nabla w \in L^2(\mathbb{R}^2) \right\},$$

$$(4.34)$$

where $r = |x|$. Recall that Δ sets an isomorphism from $W_d(\mathbb{R}^d)$ to its dual $(W_d(\mathbb{R}^d))^*$; see, for example, [255].

Define $\phi = \sum a_i (\lambda I - \mathcal{K}_B^*)^{-1}(\partial x^i / \partial \nu)$, and set $w_B = \mathcal{S}_B \phi$. Then

$$\begin{cases} \nabla \cdot (1 + (k-1)\chi(B))\nabla(w_B + f) = 0 & \text{in } \mathbb{R}^d, \\ w_B = O(|x|^{1-d}) & \text{as } |x| \to +\infty, \end{cases}$$

$$(4.35)$$

since $\int_{\partial B} \phi = 0$, which implies that for all $v \in W_d(\mathbb{R}^d)$,

$$\int_{\mathbb{R}^d} \left(1 + (k-1)\chi(B) \right)\left(\nabla w_B + (1 - \frac{1}{k})\chi(B)\nabla f \right) \cdot \nabla v = 0 .$$

$$(4.36)$$

Therefore, w_B is the minimizer of the functional

$$I_B(w) := \int_{\mathbb{R}^d} (1 + (k-1)\chi(B))\left| \nabla w + (1 - \frac{1}{k})\chi(B)\nabla f \right|^2$$

$$= \int_{\mathbb{R}^d} (1 + (k-1)\chi(B))|\nabla w|^2 + \frac{(k-1)^2}{k} \int_B |\nabla f|^2 \qquad (4.37)$$

$$+ 2(k-1) \int_B \nabla w \cdot \nabla f ,$$

namely,

$$I_B(w_B) = \inf_{w \in W_d} I_B(w).$$

We then get from (4.31) and (4.36) with $v = w_B$ the following variational characterization of M:

$$\sum_{i,j \in I} a_i a_j M_{ij} = I_B(w_B) + (1 - \frac{1}{k}) \int_B |\nabla f|^2$$

$$= \inf_{w \in W_d} I_B(w) + (1 - \frac{1}{k}) \int_B |\nabla f|^2 . \qquad (4.38)$$

Substituting $v = w_B$ in (4.36), we get

$$- \int_{\mathbb{R}^d} (1 + (k-1)\chi(B))|\nabla w_B|^2 = (k-1) \int_B \nabla f \cdot \nabla w_B.$$

Thus,

$$I_B(w_B) = - \int_{\mathbb{R}^d} (1 + (k-1)\chi(B))|\nabla w_B|^2 + \frac{(k-1)^2}{k} \int_B |\nabla f|^2 ,$$

and we therefore arrive at

$$\sum_{i,j\in I} a_i a_j M_{ij} = -\int_{\mathbb{R}^d}(1+(k-1)\chi(B))|\nabla w_B|^2 + (k-1)\int_B |\nabla f|^2 \ . \qquad (4.39)$$

Combining (4.38) and (4.39) we obtain the following theorem.

Theorem 4.13 *Assume that a_i, $i\in I$, where I is a finite index set, are constants such that $f(y)=\sum_{i\in I} a_i y^i$ is a harmonic polynomial. Then*

$$(1-\frac{1}{k})\int_B |\nabla f|^2 \le \sum_{i,j\in I} a_i a_j M_{ij}(k,B) \le (k-1)\int_B |\nabla f|^2 \ . \qquad (4.40)$$

Based on the above inequalities the harmonic moments of the inclusion B can be estimated from the GPTs. Note that we do not know whether the bounds in (4.40) are optimal. However, (4.40) yields the optimal estimates when $|i|=|j|=1$.

Corollary 4.14 *Let $M = (m_{pq})_{p,q=1}^d$ be the polarization tensor of Pólya–Szegö associated with the bounded Lipschitz domain B and conductivity $0 < k \ne 1 < +\infty$, and let κ be an eigenvalue of M. Then*

$$(1-\frac{1}{k})|B| \le \kappa \le (k-1)|B| \ . \qquad (4.41)$$

We can also find upper and lower bounds on the diagonal elements $(m_{pp})_{p=1,\ldots,d}$ using (4.31). We have

$$m_{pp} = \frac{k-1}{k+1}\left[k\int_B |\nabla \mathcal{S}_B \phi_p + e_p|^2 + \int_{\mathbb{R}^d\backslash\overline{B}} |\nabla \mathcal{S}_B \phi_p|^2 + |B|\right] \ ,$$

where $\phi_p = (\lambda I - \mathcal{K}_B^*)^{-1}(\nu_p)$. For $\tau \in \mathbb{R}$, we compute

$$\int_B |\tau\nabla(\mathcal{S}_B \phi_p + y_p) + e_p|^2$$

$$= \tau^2 \int_B |\nabla \mathcal{S}_B \phi_p + e_p|^2 + 2\tau \int_B \nabla(\mathcal{S}_B \phi_p + y_p)\cdot e_p + |B|$$

$$= \tau^2 \int_B |\nabla \mathcal{S}_B \phi_p + e_p|^2 + 2\tau \int_{\partial B}\left(\frac{\partial}{\partial\nu}\mathcal{S}_B \phi_p\Big|_{-} + \nu_p\right) y_p + |B| \ .$$

Since

$$\frac{\partial}{\partial\nu}\mathcal{S}_B \phi_p\Big|_{-} = (-\frac{1}{2}I + \mathcal{K}_B^*)\phi_p = (\lambda - \frac{1}{2})\phi_p - \nu_p \ ,$$

we obtain

$$\int_B |\nabla \mathcal{S}_B \phi_p + e_p|^2 = \frac{1}{\tau^2}\int_B |\tau\nabla(\mathcal{S}_B \phi_p + y_p) + e_p|^2 - \frac{2}{\tau}(\lambda - \frac{1}{2})m_{pp} - \frac{1}{\tau^2}|B| \ ,$$

and hence

$$\frac{m_{pp}}{k-1}\left(1+\frac{2k}{\tau(k+1)}\right)=|B|(1-\frac{k}{\tau^2})\frac{1}{k+1}$$
$$+\frac{1}{k+1}\left[\frac{k}{\tau^2}\int_B|\tau\nabla(\mathcal{S}_B\phi_p+y_p)+e_p|^2+\int_{\mathbb{R}^d\setminus\overline{B}}|\nabla\mathcal{S}_B\phi_p|^2\right].$$

Taking $\tau=-1$ in the above identity we arrive at

$$\frac{m_{pp}}{k-1}=|B|+\frac{1}{1-k}\left[k\int_B|-\nabla(\mathcal{S}_B\phi_p+y_p)+e_p|^2+\int_{\mathbb{R}^d\setminus\overline{B}}|\nabla\mathcal{S}_B\phi_p|^2\right],$$

and therefore

$$m_{pp}\le(k-1)|B|\,.$$

Taking $\tau=-k$ yields

$$m_{pp}\ge(1-\frac{1}{k})|B|\,.$$

The following optimal upper and lower bounds for the diagonal elements of the Polarization Tensor of Pólya–Szegö hold.

Lemma 4.15 *If $M=(m_{pq})_{p,q=1}^d$ is the polarization tensor of Pólya–Szegö associated with the bounded Lipschitz domain B and conductivity $0<k\ne 1<+\infty$, then*

$$(1-\frac{1}{k})|B|\le m_{pp}\le(k-1)|B|,\quad p=1,\dots,d\,. \tag{4.42}$$

The bounds (4.41) and (4.42) are optimal in the sense that they are achieved by the diagonal elements of thin ellipses (for $d=2$) and thin spheroids (for $d=3$); see (4.11) and (4.14). Later, we shall need optimal bounds on the trace of M. In this connection, we note that the bounds $d|B|(1-1/k)$ and $d|B|(k-1)$ on the trace $\mathrm{Tr}(M)$ of the matrix M, which follow directly from (4.41), are not optimal. See the next section.

4.7 Optimal Bounds for the Polarization Tensor

The aim of this section is to derive important isoperimetric inequalities satisfied by the polarization tensor of Pólya–Szegö. The following theorem was obtained by Lipton [222] and Capdeboscq and Vogelius [82, 83].

Theorem 4.16 *If M is the polarization tensor of Pólya–Szegö associated with the bounded Lipschitz domain B, and conductivity $0<k\ne 1<+\infty$, then*

$$\frac{1}{k-1}\,\mathrm{Tr}(M)\le(d-1+\frac{1}{k})|B| \tag{4.43}$$

and

$$(k-1)\,\mathrm{Tr}(M^{-1})\le\frac{d-1+k}{|B|}\,. \tag{4.44}$$

Proof. Suppose $k > 1$ and B is of unit volume, $|B| = 1$, without loss of generality. Let $\xi = (\xi_p)_{p=1}^d$, $f = \sum \xi_p x_p$, $\phi = \sum \xi_p(\lambda I - \mathcal{K}_B^*)^{-1}(\partial x_p/\partial \nu)$, and set $w_B = \mathcal{S}_B\phi$. Then by (4.38) we have

$$\sum_{p,q=1}^d m_{pq}\xi_p\xi_q = \inf_{w \in W_d} I_B(w) + (1 - \frac{1}{k})|\xi|^2, \quad d = 2, 3 \,. \tag{4.45}$$

The proof of the bounds (4.43) and (4.44) now relies on the Hashin-Shtrikman variational technique as described by Kohn and Milton [197]. Introduce a constant reference medium with conductivity $c < 1$. By writing the first term of the right-hand side of the above variational characterization of M as a maximum over "dual fields," and then interchanging the order of maximization and minimization, we obtain the following variational principle:

$$\sum_{p,q=1}^d m_{pq}\xi_p\xi_q = \sup_{v \in L^2(\mathbb{R}^d)^d} F_c(v) + (1 - \frac{1}{k})|\xi|^2 \,, \tag{4.46}$$

with

$$F_c(v) = -\int_{\mathbb{R}^d} \frac{1}{1 + (k-1)\chi(B) - c}|v|^2\,dx + c(1 - \frac{1}{c})^2|\xi|^2$$
$$+ 2(1 - \frac{1}{k})\xi \int_B v\,dx + \frac{1}{c}\int_{\mathbb{R}^d} L(v + c(1 - \frac{1}{k})\chi(B)\xi) \cdot (v + c(1 - \frac{1}{k})\chi(B)\xi) \,,$$

and L denoting the operator $L = -\nabla\Delta^{-1}\nabla\cdot$.

In fact, we have

$$I_B(w) = \int_{\mathbb{R}^d} (\gamma_B - c)\left|\nabla w + (1 - \frac{1}{k})\chi(B)\xi\right|^2 + c\int_{\mathbb{R}^d}\left|\nabla w + (1 - \frac{1}{k})\chi(B)\xi\right|^2 \,,$$

where $\gamma_B = 1 + (k-1)\chi(B)$. Since

$$(\gamma_B - c)|a|^2 \geq 2a \cdot b - \frac{1}{\gamma_B - c}|b|^2 \quad \forall a, b \in \mathbb{R}^d,$$

we get

$$\inf_{w \in W_d} I_B(w) = \inf_{w \in W_d} \sup_{v \in L^2(\mathbb{R}^d)^d} \int_{\mathbb{R}^d} \left[2(\nabla w + (1 - \frac{1}{k})\chi(B)\xi) \cdot v - \frac{1}{\gamma_B - c}|v|^2\right.$$
$$\left. + c\left|\nabla w + (1 - \frac{1}{k})\chi(B)\xi\right|^2\right]$$

$$= \sup_{v \in L^2(\mathbb{R}^d)^d} \inf_{w \in W_d} \int_{\mathbb{R}^d} \left[2(\nabla w + (1 - \frac{1}{k})\chi(B)\xi) \cdot v - \frac{1}{\gamma_B - c}|v|^2\right.$$
$$\left. + c\left|\nabla w + (1 - \frac{1}{k})\chi(B)\xi\right|^2\right] \,,$$

where the interchange of inf and sup is possible thanks to [119, Prop. 2.2]. For $v \in L^2(\mathbb{R}^d)^d$, define a functional J by

$$J(w) := \int_{\mathbb{R}^d} \left[c\left|\nabla w + (1 - \frac{1}{k})\chi(B)\xi\right|^2 + 2\nabla w \cdot v \right].$$

The minimizer $w_v \in W_d$ of J is the solution to

$$\Delta w = -\frac{1}{c}\nabla \cdot \left(v + (1 - \frac{1}{k})\chi(B)\xi \right)$$

and satisfies

$$c\int_{\mathbb{R}^d} \nabla w_v \cdot \left(\nabla w_v + (1 - \frac{1}{k})\chi(B)\xi \right) = \int_{\mathbb{R}^d} \nabla w_v \cdot v.$$

It then follows that

$$\inf_{w \in W_d} I_B(w) = \sup_{v \in L^2(\mathbb{R}^d)^d} \int_{\mathbb{R}^d} \left[-\frac{1}{c}\eta \cdot \nabla \Delta^{-1}\nabla \cdot \eta - \frac{1}{\gamma_B - c}|v|^2 \right.$$
$$\left. + 2(1 - \frac{1}{k})\chi(B)\xi \cdot v + c(1 - \frac{1}{k})^2\chi(B)|\xi|^2 \right],$$

where $\eta = v + (1 - \frac{1}{k})\chi(B)\xi$. By replacing v with $\eta - c(1 - \frac{1}{k})\chi(B)\xi$, we obtain (4.46).

Similarly, we introduce a constant reference medium with conductivity $c > k$. By writing the first term of the right-hand side of (4.45) as a minimum over "dual fields," and then interchanging the order of the two minimizations, we arrive at the variational principle

$$\sum_{p,q=1}^{d} m_{pq}\xi_p\xi_q = \inf_{v \in L^2(\mathbb{R}^d)^d} F_c(v) + (1 - \frac{1}{k})|\xi|^2 .$$

Changing variables to $\tilde{v} = v + c(1 - \frac{1}{k})\chi(B)\xi$, we get that the above variational principles are equivalent to

$$\sum_{p,q=1}^{d} (m_{pq} - \frac{1-c}{k-c}\delta_{pq})\xi_p\xi_q = \sup_{\tilde{v} \in L^2(\mathbb{R}^d)^d} G_c(\tilde{v}) \tag{4.47}$$

for $c < 1$, and

$$\sum_{p,q=1}^{d} (m_{pq} - \frac{1-c}{k-c}\delta_{pq})\xi_p\xi_q = \inf_{\tilde{v} \in L^2(\mathbb{R}^d)^d} G_c(\tilde{v}) \tag{4.48}$$

for $c > k$, with

$$G_c(\widetilde{v}) = -\int_{\mathbb{R}^d} \frac{1}{1 + (k-1)\chi(B) - c}|\widetilde{v}|^2\, dx + \frac{2k}{k-c}(1 - \frac{1}{k})\xi \int_B \widetilde{v}\, dx$$
$$+ \frac{1}{c}\int_{\mathbb{R}^d} L(\widetilde{v}) \cdot \widetilde{v}\,.$$

By only using test functions of the form $\widetilde{v} = \tau(1 - \frac{1}{k})\chi(B)\xi$ in (4.48), where τ is a constant, we obtain

$$\sum_{p,q=1}^{d}(m_{pq} - \frac{1-c}{k-c}\delta_{pq})\xi_p\xi_q \le (k-1)\left[(\frac{2}{k-c}\tau - \tau^2\frac{1}{k-c})|\xi|^2\right.$$
$$\left. +\tau^2\frac{1}{c}(1 - \frac{1}{k})^2\int_B L(\chi(B)\xi) \cdot \xi\right]\,,$$

provided $c > k$.

We claim that the trace of the symmetric tensor $\int_B L(\chi(B)\xi) \cdot \xi$ equals -1. In fact, one can easily see by taking the Fourier transform that

$$\int_B L(\chi(B)\xi) \cdot \xi = -\int_{\mathbb{R}^d} |y \cdot \widehat{\chi(B)\xi}|^2 dy\,,$$

where $\widehat{}$ denote the Fourier transform. Hence the trace of the operator $\xi \mapsto \int_B L(\chi(B)\xi) \cdot \xi$ equals -1. It then follows that

$$\mathrm{Tr}(M) \le (k-1)\min_{\tau \in \mathbb{R}}\left[d\frac{1-c}{k-c} + 2d\tau\frac{1}{k-c} - \tau^2(d\frac{1}{k-c} + \frac{1}{c})\right]$$
$$= (k-1)(d-1+\frac{1}{c})(1 + \frac{k-c}{dc})^{-1}\,,$$

provided $c > k$. In the limit as c tends to k this becomes exactly the bound (4.43).

If we only use test functions of the form $\widetilde{v} = \chi(B)\eta$, then (4.47) yields

$$\left(M - \frac{1-c}{k-c}\right)\xi \cdot \xi - 2\frac{1}{k-c}\xi \cdot \eta \ge -\frac{1}{k-c}\eta \cdot \eta + \frac{1}{c}\int_B L(\chi(B)\eta) \cdot \eta\,.$$

Insertion of

$$\xi = \frac{1}{k-c}\left(M - \frac{1-c}{k-c}\right)^{-1}\eta$$

into the above inequality gives

$$\mathrm{Tr}\left(M - \frac{1-c}{k-c}\right)^{-1} \le (k-c)(d + \frac{k}{c} - 1)\,,$$

which, in the limit as c tends to 1, becomes exactly the bound (4.44). $\square$

Suppose that B is of unit volume, $|B| = 1$. The above theorem says, in particular, that if $d = 2, k > 1$, and κ_1 and κ_2 are two eigenvalues of $M(k, B)$, then

$$\kappa_1 + \kappa_2 \leq \frac{(k-1)(k+1)}{k} \tag{4.49}$$

and

$$\frac{1}{\kappa_1} + \frac{1}{\kappa_2} \leq \frac{k+1}{k-1} \, . \tag{4.50}$$

Figure 4.1 shows these bounds graphically. The square box $[1 - 1/k, k - 1] \times [1 - 1/k, k - 1]$ in Figure 4.1 represents the estimates (4.41). This box is called a Wiener box in the composite materials community.

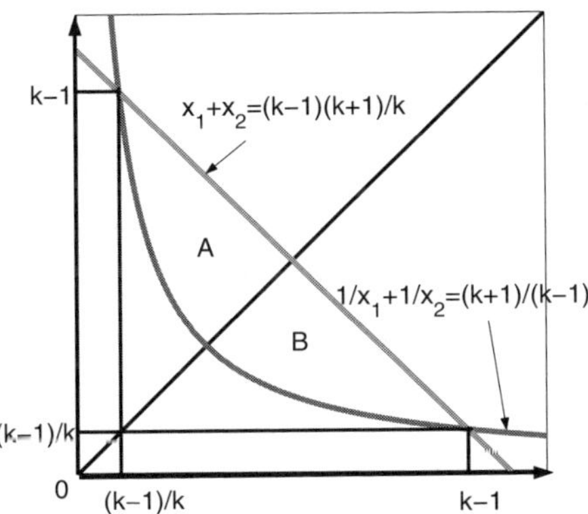

Fig. 4.1. The optimal bounds for the polarization tensor in $\mathbb{R}^2$.

The bounds in (4.43) and (4.44) are referred to as the Hashin–Shtrikman bounds after the names of the two authors who derived a similar type of bounds for composite materials using variational methods.

Capdeboscq and Vogelius showed that the bounds (4.43) and (4.44) are optimal in two dimensions in the sense that each point inside the bounds is a pair of eigenvalues of the PT associated with a domain of unit area [82]. They showed that each point inside the bounds is attained as a PT associated with a coated ellipse or a washer of elliptic shape [83]. In fact, every point on the lower bound $1/\kappa_1 + 1/\kappa_2 = (k + 1)/(k - 1)$ corresponds to an ellipse as one can see it from (4.11), and as the ellipses get thinner, the corresponding points on the lower bound move to the upper or lower corner. If we start from an ellipse corresponding to a point on the lower bound, and make confocal washers of elliptic shape, then corresponding points move toward the upper bound following a certain curve as the washers get thinner and larger. These curves make foliations and cover all regions inside the bounds except the upper bound. This result is exact, and PT for the elliptic washer can be computed using elliptic coordinates. These optimal estimates were efficiently used to estimate the size of unknown inclusions [82]; see Chapter 7.

On the other hand, it is shown numerically that each point inside the bounds is attained by a simply connected domain [16]. It turns out that, if we start from a disk-shaped domain and change it to make it look like a thin and long cross as in Figure 4.2, the corresponding eigenvalues move from the intersection point of the lower hyperbola and the line $\kappa_1 = \kappa_2$ toward the intersection point of the upper bound and the line $\kappa_1 = \kappa_2$ following the line $\kappa_1 = \kappa_2$. Note that the intersection point of the lower hyperbola and the line $\kappa_1 = \kappa_2$ is the pair of eigenvalues of the PT associated with the disk. We also note that the cross-shaped domain in Figure 4.2 is invariant under rotation by $\pi/2$, and hence the corresponding PT is of the form λI for some λ where I is the 2×2 identity-matrix. Thus by interpolating a cross-shape domain and an ellipse, we can obtain foliation of the region inside the bounds (4.49) and (4.50). It should be noted that the result of [16] is numerical; exact computation of PTs associated with cross-shape domains seems unlikely. However, it has been proved in [16] that the PT associated with a cross approaches to the upper bound as crosses get thinner and longer. In connection with this result, Capdeboscq and Kang obtained a non-trivial bound showing that, if an inclusion has finite extent and is not thin, then it cannot attain the upper HS bound on the PT [80].

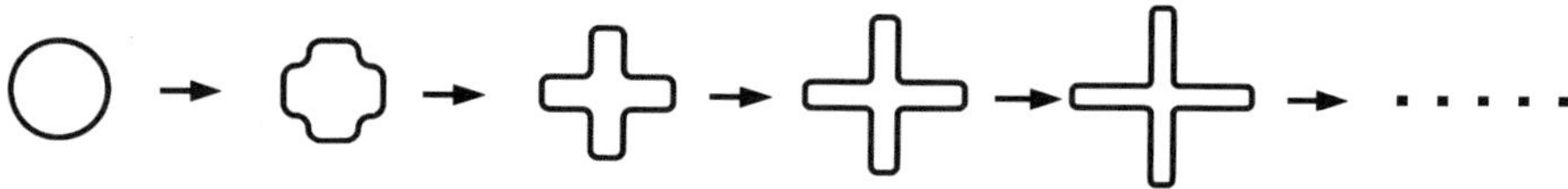

Fig. 4.2. The variation of cross-domains starting from disk.

As has been pointed out by Kozlov in [201, 202], the derivation of optimal bounds for the polarization tensor of Pólya–Szegö and the estimates of its possible values are direct analogues of the corresponding estimates for the effective conductivity matrix known in the theory of composite materials [145, 223, 248, 235]. See Chapter 8.

Finally we would like to mention the following important conjecture of Pólya–Szegö that is related to Theorem 4.16: If the polarization tensor $M(k, B)$ associated with the domain B and the conductivity k has the minimal trace or

$$\mathrm{Tr}(M(k, B)) = (k - 1)|B|\frac{d^2}{(d - 1 + k)},$$

then B is a disk in the plane and a ball in three-dimensional space.

Quite recently Kang and Milton proved that the conjecture is true in two and three dimensions [178, 179]. In fact, they showed that, if the lower Hashin–Shtrikman bound (4.44) is attained by a simply connected domain B, or in other words,

$$|B|(k - 1)\,\mathrm{Tr}(M^{-1}) \le d - 1 + k\,,$$

then B must be an ellipse or an ellipsoid. The conjecture of Pólya–Szegö follows immediately from this result since for the ellipses and the ellipsoids the polarization tensors can be computed explicitly. See (4.11).

4.8 Monotonocity

Another interesting result that can be obtained by using the variational principle (4.38) is the following: $(1/(k-1))\, M(k, B)$ is a monotonically increasing positive-definite matrix if we replace the given domain B by another B' that contains B. The following holds.

Theorem 4.17 *Let $B' \subsetneqq B$. Suppose that a_i, $i \in I$, where I is a finite index set, are constants such that $f(y) = \sum_{i \in I} a_i y^i$ is a harmonic polynomial. Then*

$$\sum_{i,j \in I} a_i a_j M_{ij}(k, B) > \sum_{i,j \in I} a_i a_j M_{ij}(k, B') \quad \text{if } k > 1 \tag{4.51}$$

and

$$\sum_{i,j \in I} a_i a_j M_{ij}(k, B) < \sum_{i,j \in I} a_i a_j M_{ij}(k, B') \quad \text{if } 0 < k < 1 . \tag{4.52}$$

Proof. Suppose that $k > 1$. We may argue in a similar way when $0 < k < 1$. We get from (4.38) that

$$\sum_{i,j \in I} a_i a_j \left(M_{ij}(k, B) - M_{ij}(k, B') \right)$$

$$= I_B(w_B) - I_{B'}(w_{B'}) + \left(1 - \frac{1}{k}\right) \int_{B \setminus \overline{B'}} |\nabla f|^2$$

$$\geq I_B(w_B) - I_{B'}(w_B) + \left(1 - \frac{1}{k}\right) \int_{B \setminus \overline{B'}} |\nabla f|^2 .$$

Making use of the second identity in (4.37), we obtain

$$\sum_{i,j \in I} a_i a_j \left(M_{ij}(k, B) - M_{ij}(k, B') \right)$$

$$\geq (k-1) \left(\int_{B \setminus \overline{B'}} |\nabla w_B|^2 + 2 \int_{B \setminus \overline{B'}} \nabla w_B \cdot \nabla f + \int_{B \setminus \overline{B'}} |\nabla f|^2 \right)$$

$$\geq (k-1) \int_{B \setminus \overline{B'}} |\nabla(w_B + f)|^2 > 0 ,$$

which yields the desired monotonicity result. $\qquad \square$

4.9 Estimates of the Center of Mass

We now investigate the relation of GPTs with the centroid of B. Assume that B is a two-dimensional disk with radius r; then, (2.21) yields

$$\mathcal{K}_B^* \phi(x) = \mathcal{K}_B \phi(x) = \frac{1}{4\pi r} \int_{\partial B} \phi(y)\, d\sigma(y) \ ,$$

which gives that $\mathcal{K}_B^*(\phi) = 0$ for all $\phi \in L_0^2(\partial B)$. Thus, if $f(y) = \sum_i a_i y^i$ is harmonic, then

$$\sum_i a_i (\lambda I - \mathcal{K}_B^*)^{-1} (\nu_y \cdot \nabla y^i)(x) = \frac{1}{\lambda} \nu_x \cdot \nabla f \ .$$

Therefore, we have

$$\sum_i a_i M_{ij} = \frac{1}{\lambda} \int_{\partial B} y^j \nu_y \cdot \nabla f \, d\sigma(y) = \frac{1}{\lambda} \int_B \nabla y^j \cdot \nabla f \, dy \ .$$

Thus, if $i = j = e_p$, $p = 1, \ldots, d$, then $M_{ij} = \lambda^{-1}|B|$, and if $i = e_p$ and $j = 2e_p$, then $M_{ij} = 2\lambda^{-1}|B|x_p^*$, where x^* is the center of the ball. Here $\{e_p\}_{p=1}^d$ is an orthonormal basis of $\mathbb{R}^d$.

Suppose now that $d = 3$ and $B = B_r(x^*)$ is a ball of center x^* and radius r. Then, by (2.22), $\mathcal{K}_B^* \phi(x) = -\frac{1}{2r} \mathcal{S}_B \phi(x)$ for all $x \in \partial B$.

Let f be a harmonic polynomial homogeneous of degree n with respect to the center x^*. Set

$$\phi(x) = \mathcal{S}_B\left(\frac{\partial f}{\partial \nu}\Big|_{\partial B}\right)(x), \quad x \in \mathbb{R}^d \setminus \overline{B} \ .$$

By (4.24) we have

$$\phi(x) = \sum_{p=1}^{+\infty} \int_{\partial B} \sum_{|j|=p} \frac{1}{j!} \partial^j \Gamma(x - x^*)(y - x^*)^j \frac{\partial f}{\partial \nu}(y)\, d\sigma(y)$$

$$= \int_{\partial B} \sum_{|j|=n} \frac{1}{j!} \partial^j \Gamma(x - x^*)(y - x^*)^j \frac{\partial f}{\partial \nu}(y)\, d\sigma(y) \ .$$

In particular, $\phi(x)$, $x \in \mathbb{R}^3 \setminus \overline{B}$, is homogeneous of degree $-n-1$ with respect to x^*.

By (2.27), we get

$$\frac{\partial \phi}{\partial \nu}\Big|_+(x) = \left(\frac{1}{2}I + \mathcal{K}_B^*\right)\left(\frac{\partial f}{\partial \nu}\Big|_{\partial B}\right)(x)$$

$$= \frac{1}{2}\frac{\partial f}{\partial \nu}(x) - \frac{1}{2r}\mathcal{S}_B\left(\frac{\partial f}{\partial \nu}\Big|_{\partial B}\right)(x), \quad x \in \partial B \ .$$

Therefore,

$$\frac{x - x^*}{r} \cdot \nabla\phi + \frac{1}{2r}\phi = \frac{1}{2}\frac{\partial f}{\partial \nu}(x) \quad \text{on } \partial B \ .$$

It then follows from the homogeneity of ϕ and f that $(x-x^*)\cdot\nabla\phi = -(n+1)\phi$, and hence,

$$\phi = -\frac{r}{2n+1}\frac{\partial f}{\partial \nu} \quad \text{on } \partial B \ .$$

So far we have proved that, if f is a harmonic polynomial homogeneous of degree n with respect to the center of the ball B, then

$$\mathcal{K}_B^* \left(\frac{\partial f}{\partial \nu}\bigg|_{\partial B}\right)(x) = -\frac{1}{2r}\mathcal{S}_B\left(\frac{\partial f}{\partial \nu}\bigg|_{\partial B}\right)(x) = \frac{1}{2(2n+1)}\frac{\partial f}{\partial \nu}(x), \quad x \in \partial B \ .$$

It then follows that

$$(\lambda I - \mathcal{K}_B^*)^{-1}\left(\frac{\partial f}{\partial \nu}\bigg|_{\partial B}\right) = \frac{(k-1)(2n+1)}{kn+n+1}\frac{\partial f}{\partial \nu} \quad \text{on } \partial B \ . \tag{4.53}$$

In particular, if $f(x) = x_p$, $p = 1, 2, 3$, then

$$\frac{\partial f}{\partial \nu} = \frac{\partial}{\partial \nu}(x_p - x_p^*) \ .$$

Thus by (4.53) we get

$$(\lambda I - \mathcal{K}_B^*)^{-1}\left(\frac{\partial f}{\partial \nu}\bigg|_{\partial B}\right) = \frac{3(k-1)}{k+2}\frac{\partial f}{\partial \nu} \quad \text{on } \partial B \ .$$

Therefore, if $|i| = 1$, then

$$M_{ij} = \frac{3(k-1)}{k+2}\int_B \nabla y^j \cdot \nabla y^i \, dy \ . \tag{4.54}$$

Observe that, if $j = 2e_p$ and $i = e_p$, $p = 1, \ldots, d$, then

$$\int_B \nabla y^j \cdot \nabla y^i \, dy = 2\int_B y_p \, dy = 2x_p^*|B| \ .$$

So far we have proved the following theorem.

Theorem 4.18 *Suppose that $B = B_r(x^*)$ is a ball in $\mathbb{R}^d$, $d = 2, 3$. Let $i_l := e_l$ and $j_l := 2e_l$, $l = 1, \ldots, d$. Then*

$$M_{i_l i_l} = \frac{d(k-1)}{k+d-1}|B|, \quad l = 1, \ldots, d \ ,$$

and

$$(M_{i_1 j_1}, \ldots, M_{i_d j_d}) = \frac{2d(k-1)}{k+d-1}|B|x^* \ .$$

For a general bounded Lipschitz domain B, we have the following theorem.

Theorem 4.19 *Let B be a bounded Lipschitz domain and x^* the center of mass of B. Let $i_l := e_l$ and $j_l := 2e_l$, $l = 1, \ldots, d$. Then C exists, which depends only on the Lipschitz character of B such that*

$$\left| \frac{M_{i_l j_l}}{M_{i_l i_l}} - 2x_l^* \right| \leq C \frac{|k-1|}{k+1} \operatorname{diam}(B) . \tag{4.55}$$

Proof.   Since

$$(\lambda I - \mathcal{K}_B^*)^{-1}(\nu_l) = \lambda^{-1} \nu_l + \lambda^{-1}(\lambda I - \mathcal{K}_B^*)^{-1} \mathcal{K}_B^*(\nu_l) ,$$

it follows from (2.44) that

$$\|(\lambda I - \mathcal{K}_B^*)^{-1}(\nu_l) - \lambda^{-1}\nu_l\|_{L^2(\partial B)} \leq C|\lambda|^{-1}\|(\lambda I - \mathcal{K}_B^*)^{-1}\mathcal{K}_B^*(\nu_l)\|_{L^2(\partial B)}$$

$$\leq C|\lambda|^{-2}\|\mathcal{K}_B^*(\nu_l)\|_{L^2(\partial B)} \leq C|\lambda|^{-2}|\partial B|^{1/2} .$$

Note that

$$M_{i_l j_l} - 2x_l^* M_{i_l i_l} = \int_{\partial B} (y_l - x_l^*)^2 (\lambda I - \mathcal{K}_B^*)^{-1}(\nu_l)(y) \, d\sigma(y) .$$

We also note that

$$\int_{\partial B} (y_l - x_l^*)^2 \nu_l(y) \, d\sigma(y) = 0 .$$

It then follows from the Cauchy–Schwarz inequality that

$$|M_{i_l j_l} - 2x_l^* M_{i_l i_l}| = \left| \int_{\partial B} (y_l - x_l^*)^2 \left[(\lambda I - \mathcal{K}_B^*)^{-1}(\nu_l)(y) - \lambda^{-1}\nu_l(y) \right] d\sigma(y) \right|$$

$$\leq C \operatorname{diam}(B)^2 |\partial B| |\lambda|^{-2} .$$

Then (4.55) follows from (4.40). This completes the proof. $\square$

Theorem 4.19 says that, if either k is close to 1 or the diameter of B is small, then $(M_{i_l j_l}/2M_{i_l i_l})_{l=1,\ldots,d}$, where $j_l = 2e_l$, is a good approximation of the centroid of B.

4.10 Polarization Tensors of Multiple Inclusions

Our goal in this section is to investigate properties of polarization tensors associated with multiple inclusions such as symmetry and positivity, which, in the most natural way, generalize those already derived for a single inclusion in the above sections. We also estimate their eigenvalues in terms of the total volume of the inclusions and explicitly compute them in the multi-disk case. These results are from [29].

Let B_s for $s = 1, \ldots, m$, be a bounded Lipschitz domain in $\mathbb{R}^d$. Throughout this section, we assume that:

(H1) Positive constants C_1 and C_2 exist such that

$$C_1 \leq \operatorname{diam} B_s \leq C_2, \quad \text{and} \quad C_1 \leq \operatorname{dist}(B_s, B_{s'}) \leq C_2, \quad s \neq s' .$$

(H2) The conductivity of the inclusion B_s for $s = 1, \ldots, m$, is equal to some positive constant $k_s \neq 1$.

4.10.1 Definition

To begin, we prove the following theorem.

Theorem 4.20 *Let H be a harmonic function in $\mathbb{R}^d$ for $d = 2$ or 3. Let u be the solution of the transmission problem*

$$\begin{cases} \nabla \cdot \left(\chi(\Omega \setminus \bigcup_{s=1}^{m} \overline{B_s}) + \sum_{s=1}^{m} k_s \chi(B_s) \right) \nabla u = 0 \quad in \ \mathbb{R}^d , \\ u(x) - H(x) = O(|x|^{1-d}) \quad as \ |x| \to +\infty . \end{cases} \tag{4.56}$$

There are unique functions $\phi^{(l)} \in L_0^2(\partial B_l)$, $l = 1, \ldots, m$, such that

$$u(x) = H(x) + \sum_{l=1}^{m} \mathcal{S}_{B_l} \phi^{(l)}(x) . \tag{4.57}$$

The potentials $\phi^{(l)}$, $l = 1, \ldots, m$, satisfy

$$(\lambda_l I - \mathcal{K}_{B_l}^*)\phi^{(l)} - \sum_{s \neq l} \frac{\partial(\mathcal{S}_{B_s} \phi^{(s)})}{\partial \nu^{(l)}} \Big|_{\partial B_l} = \frac{\partial H}{\partial \nu^{(l)}} \Big|_{\partial B_l} \quad on \ \partial B_l , \tag{4.58}$$

where $\nu^{(l)}$ denotes the outward unit normal to ∂B_l and

$$\lambda_l = \frac{k_l + 1}{2(k_l - 1)} .$$

Proof. It is easy to see from (2.27) that u defined by (4.57) and (4.58) is the solution of (4.56). Thus it is enough to show that the integral equation (4.58) has a unique solution.

Let $X := L_0^2(\partial B_1) \times \cdots \times L_0^2(\partial B_m)$. We prove that the operator $T : X \to X$ defined by

$$T(\phi^{(1)}, \cdots, \phi^{(m)}) = T_0(\phi^{(1)}, \cdots, \phi^{(m)}) + T_1(\phi^{(1)}, \cdots, \phi^{(m)})$$

$$:= \left((\lambda_1 I - \mathcal{K}_{B_1}^*)\phi^{(1)}, \cdots, (\lambda_m I - \mathcal{K}_{B_m}^*)\phi^{(m)} \right)$$

$$- \left(\sum_{s \neq 1} \frac{\partial(\mathcal{S}_{B_s} \phi^{(s)})}{\partial \nu^{(1)}} \Big|_{\partial B_1}, \cdots, \sum_{s \neq m} \frac{\partial(\mathcal{S}_{B_s} \phi^{(s)})}{\partial \nu^{(m)}} \Big|_{\partial B_m} \right)$$

is invertible. By Theorem 2.21, T_0 is invertible on X. On the other hand, since the domains B_s are a fixed distance apart, it is easy to see that T_1 is a compact operator on X. Thus, by the Fredholm alternative, it suffices to show that T is injective on X.

If $T(\phi^{(1)}, \cdots, \phi^{(m)}) = 0$, then $u(x) := \sum_{l=1}^{m} \mathcal{S}_{B_l} \phi^{(l)}(x)$, $x \in \mathbb{R}^d$ is the solution of (4.56) with $H = 0$. By the uniqueness of the solution to (4.56), we get $u \equiv 0$. In particular, $\mathcal{S}_{B_l} \phi^{(l)}$ is smooth across ∂B_l, $l = 1, \ldots, m$. Therefore,

$$\phi^{(l)} = \left. \frac{\partial(\mathcal{S}_{B_l} \phi^{(l)})}{\partial \nu^{(l)}} \right|_+ - \left. \frac{\partial(\mathcal{S}_{B_l} \phi^{(l)})}{\partial \nu^{(l)}} \right|_- = 0 \,.$$

This completes the proof. $\qquad\qquad\qquad\qquad\qquad\qquad\qquad\qquad\qquad\qquad\quad\square$

With the above theorem, we can proceed to introduce the polarization tensors of multiple inclusions.

Definition 4.21 *Let $i = (i_1, \ldots, i_d), j = (j_1, \ldots, j_d) \in \mathbb{N}^d$ be multi-indices. For $l = 1, \ldots, m$, let $\phi_i^{(l)}$ be the solution of*

$$(\lambda_l I - \mathcal{K}_{B_l}^*)\phi_i^{(l)} - \sum_{s \neq l} \frac{\partial(\mathcal{S}_{B_s} \phi_i^{(s)})}{\partial \nu^{(l)}} \Big|_{\partial B_l} = \frac{\partial x^i}{\partial \nu^{(l)}} \Big|_{\partial B_l} \quad on \; \partial B_l \,. \tag{4.59}$$

Then the generalized polarization tensor M_{ij} is defined to be

$$M_{ij} = \sum_{l=1}^{m} \int_{\partial B_l} x^j \phi_i^{(l)}(x) \, d\sigma(x) \,. \tag{4.60}$$

If $|i| = |j| = 1$, we denote M_{ij} by m_{pq}, $p, q = 1, \ldots, d$. We call $M = (m_{pq})_{p,q=1}^{d}$ the (first-order) polarization tensor.

4.10.2 Properties

Like the single inclusion case, the properties that we will present now will be derived via some integral identities.

Theorem 4.22 *Suppose that a_i and b_j are constants such that $\sum_i a_i y^i$ and $\sum_j b_j y^j$ are harmonic polynomials. Then*

$$\sum_{i,j} a_i b_j M_{ij} = \sum_{i,j} a_i b_j M_{ji} \,. \tag{4.61}$$

Proof. Reasoning as in the proof of Theorem 4.10 we put $f(y) := \sum_i a_i y^i$, $g(y) := \sum_j b_j y^j$, $\phi^{(l)} := \sum_i a_i \phi_i^{(l)}$, and $\psi^{(l)} := \sum_j b_j \phi_j^{(l)}$ to easily see that

$$\sum_{i,j} a_i b_j M_{ij} = \sum_{l=1}^{m} \int_{\partial B_l} g \phi^{(l)} \, d\sigma \quad and \quad \sum_{i,j} a_i b_j M_{ji} = \sum_{l=1}^{m} \int_{\partial B_l} f \psi^{(l)} \, d\sigma \,.$$

Observe now that

$$\sum_{l=1}^{m} \int_{\partial B_l} \Psi \left. \frac{\partial(\mathcal{S}_{B_l}\phi^{(l)})}{\partial \nu}\right|_{+} d\sigma = \sum_{s,l} \int_{\partial B_l} \mathcal{S}_{B_s}\psi^{(s)} \left. \frac{\partial(\mathcal{S}_{B_l}\phi^{(l)})}{\partial \nu}\right|_{+} d\sigma$$

$$= -\sum_{l=1}^{m} \int_{\mathbb{R}^d \setminus \overline{B_l}} \nabla \mathcal{S}_{B_l}\psi^{(l)} \cdot \nabla \mathcal{S}_{B_l}\phi^{(l)} \, dx$$

$$-\frac{1}{2} \sum_{l \neq s} \int_{\mathbb{R}^d \setminus \overline{B_l \cup B_s}} \nabla \mathcal{S}_{B_s}\psi^{(s)} \cdot \nabla \mathcal{S}_{B_l}\phi^{(l)} \, dx \, ,$$

and on the other hand,

$$\sum_{l=1}^{m} \int_{\partial B_l} \Psi \left. \frac{\partial(\mathcal{S}_{B_l}\phi^{(l)})}{\partial \nu}\right|_{-} d\sigma = \sum_{s,l} \int_{B_l} \nabla \mathcal{S}_{B_s}\psi^{(s)} \cdot \nabla \mathcal{S}_{B_l}\phi^{(l)} \, dx$$

$$= \sum_{l=1}^{m} \int_{B_l} \nabla \mathcal{S}_{B_l}\psi^{(l)} \cdot \nabla \mathcal{S}_{B_l}\phi^{(l)} \, dx + \frac{1}{2} \sum_{s \neq l} \int_{B_l \cup B_s} \nabla \mathcal{S}_{B_s}\psi^{(s)} \cdot \nabla \mathcal{S}_{B_l}\phi^{(l)} \, dx \, .$$

Then we finally obtain

$$\begin{aligned}
\sum_{i,j} a_i b_j M_{ij} &= \sum_{l=1}^{m} (k_l - 1)\langle (g+\Psi), (f+\Phi)\rangle_{B_l} \\
&+ \sum_{l=1}^{m} \langle \mathcal{S}_{B_l}\psi^{(l)}, \mathcal{S}_{B_l}\phi^{(l)}\rangle_{\mathbb{R}^d} + \frac{1}{2}\sum_{s \neq l}\langle \mathcal{S}_{B_s}\psi^{(s)}, \mathcal{S}_{B_l}\phi^{(l)}\rangle_{\mathbb{R}^d} \, .
\end{aligned} \tag{4.65}$$

Here, the notation $\langle u, v\rangle_D := \int_D \nabla u \cdot \nabla v \, dx$ has been used. The symmetry (4.61) follows immediately from (4.65) and the proof is complete. $\qquad\square$

Theorem 4.23 *Suppose that either $k_l - 1 > 0$ or $k_l - 1 < 0$ for all $l = 1, \ldots, m$. Let*

$$\kappa := \max_{1 \leq l \leq m} \left| 1 - \frac{1}{k_l}\right| .$$

For any a_i such that $\sum_i a_i y^i$ is harmonic,

$$\left| \sum_{i,j} a_i a_j M_{ij}\right| \geq \frac{|\kappa - 1|}{m+1}\sum_{l=1}^{m} |k_l - 1| \int_{B_l} \left| \nabla\left(\sum_i a_i y^i\right)\right|^2 dy \, . \tag{4.66}$$

In particular, if $k_l - 1 > 0$ (resp. < 0) for all $l = 1, \ldots, m$, then $M = (m_{pq})_{p,q=1}^{d}$ is positive (resp. negative) definite and if $\sum_{p=1}^{d} a_p^2 = 1$, then

$$\left| \sum_{p,q=1}^{d} a_p a_q m_{pq}\right| \geq \frac{|\kappa - 1|}{m+1}\sum_{l=1}^{m} |k_l - 1| \, |B_l| \, .$$

We also put

$$\Phi(x) := \sum_{l=1}^{m} \mathcal{S}_{B_l}\phi^{(l)} \quad \text{and} \quad \Psi(x) := \sum_{l=1}^{m} \mathcal{S}_{B_l}\psi^{(l)} \ .$$

From the definition of $\phi_i^{(l)}$, one can readily get

$$k_l \frac{\partial(f+\Phi)}{\partial\nu^{(l)}}\bigg|_{-} = \frac{\partial(f+\Phi)}{\partial\nu^{(l)}}\bigg|_{+} \quad \text{on } \partial B_l \ , \tag{4}$$

and the same relation for $g + \Psi$ holds. From (4.59) we obtain

$$\frac{\partial(\mathcal{S}_{B_l}\phi^{(l)})}{\partial\nu^{(l)}}\bigg|_{+} - k_l \frac{\partial(\mathcal{S}_{B_l}\phi^{(l)})}{\partial\nu^{(l)}}\bigg|_{-} = \sum_i a_i \left[\frac{\partial(\mathcal{S}_{B_l}\phi_i^{(l)})}{\partial\nu^{(l)}}\bigg|_{+} - k_l \frac{\partial(\mathcal{S}_{B_l}\phi_i^{(l)})}{\partial\nu^{(l)}}\bigg|_{-} \right]$$

$$= (k_l - 1)\sum_i a_i \frac{\partial}{\partial\nu^{(l)}} \left[x^i + \sum_{s \neq l} \mathcal{S}_{B_s}\phi_i^{(s)} \right]$$

$$= (k_l - 1)\frac{\partial}{\partial\nu^{(l)}} \left[f + \sum_{s \neq l} \mathcal{S}_{B_s}\phi_i^{(s)} \right] \quad \text{on } \partial B_l \ .$$

Thus, it follows from (4.63) that

$$\phi^{(l)} = \frac{\partial(\mathcal{S}_{B_l}\phi^{(l)})}{\partial\nu^{(l)}}\bigg|_{+} - \frac{\partial(\mathcal{S}_{B_l}\phi^{(l)})}{\partial\nu^{(l)}}\bigg|_{-} = (k_l - 1)\frac{\partial(f+\Phi)}{\partial\nu^{(l)}}\bigg|_{-} \quad \text{on } \partial B_l \ . \tag{4.64}$$

Therefore, we get

$$\sum_{i,j} a_i b_j M_{ij} = \sum_{l=1}^{m}(k_l - 1)\int_{\partial B_l} g\frac{\partial(f+\Phi)}{\partial\nu}\bigg|_{-} d\sigma$$

$$= \sum_{l=1}^{m}(k_l - 1)\int_{\partial B_l} (g+\Psi)\frac{\partial(f+\Phi)}{\partial\nu}\bigg|_{-} d\sigma$$

$$- \sum_{l=1}^{m}(k_l - 1)\int_{\partial B_l} \Psi\frac{\partial(f+\Phi)}{\partial\nu}\bigg|_{-} d\sigma$$

$$= \sum_{l=1}^{m}(k_l - 1)\int_{\partial B_l} (g+\Psi)\frac{\partial(f+\Phi)}{\partial\nu}\bigg|_{-} d\sigma$$

$$- \sum_{l=1}^{m}\int_{\partial B_l} \Psi \left[\frac{\partial(\mathcal{S}_{B_l}\phi^{(l)})}{\partial\nu}\bigg|_{+} - \frac{\partial(\mathcal{S}_{B_l}\phi^{(l)})}{\partial\nu}\bigg|_{-} \right] d\sigma \ .$$

Proof.   Suppose that either $k_l - 1 > 0$ or $k_l - 1 < 0$ for all $l = 1, \ldots, m$. Recall that the quadratic form $Q_D(u)$ is defined by $Q_D(u) := \langle u, u \rangle_D$. It then follows from (4.65) that

$$
\begin{aligned}
\sum_{i,j} a_i a_j M_{ij} &= \sum_{l=1}^{m} (k_l - 1) Q_{B_l}(f + \Phi) + \sum_{l=1}^{m} Q_{\mathbb{R}^d}(\mathcal{S}_{B_l} \phi^{(l)}) \\
&\quad + \frac{1}{2} \sum_{s \neq l} \langle \mathcal{S}_{B_s} \phi^{(s)}, \mathcal{S}_{B_l} \phi^{(l)} \rangle_{\mathbb{R}^d} \\
&= \sum_{l=1}^{m} (k_l - 1) Q_{B_l}(f + \Phi) + Q_{\mathbb{R}^d}(\Phi) ,
\end{aligned}
\tag{4.67}
$$

where Φ is defined in (4.62). On the other hand, because of (4.63), we get

$$
(k_l - 1) \frac{\partial f}{\partial \nu^{(l)}} = \left. \frac{\partial \Phi}{\partial \nu^{(l)}} \right|_{+} - k_l \left. \frac{\partial \Phi}{\partial \nu^{(l)}} \right|_{-} \quad \text{on } \partial B_l, \quad l = 1, \ldots, m .
$$

Thus, it follows from (4.64) that

$$
\begin{aligned}
\sum_{i,j} a_i a_j M_{ij} &= \sum_{l=1}^{m} (k_l - 1) \int_{\partial B_l} f \left. \frac{\partial (f + \Phi)}{\partial \nu} \right|_{-} d\sigma \\
&= \sum_{l=1}^{m} (k_l - 1) Q_{B_l}(f) + \sum_{l=1}^{m} (k_l - 1) \int_{\partial B_l} \frac{\partial f}{\partial \nu} \Phi \, d\sigma \\
&= \sum_{l=1}^{m} (k_l - 1) Q_{B_l}(f) + \sum_{l=1}^{m} \int_{\partial B_l} \left. \frac{\partial \Phi}{\partial \nu} \right|_{+} \Phi \, d\sigma - \sum_{l=1}^{m} k_l \int_{\partial B_l} \left. \frac{\partial \Phi}{\partial \nu} \right|_{-} \Phi \, d\sigma \\
&= \sum_{l=1}^{m} (k_l - 1) Q_{B_l}(f) - \sum_{l=1}^{m} Q_{\mathbb{R}^d}(\Phi) - \sum_{l=1}^{m} (k_l - 1) Q_{B_l}(\Phi) .
\end{aligned}
\tag{4.68}
$$

By equating (4.67) and (4.68), we have

$$
\begin{aligned}
&\sum_{l=1}^{m} (k_l - 1) Q_{B_l}(f + \Phi) + Q_{\mathbb{R}^d}(\Phi) \\
&= \sum_{l=1}^{m} (k_l - 1) Q_{B_l}(f) - \sum_{l=1}^{m} Q_{\mathbb{R}^d}(\Phi) - \sum_{l=1}^{m} (k_l - 1) Q_{B_l}(\Phi) ,
\end{aligned}
\tag{4.69}
$$

and consequently, one gets

$$
\sum_{l=1}^{m} (k_l - 1) Q_{B_l}(f) \geq \sum_{l=1}^{m} k_l Q_{B_l}(\Phi) .
\tag{4.70}
$$

It also follows from (4.69) that

$$Q_{\mathbb{R}^d}(\Phi) = \frac{1}{m+1} \sum_{l=1}^{m} (k_l - 1)\left[Q_{B_l}(f) - Q_{B_l}(f + \Phi) - Q_{B_l}(\Phi) \right]. \qquad (4.71)$$

Substituting (4.71) into (4.67), we obtain

$$\sum_{i,j} a_i a_j M_{ij} = \frac{m}{m+1} \sum_{l=1}^{m} (k_l - 1) Q_{B_l}(f + \Phi)$$

$$+ \frac{1}{m+1} \sum_{l=1}^{m} (k_l - 1)\left[Q_{B_l}(f) - Q_{B_l}(\Phi) \right],$$

and hence

$$\sum_{i,j} a_i a_j M_{ij} \geq \frac{1}{m+1} \sum_{l=1}^{m} (k_l - 1)\left[Q_{B_l}(f) - Q_{B_l}(\Phi) \right]. \qquad (4.72)$$

But by (4.70), we get

$$\sum_{l=1}^{m} (k_l - 1) Q_{B_l}(\Phi) = \sum_{l=1}^{m} \frac{(k_l - 1)}{k_l} k_l Q_{B_l}(\Phi)$$

$$\leq \kappa \sum_{l=1}^{m} k_l Q_{B_l}(\Phi) \leq \kappa \sum_{l=1}^{m} (k_l - 1) Q_{B_l}(f),$$

and hence, (4.66) follows immediately from (4.72). This completes the proof. $\qquad \square$

Based on the definition (4.60), polarization tensors associated with multiple disks and balls are explicitly computed in [29, 220]. We only give in the next section these calculations in the two-dimensional case. It should also be noted that Cheng and Greengard gave in Theorem 2.2 of their interesting paper [91] a solution to the two- and three-disk conductivity problem based on a method of images.

4.11 Explicit Formulae for the Polarization Tensor of Multiple Disks

In this section, we explicitly compute the solution $\phi^{(l)}$ of the integral equation (4.58) in the case where all domains B_l are two-dimensional disks. These calculations are from [29].

Let $B_l = B_{r_l}(z_l)$ be the disk with center z_l and radius r_l for $l = 1, \ldots, m$. Let R_l, $l = 1, \ldots, m$, be the reflection with respect to the disk B_l; i.e.,

$$R_l(x) := \frac{r_l^2(x - z_l)}{|x - z_l|^2} + z_l .$$

We also define the reflection of a function f by

$$(R_l f)(x) = f(R_l(x)), \quad x \in \mathbb{R}^2, \quad l = 1, \ldots, m .$$

The following lemma will be useful later.

Lemma 4.24 *For a function u harmonic in $\overline{B_l}$, we have*

$$\mathcal{S}_{B_l}\left(\frac{\partial u}{\partial \nu^{(l)}}\Big|_{\partial B_l}\right)(x) = -\frac{1}{2} R_l u(x) + \frac{1}{2} u(z_l), \quad x \in \mathbb{R}^2 \setminus \overline{B_l} . \tag{4.73}$$

Proof. By (2.27), we have

$$\frac{\partial}{\partial \nu^{(l)}} \mathcal{S}_{B_l}\left(\frac{\partial u}{\partial \nu^{(l)}}\Big|_{\partial B_l}\right)\Big|_+ (x) = (\frac{1}{2} I + \mathcal{K}_{B_l}^*)\left(\frac{\partial u}{\partial \nu^{(l)}}\Big|_{\partial B_l}\right)(x), \quad x \in \partial B_l .$$

Since B_l is a disk and $\int_{\partial B_l} \frac{\partial u}{\partial \nu^{(l)}} d\sigma = 0$, one can get that $\mathcal{K}_{B_l}^*(\frac{\partial u}{\partial \nu^{(l)}}\big|_{\partial B_l}) = 0$ on ∂B_l. Therefore, we get

$$\frac{\partial}{\partial \nu^{(l)}} \mathcal{S}_{B_l}\left(\frac{\partial u}{\partial \nu^{(l)}}\Big|_{\partial B_l}\right)\Big|_+ (x) = \frac{1}{2} \frac{\partial u}{\partial \nu^{(l)}}\Big|_{\partial B_l}(x) ,$$

and thus

$$\mathcal{S}_{B_l}\left(\frac{\partial u}{\partial \nu^{(l)}}\Big|_{\partial B_l}\right)(x) = -\frac{1}{2} R_l u(x) + C$$

for some constant C. Since $\int_{\partial B_l} \frac{\partial u}{\partial \nu^{(l)}} d\sigma = 0$ and hence $\mathcal{S}_{B_l}(\frac{\partial u}{\partial \nu^{(l)}}\big|_{\partial B_l})(x) \to 0$ as $|x| \to +\infty$, we have $C = (1/2)\, u(z_l)$. This completes the proof. $\square$

Our main result in this section is the following theorem.

Theorem 4.25 *For $l = 1, \ldots, m$, let*

$$S_l = \{\Theta = (p_1, \cdots, p_n), n \in \mathbb{N}, p_s \in \{1, \cdots, m\} : p_1 \neq l, p_s \neq p_{s+1}\} .$$

For $\Theta = (p_1, \ldots, p_n) \in S_l$, let

$$R_\Theta = R_{p_1} R_{p_2} \cdots R_{p_n} \quad and \quad \Lambda_\Theta = \prod_{s=1}^{n}\left(-\frac{1}{2\lambda_{p_s}}\right) .$$

Then, for a given harmonic function H, the solution of (4.58) is given by

$$\phi^{(l)} = \frac{1}{\lambda_l} \sum_{\Theta \in S_l} \Lambda_\Theta \frac{\partial}{\partial \nu^{(l)}}(R_\Theta H)\Big|_{\partial B_l} + \frac{1}{\lambda_l} \frac{\partial H}{\partial \nu^{(l)}}\Big|_{\partial B_l}, \quad l = 1, \cdots, m , \tag{4.74}$$

provided that

$$\min_{1 \leq s \neq s' \leq m} dist(B_s, B_{s'}) > (\sqrt{m-1} - 1) \max_{1 \leq s \leq m} r_s . \tag{4.75}$$

The series in (4.74) converges absolutely.

Proof. We first prove that the series in (4.74) converges absolutely on ∂B_l. Observe that

$$|\nabla(R_\Theta H)(x)| \le |R_\Theta \nabla H(x)| \prod_{s=1}^{n} \left| DR_{p_s}(R_{p_{s-1}} \cdots R_{p_1}(x)) \right| . \qquad (4.76)$$

Assuming (4.75) and using

$$|DR_s(x)| \le \frac{r_s^2}{|x - z_s|^2}, \quad x \in \mathbb{R}^2 \setminus B_s, \quad s = 1, \ldots, m , \qquad (4.77)$$

it follows from (4.76) that for $x \in \partial B_l$ we have

$$|\nabla(R_\Theta H)(x)| \le \Lambda \prod_{s=1}^{n} \frac{r_{p_s}^2}{(c + r_{p_s})^2} \le \Lambda \left(\frac{r_{max}}{(c + r_{max})} \right)^{2n} < \Lambda \left(\frac{\delta}{m-1} \right)^n \qquad (4.78)$$

for some $\delta < 1$, where

$$c = \min_{1 \le s \ne s' \le m} \mathrm{dist}(B_s, B_{s'}), \quad r_{max} = \max_{1 \le s \le m} r_s, \quad \text{and } \Lambda = \|\nabla H\|_{L^\infty(\bigcup_{s=1}^m \overline{B_s})} .$$

Note that the number of those Θ's, which have n components, is $(m-1)^n$. It can be deduced from (4.78) that for $x \in \partial B_l$,

$$\sum_{\Theta \in S_l} \left| \Lambda_\Theta \frac{\partial}{\partial \nu^{(l)}}(R_\Theta H)(x) \right| \le \Lambda \sum_{n=1}^{+\infty} \left(\frac{\delta}{m-1} \right)^n (m-1)^n < C ,$$

for some constant C independent of x.

We now prove that $\phi^{(l)}$ satisfies (4.58). Let us first observe the following: For each $l = 1, \ldots, m$,

$$\bigcup_{s \ne l} \left\{ (s, \Theta), \ (s) \mid \Theta \in S_s \right\} = S_l . \qquad (4.79)$$

Recalling that $\mathcal{K}_{B_l}^* \phi^{(l)} = 0$, $l = 1, \ldots, m$, and using (4.73), (4.74), and (4.79), we arrive at

$$\sum_{s \ne l} \frac{\partial(\mathcal{S}_{B_s}\phi^{(s)})}{\partial \nu^{(l)}}\Big|_{\partial B_l} = \sum_{s \ne l} \frac{\partial}{\partial \nu^{(l)}} \left(\frac{-1}{2\lambda_s} R_s \left[\sum_{\Theta \in S_s} \Lambda_\Theta(R_\Theta H) + H \right] \right)$$

$$= \sum_{\Theta \in S_l} \Lambda_\Theta \frac{\partial}{\partial \nu^{(l)}}(R_\Theta H)$$

$$= \lambda_l \phi^{(l)} - \frac{\partial H}{\partial \nu^{(l)}}\Big|_{\partial B_l} ,$$

which is exactly the desired result. $\square$

An immediate application of the above theorem is the derivation of the explicit form of the first-order polarization tensor.

Theorem 4.26 *Suppose $d = 2$. The first-order polarization tensor $(m_{pq})_{p,q=1,2}$ is given by*

$$m_{pq} = \sum_{l=1}^{m} |B_l| \frac{1}{\lambda_l} \left[\sum_{\Theta \in S_l} \Lambda_\Theta \frac{\partial}{\partial x_q} (R_\Theta(x_p))(z_l) + \delta_{pq} \right], \quad p, q = 1, 2, \quad (4.80)$$

provided that (4.75) is fulfilled.

Proof. Let $H(x) = x_p$ and $\phi_p^{(l)}$ be the corresponding solution of (4.58). Then by (4.74), we have

$$\phi_p^{(l)} = \frac{1}{\lambda_l} \frac{\partial}{\partial \nu^{(l)}} \left[\sum_{\Theta \in S_l} \Lambda_\Theta(R_\Theta(x_p)) + H \right], \quad p = 1, 2, \; l = 1, \cdots, m.$$

It then follows from the divergence theorem and the mean value property of harmonic functions that

$$\int_{\partial B_l} x_q \phi_p^{(l)} d\sigma = \frac{1}{\lambda_l} \left[\sum_{\Theta \in S_l} \Lambda_\Theta \int_{\partial B_l} x_q \frac{\partial}{\partial \nu^{(l)}} (R_\Theta(x_p))(x) \, d\sigma + \int_{\partial B_l} x_q \frac{\partial x_p}{\partial \nu^{(l)}} \, d\sigma \right]$$

$$= \frac{1}{\lambda_l} \left[\sum_{\Theta \in S_l} \Lambda_\Theta \int_{B_l} \frac{\partial}{\partial x_q} (R_\Theta(x_p))(x) \, dv + \delta_{pq} |B_l| \right]$$

$$= |B_l| \frac{1}{\lambda_l} \left[\sum_{\Theta \in S_l} \Lambda_\Theta \frac{\partial}{\partial x_q} (R_\Theta(x_p))(z_l) + \delta_{pq} \right].$$

Thus we get the explicit expression (4.80) as desired. $\qquad\square$

Let us now write formulae (4.74) and (4.80) in a more explicit way assuming that there are only two disk-shaped inclusions. We note that in this case the assumption (4.75) is trivially fulfilled. If $m = 2$, then R_Θ for $\Theta \in S_1$ takes the form

$$R_\Theta = (R_2 R_1)^s R_2 R_1^n \quad \text{for some } s = 0, 1, \ldots, \text{ and } n = 0, 1, \quad (4.81)$$

and R_Θ for $\Theta \in S_2$ becomes

$$R_\Theta = (R_1 R_2)^s R_1 R_2^n \quad \text{for some } s = 0, 1, \ldots, \text{ and } n = 0, 1. \quad (4.82)$$

Here $R_p^0 = I$, $p = 1, 2$.

Corollary 4.27 *If $m = 2$, then the solution $(\phi^{(1)}, \phi^{(2)})$ of the integral equation (4.58) is given by*

$$\phi^{(1)} = \frac{1}{\lambda_1} \sum_{s=0}^{+\infty} \frac{1}{(4\lambda_1\lambda_2)^s} \frac{\partial}{\partial \nu^{(1)}} \left[(R_2 R_1)^s (I - \frac{1}{2\lambda_2} R_2) H \right] \Big|_{\partial B_1},$$

$$\phi^{(2)} = \frac{1}{\lambda_2} \sum_{s=0}^{+\infty} \frac{1}{(4\lambda_1\lambda_2)^s} \frac{\partial}{\partial \nu^{(2)}} \left[(R_1 R_2)^s (I - \frac{1}{2\lambda_1} R_1) H \right] \Big|_{\partial B_2}.$$

$$(4.83)$$

Proof. It follows from (4.74), (4.81), and (4.82) that

$$\phi^{(1)} = \frac{1}{\lambda_1}\frac{\partial}{\partial\nu^{(1)}}$$
$$\times \left[\sum_{s=0}^{+\infty}\frac{1}{(4\lambda_1\lambda_2)^s}(R_2R_1)^s\left(-\frac{1}{2\lambda_2}R_2 + \frac{1}{4\lambda_1\lambda_2}R_2R_1\right)H + H\right]\Bigg|_{\partial B_1},$$

$$\phi^{(2)} = \frac{1}{\lambda_2}\frac{\partial}{\partial\nu^{(2)}}$$
$$\times \left[\sum_{s=0}^{+\infty}\frac{1}{(4\lambda_1\lambda_2)^s}(R_1R_2)^s\left(-\frac{1}{2\lambda_1}R_1 + \frac{1}{4\lambda_1\lambda_2}R_1R_2\right)H + H\right]\Bigg|_{\partial B_2}.$$

By rearranging the summations, we get (4.83). $\square$

Corollary 4.28 *Let $m = 2$. Suppose that the centers of the disks B_1 and B_2 are on the x_1-axis. Then the polarization tensor m_{pq} is given by*

$$m_{12} = m_{21} = 0\,,$$

$$m_{11} = \frac{|B_1|}{\lambda_1} + \frac{|B_2|}{\lambda_2}$$
$$+ \frac{|B_1|}{\lambda_1}\sum_{s=0}^{+\infty}\frac{1}{(4\lambda_1\lambda_2)^s}\left[(R_2R_1)^s\left(\frac{1}{2\lambda_2}g_2\right.\right.$$
$$+ \left.\left.\frac{1}{4\lambda_1\lambda_2}R_2(g_1)g_2\right)\prod_{s'=0}^{s-1}(R_2R_1)^{s'}(R_2(g_1)g_2)\right](z_1)$$
$$+ \frac{|B_2|}{\lambda_2}\sum_{s=0}^{+\infty}\frac{1}{(4\lambda_1\lambda_2)^s}\left[(R_1R_2)^s\left(\frac{1}{2\lambda_1}g_1\right.\right.$$
$$+ \left.\left.\frac{1}{4\lambda_1\lambda_2}R_1(g_2)g_1\right)\prod_{s'=0}^{s-1}(R_1R_2)^{s'}(R_1(g_2)g_1)\right](z_2)\,,$$

$$m_{22} = \frac{|B_1|}{\lambda_1} + \frac{|B_2|}{\lambda_2}$$
$$+ \frac{|B_1|}{\lambda_1}\sum_{s=0}^{+\infty}\frac{1}{(4\lambda_1\lambda_2)^s}\left[(R_2R_1)^s\left(-\frac{1}{2\lambda_2}g_2\right.\right.$$
$$+ \left.\left.\frac{1}{4\lambda_1\lambda_2}R_2(g_1)g_2\right)\prod_{s'=0}^{s-1}(R_2R_1)^{s'}(R_2(g_1)g_2)\right](z_1)$$
$$+ \frac{|B_2|}{\lambda_2}\sum_{s=0}^{+\infty}\frac{1}{(4\lambda_1\lambda_2)^s}\left[(R_1R_2)^s\left(-\frac{1}{2\lambda_1}g_1\right.\right.$$
$$+ \left.\left.\frac{1}{4\lambda_1\lambda_2}R_1(g_2)g_1\right)\prod_{s'=0}^{s-1}(R_1R_2)^{s'}(R_1(g_2)g_1)\right](z_2)\,,$$

where the functions g_1 and g_2 are defined by

$$g_p(x) := \frac{r_p^2}{|x - z_p|^2}, \quad x \in \mathbb{R}^2 \setminus \overline{B_p}, p = 1, 2 .$$

Proof.   By Theorem 4.26, (4.81), and (4.82), we have

$$m_{pq} = \frac{|B_1|}{\lambda_1}\left[\sum_{s=0}^{+\infty}(4\lambda_1\lambda_2)^{-s}\frac{\partial}{\partial x_q}\left((R_2R_1)^s(-\frac{1}{2\lambda_2}R_2\right.\right.$$
$$\left.\left.+ \frac{1}{4\lambda_1\lambda_2}R_2R_1)(x_p)\right)(z_1) + \delta_{pq}\right]$$
$$+ \frac{|B_2|}{\lambda_2}\left[\sum_{s=0}^{+\infty}(4\lambda_1\lambda_2)^{-s}\frac{\partial}{\partial x_q}\left((R_1R_2)^s(-\frac{1}{2\lambda_1}R_1\right.\right.$$
$$\left.\left.+ \frac{1}{4\lambda_1\lambda_2}R_1R_2)(x_p)\right)(z_2) + \delta_{pq}\right] .$$

Easy computations show that for x on the x_1-axis,

$$DR_p(x) = g_p(x)\begin{pmatrix} -1 & 0 \\ 0 & 1 \end{pmatrix}, \quad p = 1, 2 ,$$

and

$$\nabla R_p f(x) = g_p(x)\begin{pmatrix} -1 & 0 \\ 0 & 1 \end{pmatrix} \cdot (R_p\nabla f)(x), \quad p = 1, 2 .$$

Therefore we get for $H = x_p$,

$$\nabla\left((R_2R_1)^s R_2(H)\right)(x)$$
$$= \left[(R_2R_1)^s g_2(x)\prod_{s'=0}^{s-1}(R_2R_1)^{s'}(R_2(g_1)g_2)(x)\right]\begin{pmatrix} -1 & 0 \\ 0 & 1 \end{pmatrix} \cdot \nabla H ,$$
$$\nabla\left((R_2R_1)^s R_2R_1(H)\right)(x) = \left[\prod_{s'=0}^{s}(R_2R_1)^{s'}(R_2(g_1)g_2)(x)\right]\begin{pmatrix} 1 & 0 \\ 0 & 1 \end{pmatrix} \cdot \nabla H .$$

One can get similar formulae for $\nabla((R_1R_2)^s R_1(H))$ and $\nabla((R_1R_2)^s R_1R_2(H))$. By substituting these formulae into the first equation of the proof, we obtain Corollary 4.28. $\square$

4.11.1 Representation by Equivalent Ellipses

Suppose $d = 2$, and let $M = (m_{pq})_{p,q=1}^2$ be the first-order polarization tensor of the inclusions $\cup_{s=1}^m B_s$. We define the overall conductivity $\overline{k}$ of $B = \cup_{s=1}^m B_s$ by

$$\frac{\overline{k} - 1}{\overline{k} + 1}\sum_{s=1}^m |B_s| := \sum_{s=1}^m \frac{k_s - 1}{k_s + 1}|B_s| \qquad (4.84)$$

and its *center* $\overline{z}$ by

$$\frac{\overline{k}-1}{\overline{k}+1}\overline{z}\sum_{s=1}^{m}|B_s| = \sum_{s=1}^{m}\frac{k_s-1}{k_s+1}\int_{B_s} x\,dx\;. \qquad (4.85)$$

Note that, if k_s is the same for all s, then $\overline{k}=k_s$ and $\overline{z}$ is the center of mass of B.

In this section we represent and visualize the multiple inclusions $\cup_{s=1}^{m}B_s$ by means of an ellipse $\mathcal{E}$ of center $\overline{z}$ with the same polarization tensor. We call $\mathcal{E}$ the equivalent ellipse of $\cup_{s=1}^{m}B_s$.

At this point let us review a method to find an ellipse from a given first-order polarization tensor. This method is due to Brühl, Hanke, and Vogelius [73] and is based on Proposition 4.6. Let $\mathcal{E}'$ be an ellipse whose semi-axes are on the x_1- and x_2-axes and of length a and b, respectively. Let $\mathcal{E}=R\mathcal{E}'$, where $R=\begin{pmatrix}\cos\theta & -\sin\theta\\ \sin\theta & \cos\theta\end{pmatrix}$ and $\theta\in[0,\pi]$. Let M be the polarization tensor of $\mathcal{E}$. We want to recover a, b, and θ from M knowing the conductivity $k=\overline{k}$.

Recall that the polarization tensor M' for $\mathcal{E}'$ takes the form

$$M' = (k-1)|\mathcal{E}'|\begin{pmatrix}\dfrac{a+b}{a+kb} & 0\\[2mm] 0 & \dfrac{a+b}{b+ka}\end{pmatrix},$$

and that of $\mathcal{E}$ is given by $M=RM'R^{T}$. Suppose that the eigenvalues of M are κ_1 and κ_2 and corresponding eigenvectors of unit length are $(e_{11},e_{12})^{T}$ and $(e_{21},e_{22})^{T}$. Then it can be shown that

$$a=\sqrt{\frac{p}{\pi q}},\quad b=\sqrt{\frac{pq}{\pi}},\quad \theta=\arctan\frac{e_{21}}{e_{11}}\;,$$

where

$$\frac{1}{p}=\frac{k-1}{k+1}\left(\frac{1}{\kappa_1}+\frac{1}{\kappa_2}\right)\quad\text{and}\quad q=\frac{\kappa_2-k\kappa_1}{\kappa_1-k\kappa_2}\;.$$

We now show some numerical examples of equivalent ellipses. We represent the set of inclusions $B=\cup_{s=1}^{m}B_s$ by an equivalent ellipse of center $\overline{z}$ and conductivity $\overline{k}$. We assume that the inclusion B_s takes the following form:

$$\partial B_s = \left\{\left(a_0^s+a_1^s\cos(t)+a_2^s\cos(2t),\, b_0^s+b_1^s\sin(t)+b_2^s\sin(2t)\right),\, 0\le t<2\pi\right\}.$$

In order to evaluate the first-order polarization tensor of multiple inclusions, we solve the integral equation (2.65) with $H(x)=x_p$ to find $\phi_p^{(s)}$ for $p=1,2$ and $s=1,\ldots,m$, and then we calculate

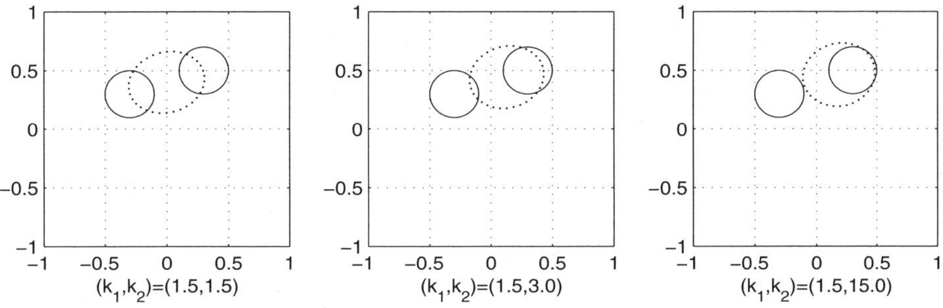

$a_0^i, a_1^i, a_2^i, b_0^i, b_1^i, b_2^i$	k_i	$\overline{k}$	a	b	θ	$\overline{z}$
	1.5	1.5	0.313	0.256	0.322	(-0.000, 0.400)
	1.5					
-0.3,0.2,0, 0.3,0.2,0	1.5	2.077	0.307	0.261	0.322	(0.129, 0.443)
0.3,0.2,0, 0.5,0.2,0	3					
	1.5	3.324	0.301	0.266	0.322	(0.188, 0.463)
	15					

Fig. 4.3. When the two disks have the same radius and the conductivity of the one on the right-hand side is increasing, the equivalent ellipse moves toward the right inclusion. In the table $\overline{k}$ and $\overline{z}$ are the overall conductivity and center defined by (4.84) and (4.85) and a, b, θ are the semi-axes lengths and angle of orientation measured in radians of the equivalent ellipse.

$$m_{pq} = \sum_{s=1}^{m} \int_{\partial B_s} x_q \phi_p^{(s)}(x) \, d\sigma(x) \ .$$

Figures 4.3 and 4.4 show how the equivalent ellipse changes as the conductivities and the sizes of the inclusions B_s vary. The solid line represents the actual inclusions, and the dashed lines are the equivalent ellipses.

The above calculation extends to the three-dimensional case. Based on the analytical expression (4.14), the parameters a, b, and c of an ellipsoid B can be recovered from the eigenvalues of its polarization tensor $M(k, B)$.

4.12 Anisotropic Polarization Tensors

In this section we define and prove some important properties of the (generalized) anisotropic polarization tensors (APTs) associated with an anisotropic inclusion embedded in an anisotropic background.

Let B be a bounded Lipschitz domain in $\mathbb{R}^d$, $d = 2, 3$. Suppose that the conductivity of B is $\widetilde{A}$ and that of $\mathbb{R}^d \setminus \overline{B}$ is A, where A and $\widetilde{A}$ are constant

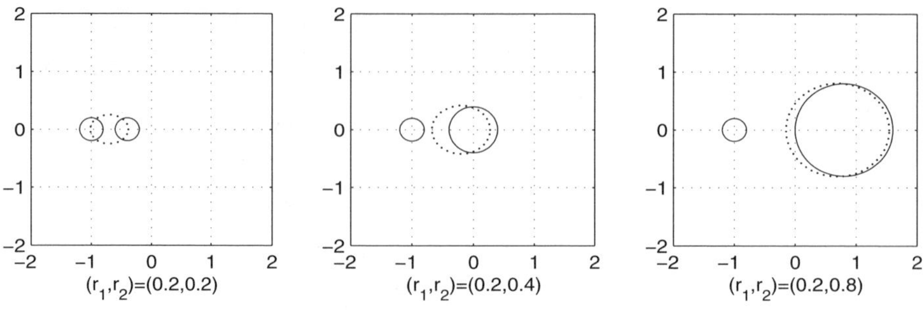

k_i	$a_0^i, a_1^i, a_2^i, b_0^i, b_1^i, b_2^i$	$\overline{k}$	a	b	θ	$\overline{z}$
	-1,0.2,0, 0,0.2,0 -0.4,0.2,0, 0,0.2,0	1.5	0.317	0.254	0	(-0.700 , 0.000)
1.5 1.5	-1,0.2,0, 0,0.2,0 0,0.2,0, 0,0.2,0	1.5	0.478	0.420	0	(-0.200, 0.000)
	-1,0.2,0, 0,0.2,0 0.8,0.2,0, 0,0.2,0	1.5	0.844	0.806	0	(0.694, 0.000)

Fig. 4.4. When the conductivities of the two disks are the same and the radius of the disk on the right-hand side is increasing, the equivalent ellipse moves toward the right inclusion.

$d \times d$ positive-definite symmetric matrices with $A \neq \widetilde{A}$. The matrix $\widetilde{A} - A$ is assumed to be either positive-definite or negative-definite. The conductivity profile of B is

$$\gamma_B := \chi(\mathbb{R}^d \setminus \overline{B})A + \chi(B)\widetilde{A} .$$

We now define APT, as follows.

Definition 4.29 *For a multi-index $i \in \mathbb{N}^d$ with $|i| \geq 1$, let $(f_i, g_i) \in L^2(\partial B) \times L^2(\partial B)$ be the unique solution to*

$$\begin{cases} \mathcal{S}_B^{\widetilde{A}} f_i - \mathcal{S}_B^A g_i = x^i \\ \nu \cdot \widetilde{A} \nabla \mathcal{S}_B^{\widetilde{A}} f_i|_- - \nu \cdot A \nabla \mathcal{S}_B^A g_i|_+ = \nu \cdot A \nabla x^i \end{cases} \quad on \ \partial B . \qquad (4.86)$$

For a pair of multi-indices $i, j \in \mathbb{N}^d$, define the generalized anisotropic polarization tensors associated with the domain B and anisotropic conductivities $\widetilde{A}$ and A, or the conductivity profile γ_B, by

$$M_{ij} = M_{ij}(A, \widetilde{A}, B) = \int_{\partial B} x^j g_i(x) \, d\sigma(x) .$$

When $i = e_p$ and $j = e_q$ for $p, q = 1, \cdots, d$, where $(e_1, \ldots, e_d)$ is the standard basis for $\mathbb{R}^d$, denote M_{ij} by $M := (m_{pq})_{p,q=1,\ldots,d}$ with

$$m_{pq} = \int_{\partial B} x_q g_p(x)\, d\sigma(x)\,.$$

Here $g_p = g_i$ for $i = e_p$.

We note that the first-order APT was first introduced in [175] and it is proved there that M is symmetric and positive (negative, resp.) definite if $\widetilde{A} - A$ is positive (negative, resp.) definite. The generalized APTs enjoy the same properties.

Before establishing these properties, we first demonstrate that the APTs are a natural extension of the generalized polarization tensors for the isotropic case.

For a multi-index $i \in \mathbb{N}^d$ with $|i| \geq 1$, let

$$\theta_i := (\mathcal{S}_B^{\widetilde{A}} f_i)\chi(B) + (\mathcal{S}_B^A g_i)\chi(\mathbb{R}^d \setminus \overline{B})\,.$$

Then θ_i is the solution to the following transmission problem:

$$\begin{cases} \nabla \cdot (A\nabla\theta_i) = 0 & \text{in } \mathbb{R}^d \setminus \overline{B}\,, \\ \nabla \cdot (\widetilde{A}\nabla\theta_i) = 0 & \text{in } B\,, \\ \theta_i|_- - \theta_i|_+ = x^i & \text{on } \partial B\,, \\ \nu \cdot \widetilde{A}\nabla\theta_i|_- - \nu \cdot A\nabla\theta_i|_+ = \nu \cdot A\nabla x^i & \text{on } \partial B\,, \\ \theta_i(x) \to 0 & \text{as } |x| \to +\infty \text{ if } d = 3\,, \\ \theta_i(x) - \dfrac{1}{2\pi\sqrt{\det(A)}} \ln \|A_* x\| \displaystyle\int_{\partial B} \theta_i(y)\, d\sigma(y) \to 0 \text{ as } |x| \to +\infty \text{ if } d = 2\,. \end{cases}$$

$$(4.87)$$

It then follows from (2.85) and (4.86) that for any pair of multi-indices i, j,

$$\begin{aligned} M_{ij} &= \int_{\partial B} x^j g_i\, d\sigma \\ &= \int_{\partial B} x^j (\nu \cdot A\nabla\mathcal{S}_B^A g_i|_+ - \nu \cdot A\nabla\mathcal{S}_B^A g_i|_-)\, d\sigma \\ &= \int_{\partial B} x^j (\nu \cdot \widetilde{A}\nabla\mathcal{S}_B^{\widetilde{A}} f_i|_- - \nu \cdot A\nabla x^i)\, d\sigma - \int_{\partial B} \nu \cdot A\nabla x^j (\mathcal{S}_B^{\widetilde{A}} f_i - x^i)\, d\sigma \\ &= \int_{\partial B} (\nu \cdot (\widetilde{A} - A)\nabla x^j)\theta_i|_-\, d\sigma\,. \end{aligned}$$

In particular, if A and $\widetilde{A}$ are isotropic, or $A = I$ and $\widetilde{A} = kI$, where I is the identity matrix, then

$$M_{ij} = (k-1)\int_{\partial B} \frac{\partial x^j}{\partial \nu}\theta_i\, d\sigma = (k-1)\left[\int_{\partial B} x^j \frac{\partial x^i}{\partial \nu} + \int_{\partial B} x^j \frac{\partial \theta_i}{\partial \nu}\Big|_+ d\sigma\right]\,,$$

which is exactly (up to a multiplicative constant) the isotropic generalized polarization tensor as defined in (4.10), since

$$\theta_i = \begin{cases} (k-1)\psi_i & \text{in } \mathbb{R}^d \setminus \overline{B} , \\ (k-1)\psi_i + x^i & \text{in } B , \end{cases}$$

where ψ_i is the solution of (4.6).

Next, we write a transformation formula for the first-order APT. We denote the first-order APT, $M = (m_{pq})_{1 \leq p,q \leq d}$, which is associated with the conductivity distribution γ_B by $M(A, \widetilde{A}; B)$. Then the following lemma can be proved by a simple change of variables.

Lemma 4.30 *For any unitary transformation R, the following holds:*

$$M(A, \widetilde{A}; B) = RM(R^T AR, R^T \widetilde{A}R; R^{-1}(B))R^T ,$$

where T denotes the transpose.

Finally, we derive an explicit formula for the first-order APT $M(I, \widetilde{A}; B)$ due to Kang and Kim [176]. Define $(f, g) \in L^2(\partial B) \times L^2(\partial B)$ as the solution of

$$\begin{cases} \mathcal{S}_B^{\widetilde{A}} f - \mathcal{S}_B g = x \\ \nu \cdot \widetilde{A} \nabla \mathcal{S}_B^{\widetilde{A}} f|_- - \nu \cdot \nabla \mathcal{S}_B g|_+ = \nu \cdot \nabla x \end{cases} \quad \text{on } \partial B .$$

As in the derivation of formula (4.13), we write

$$\begin{aligned} M(I, \widetilde{A}; B) &= \int_{\partial B} x g(x) \, d\sigma(x) \\ &= \int_{\partial B} x \left(\nu \cdot \nabla \mathcal{S}_B g|_+ - \nu \cdot \nabla \mathcal{S}_B g|_- \right)(x) \, d\sigma(x) \\ &= \int_{\partial B} x \nu \cdot \left(\widetilde{A} \nabla \mathcal{S}_B^{\widetilde{A}} f|_- - \nabla x - \nabla \mathcal{S}_B g|_- \right)(x) \, d\sigma(x) . \end{aligned}$$

Since $\nabla \cdot (\widetilde{A} \nabla x) = 0$, by integrating by parts, we see that

$$\int_{\partial B} x \nu \cdot \widetilde{A} \nabla \mathcal{S}_B^{\widetilde{A}} f|_-(x) \, d\sigma(x) = \int_{\partial B} \nu \cdot \nabla(\widetilde{A}x) \mathcal{S}_B^{\widetilde{A}} f(x) \, d\sigma(x) ,$$

and hence, a straightforward calculation shows that

$$M(I, \widetilde{A}; B) = (\widetilde{A} - I) \int_{\partial B} x(-\frac{1}{2} I + \mathcal{K}_B^*)(g)(x) \, d\sigma(x) + (\widetilde{A} - I)|B| .$$

Using (2.23), we obtain the formula below.

Proposition 4.31 *If B is an ellipse whose semi-axes are on the x_1-and x_2-axes and of length a and b, respectively, then its first-order APT $M(I, \widetilde{A}; B)$ takes the form*

$$M(I, \widetilde{A}; B) = |B| \left(I + (\widetilde{A} - I)(\frac{1}{2} I - C) \right)^{-1} (\widetilde{A} - I) ,$$

where the matrix

$$C = \frac{a-b}{2(a+b)} \begin{pmatrix} 1 & 0 \\ 0 & -1 \end{pmatrix} .$$

In particular, if B is a disk, then

$$M(I, \widetilde{A}; B) = 2|B|(\widetilde{A} + I)^{-1}(\widetilde{A} - I) . \tag{4.88}$$

For an arbitrary ellipse whose semi-axes are not aligned with the coordinate axes, one can use Lemma 4.30 to compute its first-order APT.

We are now ready to prove some important properties of the APT such as symmetry and positivity. For the first-order APT these properties were obtained in [175]. The estimates for positivity of generalized APTs established in [28] give better results than the ones in [175].

With definition 2.43, we state and prove the following result.

Theorem 4.32 (Symmetry) *Let I and J be finite sets of multi-indices, and let $\{a_i | i \in I\}$ and $\{b_j | j \in J\}$ be such that $\sum_{i \in I} a_i x^i$ and $\sum_{j \in J} b_j x^j$ are A-harmonic. Then*

$$\sum_{i \in I} \sum_{j \in J} a_i b_j M_{ij} = \sum_{i \subset I} \sum_{j \in J} a_i b_j M_{ji} . \tag{4.89}$$

In particular, $m_{pq} = m_{qp}$, $p, q = 1, \cdots, d$.

Proof.   Let

$$v_1(x) = \sum_{i \in I} a_i x^i , \quad v_2(x) = \sum_{j \in J} b_j x^j ,$$

$$\psi_1(x) = \sum_{i \in I} a_i f_i(x) , \quad \psi_2(x) = \sum_{j \in J} b_j f_j(x) ,$$

$$\phi_1(x) = \sum_{i \in I} a_i g_i(x), \quad \phi_2(x) = \sum_{j \in J} b_j g_j(x) ,$$

where (f_i, g_i) is the solution to (4.86). Then, we get

$$\sum_{i \in I} \sum_{j \in J} a_i b_j M_{ij} = \int_{\partial B} \Big(\sum_{j \in J} b_j x^j \Big) \Big(\sum_{i \in I} a_i g_i(x) \Big) \, d\sigma = \int_{\partial B} v_2(x)\phi_1(x) \, d\sigma .$$

One can see from the linearity of the integral equation that (ψ_p, ϕ_p), $p = 1, 2$, is the solution to

$$\begin{cases} \mathcal{S}_B^{\widetilde{A}}\psi_p - \mathcal{S}_B^A \phi_p = v_p \\ \nu \cdot \widetilde{A}\nabla\mathcal{S}_B^{\widetilde{A}}\psi_p|_- - \nu \cdot A\nabla\mathcal{S}_B^A\phi_p|_+ = \nu \cdot A\nabla v_p \end{cases} \quad \text{on } \partial B . \tag{4.90}$$

It then follows from (4.90) and the jump relations that

$$\sum_{i\in I}\sum_{j\in J} a_i b_j M_{ij} = \int_{\partial B} v_2 \left(\nu \cdot A\nabla \mathcal{S}_B^A \phi_1|_+ - \nu \cdot A\nabla \mathcal{S}_B^A \phi_1|_-\right)$$

$$= \int_{\partial B} v_2 \left(\nu \cdot \widetilde{A}\nabla \mathcal{S}_B^{\widetilde{A}} \psi_1|_- - \nu \cdot A\nabla v_1\right) - \int_{\partial B} v_2 \nu \cdot A\nabla \mathcal{S}_B^A \phi_1|_-$$

$$= \int_{\partial B} (\mathcal{S}_B^{\widetilde{A}} \psi_2 - \mathcal{S}_B^A \phi_2)\nu \cdot \widetilde{A}\nabla \mathcal{S}_B^{\widetilde{A}} \psi_1|_- - \int_{\partial B} v_2 \nu \cdot A\nabla v_1 - \int_{\partial B} \mathcal{S}_B^A \phi_1 \nu \cdot A\nabla v_2$$

$$= \int_{\partial B} \mathcal{S}_B^{\widetilde{A}} \psi_2 \nu \cdot \widetilde{A}\nabla \mathcal{S}_B^{\widetilde{A}} \psi_1|_- - \int_{\partial B} \mathcal{S}_B^A \phi_2 \left(\nu \cdot A\nabla \mathcal{S}_B^A \phi_1|_+ + \nu \cdot A\nabla v_1\right)$$

$$- \int_{\partial B} v_2 \nu \cdot A\nabla v_1 - \int_{\partial B} \mathcal{S}_B^A \phi_1 \nu \cdot A\nabla v_2 \,.$$

Thus we arrive at

$$\sum_{i\in I}\sum_{j\in J} a_i b_j M_{ij} = \int_{B} \widetilde{A}\nabla \mathcal{S}_B^{\widetilde{A}} \psi_1 \cdot \nabla \mathcal{S}_B^{\widetilde{A}} \psi_2 + \int_{\mathbb{R}^d \setminus \overline{B}} A\nabla \mathcal{S}_B^A \phi_1 \cdot \nabla \mathcal{S}_B^A \phi_2$$

$$- \int_{B} A\nabla v_1 \cdot \nabla v_2 - \int_{\partial B} \left(\mathcal{S}_B^A \phi_2 \nu \cdot A\nabla v_1 + \mathcal{S}_B^A \phi_1 \nu \cdot A\nabla v_2\right) \,. \tag{4.91}$$

Similarly, we get

$$\sum_{i\in I}\sum_{j\in J} a_i b_j M_{ji} = \int_{B} \widetilde{A}\nabla \mathcal{S}_B^{\widetilde{A}} \psi_2 \cdot \nabla \mathcal{S}_B^{\widetilde{A}} \psi_1 + \int_{\mathbb{R}^d \setminus \overline{B}} A\nabla \mathcal{S}_B^A \phi_2 \cdot \nabla \mathcal{S}_B^A \phi_1$$

$$- \int_{B} A\nabla v_2 \cdot \nabla v_1 - \int_{\partial B} \left(\mathcal{S}_B^A \phi_1 \nu \cdot A\nabla v_2 + \mathcal{S}_B^A \phi_2 \nu \cdot A\nabla v_1\right) \,. \tag{4.92}$$

Since A and $\widetilde{A}$ are symmetric matrices, the proof is completed. $\qquad\square$

The formula (4.91) says, in particular, that

$$\sum_{i,j\in I} a_i a_j M_{ij} = \int_{B} \widetilde{A}\nabla \mathcal{S}_B^{\widetilde{A}} \psi \cdot \nabla \mathcal{S}_B^{\widetilde{A}} \psi + \int_{\mathbb{R}^d \setminus \overline{B}} A\nabla \mathcal{S}_B^A \phi \cdot \nabla \mathcal{S}_B^A \phi$$

$$- \int_{B} A\nabla v \cdot \nabla v - 2 \int_{\partial B} \mathcal{S}_B^A \phi \nu \cdot A\nabla v \, d\sigma \,, \tag{4.93}$$

where $\psi := \psi_1 = \psi_2$, $\phi := \phi_1 = \phi_2$, and $v = v_1 = v_2$ in the proof of Theorem 4.32. Define

$$w = \begin{cases} \mathcal{S}_B^{\widetilde{A}} \psi - v & \text{in } B \,, \\ \mathcal{S}_B^A \phi & \text{in } \mathbb{R}^d \setminus \overline{B} \,. \end{cases} \tag{4.94}$$

It then follows from (4.93) that

$$\sum_{i,j\in J} a_i a_j M_{ij} = \int_B \widetilde{A}\nabla(w+v)\cdot\nabla(w+v) + \int_{\mathbb{R}^d\setminus\overline{B}} A\nabla w\cdot\nabla w$$

$$- \int_B A\nabla v\cdot\nabla v - 2\int_{\partial B} w\nu\cdot A\nabla v\, d\sigma$$

$$= \int_{\mathbb{R}^d} \gamma_B\nabla w\cdot\nabla w + 2\int_B(\widetilde{A}-A)\nabla w\cdot\nabla v + \int_B(\widetilde{A}-A)\nabla v\cdot\nabla v\,. \qquad (4.95)$$

Observe from (4.90) that w satisfies

$$\begin{cases} \nabla\cdot(\gamma_B\nabla(w+v)) = 0 & \text{in } \mathbb{R}^d\,, \\ w(x) = O(|x|^{1-d}) & \text{as } |x|\to+\infty\,. \end{cases} \qquad (4.96)$$

Since $\nu\cdot A\nabla v|_+ = \nu\cdot A\nabla v|_-$ on ∂B, it follows from (4.96) that

$$\int_{\mathbb{R}^d} \gamma_B(\nabla w + \chi(B)(I - \widetilde{A}^{-1}A)\nabla v)\cdot\nabla f \qquad (4.97)$$

$$= \int_B\left(\widetilde{A}\nabla w + (\widetilde{A}-A)\nabla v\right)\cdot\nabla f + \int_{\mathbb{R}^d\setminus\overline{B}} A\nabla w\cdot\nabla f$$

$$= \int_{\partial B}\left(\nu\cdot\widetilde{A}\nabla(w+v)|_- - \nu\cdot A\nabla(w+v)|_+\right)f\, d\sigma = 0\,,$$

for all $f\in W_d(\mathbb{R}^d)$. Hence (4.97) yields that w is the minimizer of the functional

$$I_B(f) = \int_{\mathbb{R}^d} \gamma_B(\nabla f + \chi(B)(I-\widetilde{A}^{-1}A)\nabla v)\cdot(\nabla f + \chi(B)(I-\widetilde{A}^{-1}A)\nabla v)\,, \qquad (4.98)$$

namely,

$$I_B(w) = \inf_{f\in W_d(\mathbb{R}^d)} I_B(f)\,. \qquad (4.99)$$

Moreover, by substituting w in place of f in (4.97), we get

$$\int_B(\widetilde{A}-A)\nabla w\cdot\nabla v = -\int_{\mathbb{R}^d} \gamma_B\nabla w\cdot\nabla w\,, \qquad (4.100)$$

and hence

$$I_B(w) = \int_{\mathbb{R}^d} \gamma_B(\nabla w + \chi(B)(I-\widetilde{A}^{-1}A)\nabla v)\cdot(\nabla w + \chi(B)(I-\widetilde{A}^{-1}A)\nabla v)$$

$$= \int_{\mathbb{R}^d} \gamma_B\nabla w\cdot\nabla w + 2\int_{\mathbb{R}^d} \gamma_B\nabla w\cdot\chi(B)(I-\widetilde{A}^{-1}A)\nabla v$$

$$+ \int_B(\widetilde{A}-A)\nabla v\cdot(I-\widetilde{A}^{-1}A)\nabla v$$

$$= -\int_{\mathbb{R}^d} \gamma_B\nabla w\cdot\nabla w + \int_B(\widetilde{A}-A)\nabla v\cdot(I-\widetilde{A}^{-1}A)\nabla v\,. \qquad (4.101)$$

It then follows from (4.95), (4.100), and (4.101) that

$$\sum_{i,j \in J} a_i a_j M_{ij} = -\int_{\mathbb{R}^d} \gamma_B \nabla w \cdot \nabla w + \int_B (\widetilde{A} - A)\nabla v \cdot \nabla v$$

$$= I_B(w) + \int_B (\widetilde{A} - A)\nabla v \cdot \widetilde{A}^{-1} A \nabla v .$$

In conclusion, we obtain

$$\sum_{i,j \in J} a_i a_j M_{ij} = \inf_{f \in W_d(\mathbb{R}^d)} I_B(f) + \int_B (\widetilde{A} - A)\nabla v \cdot \widetilde{A}^{-1} A \nabla v . \qquad (4.102)$$

Theorem 4.33 *Let $\{a_i | i \in J\}$ be a set of coefficients such that $v(x) = \sum_{i \in J} a_i x^i$ is A-harmonic. Then we obtain the following bounds:*

$$\int_B (\widetilde{A} - A)\nabla v \cdot \widetilde{A}^{-1} A \nabla v \leq \sum_{i,j \in J} a_i a_j M_{ij} \leq \int_B (\widetilde{A} - A)\nabla v \cdot \nabla v . \qquad (4.103)$$

Proof. We obtain the first inequality since $I_B(f) \geq 0$ for all $f \in W_d(\mathbb{R}^d)$ and the second one by applying $f = 0$. $\qquad\square$

By taking $v(x) = \xi \cdot x$ for $\xi \in \mathbb{R}^d$, we get the following corollary for the first-order APT.

Corollary 4.34 *Let $M = (M_{ij})_{|i|=|j|=1}$ be the matrix of the first-order APT. Then*

$$|B|(\widetilde{A} - A)\xi \cdot \widetilde{A}^{-1} A\xi \leq M\xi \cdot \xi \leq |B|(\widetilde{A} - A)\xi \cdot \xi, \quad \xi \in \mathbb{R}^d . \qquad (4.104)$$

In particular, M is positive (negative, resp.) definite if $\widetilde{A} - A$ is positive (negative, resp.) definite.

As an immediate consequence of (4.103), we obtain the following estimates for the isotropic case.

Corollary 4.35 *Let $A = \gamma I$ and $\widetilde{A} = \widetilde{\gamma} I$ for positive constants γ and $\widetilde{\gamma}$ with $\gamma \neq \widetilde{\gamma}$, and let $\{a_i | i \in J\}$ be a set of coefficients such that $v = \sum_{i \in I} a_i x^i$ is harmonic, where J is a set of multi-indices. Then we get the following inequalities:*

$$\frac{\gamma}{\widetilde{\gamma}}(\widetilde{\gamma} - \gamma) \int_B |\nabla v|^2 \leq \sum_{i,j \in J} a_i a_j M_{ij} \leq (\widetilde{\gamma} - \gamma) \int_B |\nabla v|^2 . \qquad (4.105)$$

In particular, if κ is an eigenvalue of the polarization tensor $M = (m_{ij})_{|i|=|j|=1}$, then

$$\frac{\gamma}{\widetilde{\gamma}}(\widetilde{\gamma} - \gamma)|B| \leq \kappa \leq (\widetilde{\gamma} - \gamma)|B| . \qquad (4.106)$$

Taking $\gamma = 1$ and $\widetilde{\gamma} = k$, we return once again to the estimate in Lemma 4.14.

4.13 Further Results and Open Problems

In this chapter we have examined symmetry, positivity, isoperimetric inequalities, and monotonicity properties of the GPTs along with their relationship to the harmonic moments of the inclusion. It has also been observed that the knowledge of all the GPTs uniquely determines the DtN map and, hence, the shape and the conductivity of the inclusion. Many important questions remain. In particular, it would be interesting to know how much information one can get from the knowledge of a finite number of these GPTs. Of similar importance would be the question of the quantification of the stability of the inverses of the maps $(k, B) \to M_{ij}(k, B)$ and $(A, \widetilde{A}, B) \to M_{ij}(A, \widetilde{A}, B)$.

In the interesting work of Capdeboscq and Vogelius [81, 82, 83], a (first-order) polarization tensor concerning bounded measurable sets ω_ϵ of small Lebesgue measure has been introduced. In the particular case for which $\omega_\epsilon = \sum_{s=1}^m \epsilon B_s + z_s$, where $\{z_s\}$ is a set of m distinct points, and each $B_s \in \mathbb{R}^d$ is a bounded, Lipschitz domain containing the origin, their polarization reduces to the one studied in this chapter. As pointed out in [81], it may be impossible to construct higher-order polarization tensors in the general setting provided by Capdeboscq and Vogelius.

5

Full Asymptotic Formula for the Potentials

Introduction

In this chapter we derive full asymptotic expansions of the steady-state voltage potentials in the presence of a finite number of diametrically small inclusions with conductivities different from the background conductivity. The derivations are rigorous and based on layer potential techniques and the decomposition formulae (2.63) and (2.89) of the steady-state voltage potentials into a harmonic part and a refraction part. The asymptotic expansions in this chapter are valid for inclusions with Lipschitz boundaries and those with extreme conductivities (zero or infinite conductivity).

One of the main results of this chapter is the full asymptotic expansion of the solution u of

$$
\begin{cases}
\nabla \cdot \left(\chi \left(\Omega \setminus \bigcup_{s=1}^{m} \overline{D_s} \right) + \sum_{s=1}^{m} k_s \chi(D_s) \right) \nabla u = 0 & \text{in } \Omega , \\
\left. \dfrac{\partial u}{\partial \nu} \right|_{\partial \Omega} = g .
\end{cases}
\tag{5.1}
$$

The leading-order term in this asymptotic formula, which expresses that the conductivity inclusion can be modeled by a dipole has been derived by Cedio-Fengya, Moskow, and Vogelius [84]; see also the prior work of Friedman and Vogelius [132] for the case of perfectly conducting or insulating inclusions. A very general representation formula for the boundary voltage perturbations caused by the internal conductivity inclusions of small volume fraction has been obtained by Capdeboscq and Vogelius [81].

Theorem 5.1 *Suppose that the inclusion consists of a single component, $D = \epsilon B + z$, and let u be the solution of (5.1). The following pointwise asymptotic expansion on $\partial \Omega$ holds for $d = 2, 3$:*

$$u(x) = U(x) - \epsilon^{d-2} \sum_{|i|=1}^{n} \sum_{|j|=1}^{n-|i|+1} \frac{\epsilon^{|i|+|j|}}{i!j!}$$

$$\times \left[\left(\left(I + \sum_{p=1}^{n+2-|i|-|j|-d} \epsilon^{d+p-1} \mathcal{Q}_p \right) (\partial^l U(z)) \right)_i M_{ij} \partial_z^j N(x,z) \right] \tag{5.2}$$

$$+ O(\epsilon^{d+n}) \,,$$

where the remainder $O(\epsilon^{d+n})$ is dominated by $C\epsilon^{d+n}\|g\|_{L^2(\partial\Omega)}$ for some C independent of $x \in \partial\Omega$. Here U is the background solution; $N(x,z)$ is the Neumann function, that is, the solution to (2.49); M_{ij}, $i,j \in \mathbb{N}^d$, are the generalized polarization tensors introduced in (4.4); and the matrix $\mathcal{Q}_p$ is defined in (5.18).

In particular, if $n = d$, then we simplify formula (5.2) to obtain:

$$u(x) = U(x) - \sum_{|i|=1}^{d} \sum_{|j|=1}^{d-|i|+1} \frac{\epsilon^{|i|+|j|+d-2}}{i!j!} \partial^i U(z) M_{ij} \partial_z^j N(x,z) + O(\epsilon^{2d}) \,. \tag{5.3}$$

We have a similar expansion for the solutions of the Dirichlet problem (Theorem 5.7).

In the expression (5.3), the remainder $O(\epsilon^{2d})$ is dominated by $C'\epsilon^{2d}$, where the constant C' can be precisely quantified in terms of the Lipschitz character of B and $\mathrm{dist}(D, \partial\Omega)$; see [43, 13].

The constant C' blows up if $\mathrm{dist}(D, \partial\Omega) \to 0$ or B has a "bad" Lipschitz character; i.e., the constant C in (2.43) goes to $+\infty$ (or, in view of Lemma 2.22, $\delta(B) = \min_{x \in \partial B}\langle x, \nu_x \rangle \to 0$ if B is a star-shaped domain with respect to the origin in two-dimensional space).

When B has a "bad" Lipschitz character we must use, in place of (5.3), the asymptotic formula corresponding to a small thin inclusion, which has been formally derived by Beretta, Mukherjee, and Vogelius in [65] and rigorously justified by Beretta, Francini, and Vogelius in their recent paper [64]; see also [63].

In the case where the small inclusion is nearly touching the boundary $(\mathrm{dist}(D, \partial\Omega) \to 0)$ a more complicated asymptotic formula first established in [13] should be used instead of (5.3). The dipole-type expansion (5.3) is valid when the potential u within the inclusion D is nearly constant. On decreasing $\mathrm{dist}(D, \partial\Omega)$, this assumption begins to fail because higher-order multi-poles become significant due to the interaction between D and $\partial\Omega$. Chapter 6 will provide some essential insight for understanding this interaction.

The derivation of the asymptotic expansions for any fixed number m of well-separated inclusions (these are a fixed distance apart) follows by iteration of the arguments that we will present for the case $m = 1$. In other words, we may develop asymptotic formulae involving the difference between the fields u and U on $\partial\Omega$ with s inclusions and those with $s - 1$ inclusions, $s = m, \ldots, 1$, and then at the end essentially form the sum of these m formulae (the reference fields change, but that may easily be remedied). The derivation of each of the m formulae is virtually identical. Suppose D takes the form $D = \cup_{s=1}^{m}(\epsilon_s B_s + z_s)$, and the conductivity of the inclusion $\epsilon_s B_s + z_s$ is k_s, $s = 1, \ldots, m$, then by iterating the formula (5.3) we can derive the following expansion in the case when there are several well-separated inclusions:

$$u(x) = U(x) - \sum_{s=1}^{m}\sum_{|i|=1}^{d}\sum_{|j|=1}^{d-|i|+1}\frac{\epsilon_s^{|i|+|j|+d-2}}{i!j!}\partial^i U(z_s)M_{ij}(k_s, B_s)\partial_z^j N(x, z_s)$$

$$+ O(\epsilon^{2d}) \, . \tag{5.4}$$

5.1 Energy Estimates

Let us begin with the following estimate of the trace of $u - U$ on the boundary $\partial\Omega$.

Proposition 5.2 *If $\partial\Omega$ and ∂D are Lipschitz boundaries, then a positive constant C exists independent of $\epsilon, k,$ and g such that, for ϵ small enough,*

$$\|u - U\|_{L^2(\partial\Omega)} \leq \begin{cases} C(k-1)\,\|g\|_{L^2(\partial\Omega)}\epsilon^d & \text{if } k > 1 \, , \\ C(\frac{1}{k} - 1)\,\|g\|_{L^2(\partial\Omega)}\epsilon^d & \text{if } 0 < k < 1 \, . \end{cases}$$

Proof. We first observe that

$$\mathcal{D}_\Omega(u - U)(x) = H(x) \, , \quad x \in \mathbb{R}^d \setminus \overline{\Omega} \, , \tag{5.5}$$

which follows immediately from the fact that $\mathcal{D}_\Omega(U|_{\partial\Omega})(x) - \mathcal{S}_\Omega(g)(x) = 0$ for $x \in \mathbb{R}^d \setminus \overline{\Omega}$.

Recall that according to (2.43), a positive constant C exists that depends only on the Lipschitz character of Ω such that

$$\|f\|_{L^2(\partial\Omega)} \leq C\left\|(-\frac{1}{2}I + \mathcal{K}_\Omega)f\right\|_{L^2(\partial\Omega)} \quad \forall\, f \in L_0^2(\partial\Omega) \, . \tag{5.6}$$

Employing this inequality, we write

$$\|u - U\|_{L^2(\partial\Omega)}^2 \leq C\|(-\frac{1}{2}I + \mathcal{K}_\Omega)(u - U)\|_{L^2(\partial\Omega)}^2 \, .$$

It then follows from the jump formula (2.28) that

$$\|u - U\|_{L^2(\partial\Omega)}^2 \leq C \lim_{t \to 0^+} \int_{\partial\Omega} \left|\mathcal{D}_\Omega(u - U)(x + t\nu_x)\right|^2 d\sigma(x) \, ,$$

which gives with the help of (2.71) and (5.5) that

$$\|u - U\|_{L^2(\partial\Omega)}^2 \leq C(k-1)^2 \int_{\partial\Omega} \left| \int_D \nabla_y \Gamma(x-y) \cdot \nabla u(y)\, dy \right|^2 d\sigma(x) \, .$$

Thus we get by the Cauchy–Schwarz inequality

$$\|u - U\|_{L^2(\partial\Omega)}^2 \leq C(k-1)^2 \left(\int_D |\nabla u(y)|^2\, dy \right) \int_{\partial\Omega} \left(\int_D |\nabla_y \Gamma(x-y)|^2\, dy \right) d\sigma(x) \, .$$

$$(5.7)$$

If $k > 1$, then using the energy identity (2.82), we arrive at

$$\|u - U\|_{L^2(\partial\Omega)} \leq C(k-1)\|g\|_{L^2(\partial\Omega)} \int_{\partial\Omega} \left(\int_D |\nabla_y \Gamma(x-y)|^2\, dy \right) d\sigma(x) \, .$$

But a positive constant C exists depending only on $|B|$ and $\mathrm{dist}(D, \partial\Omega)$ such that

$$\int_{\partial\Omega} \left(\int_D |\nabla_y \Gamma(x-y)|^2\, dy \right) d\sigma(x) \leq C\epsilon^d \, ,$$

for ϵ small enough. Inserting this into the above inequality immediately yields the desired estimate for $k > 1$.

If $0 < k < 1$, then by using (2.83), we have

$$\int_D |\nabla u(y)|^2\, dy \leq 2 \int_D |\nabla(u-U)(y)|^2\, dy + 2 \int_D |\nabla U(y)|^2\, dy$$

$$\leq \frac{2}{k} \int_\Omega \left(1 + (k-1)\chi(D) \right) |\nabla(u-U)(y)|^2\, dy + 2 \int_D |\nabla U(y)|^2\, dy$$

$$\leq \frac{2}{k(1-k)} \|u - U\|_{L^2(\partial\Omega)} \|g\|_{L^2(\partial\Omega)} \, .$$

Here we have used the energy identity (2.83). Combining (5.7) with the above estimate, we deduce that for $0 < k < 1$ the desired estimate holds and the proof of the proposition is then complete. $\square$

As a direct consequence of Proposition 5.2 and its proof, we get the following corollary.

Corollary 5.3 *Let $0 < k \neq 1 < +\infty$. A constant $C(k)$ exists independent of ϵ such that*

$$\|\nabla u\|_{L^2(D)} \leq C(k)\, \epsilon^{\frac{d}{2}} \, .$$

Next we employ the Rellich identity stated in Lemma 2.19 to estimate the L^2-norm of the tangential derivative of $u - U$ on the boundary $\partial\Omega$ as ϵ goes to zero.

Lemma 5.4 *Let T be the tangent vector to $\partial\Omega$ at x. If Ω is a Lipschitz domain, then a positive constant C exists depending only on the Lipschitz character of Ω such that*

$$\left\| \frac{\partial}{\partial T}(u-U) \right\|_{L^2(\partial\Omega)} \leq C\, \|g\|_{L^2(\partial\Omega)} \epsilon^{\frac{d}{2}} \, . \tag{5.8}$$

Proof.   Let

$$\Omega_\epsilon = \left\{ x \in \Omega, \operatorname{dist}(x, \partial\Omega) > \left(C - \max_{x\in\partial B} |x|\right)\epsilon \right\}$$

and $\boldsymbol{\alpha}$ be a smooth vector field such that the support of $\boldsymbol{\alpha}$ lies in $\mathbb{R}^d \setminus \overline{\Omega_\epsilon}$ and $\langle \boldsymbol{\alpha}, \nu \rangle > c_1 > 0$ on $\partial\Omega$ (here, c_1 depends only on the Lipschitz character of $\partial\Omega$). Using the Rellich identity (2.35) with this $\boldsymbol{\alpha}$, we obtain

$$\int_{\partial\Omega} \langle \boldsymbol{\alpha}, \nu \rangle \left| \frac{\partial}{\partial T}(u-U) \right|^2 = \int_{\Omega} -2\langle \nabla\boldsymbol{\alpha}\nabla(u-U), \nabla(u-U)\rangle + (\nabla\cdot\boldsymbol{\alpha})|\nabla(u-U)|^2 ,$$

since $\partial(u - U)/\partial\nu = 0$ on $\partial\Omega$. Hence

$$\int_{\partial\Omega} \langle \boldsymbol{\alpha}, \nu \rangle \left| \frac{\partial}{\partial T}(u - U) \right|^2 \leq C \int_{\Omega} |\nabla(u - U)|^2. \tag{5.9}$$

Combining the energy identity (2.82) together with Proposition 5.2 leads us to the estimates

$$\begin{aligned}
\int_{\Omega} |\nabla(u - U)|^2 &\leq \int_{\partial\Omega} (U - u)y \\
&\leq \|U - u\|_{L^2(\partial\Omega)} \|g\|_{L^2(\partial\Omega)} \\
&\leq C\epsilon^d \|g\|_{L^2(\partial\Omega)}^2 .
\end{aligned}$$

Therefore (5.9) implies that the estimate (5.8) holds. $\qquad\square$

Proposition 5.5 *If $\partial\Omega$ is of class $\mathcal{C}^2$, then a positive constant C exists that is independent of $\epsilon, k,$ and g such that*

$$\|u - U\|_{L^\infty(\partial\Omega)} \leq C \, |k - 1| \, \|g\|_{L^2(\partial\Omega)}\epsilon^d ,$$

for ϵ small enough.

Proof.   Since $\partial\Omega$ is of class $\mathcal{C}^2$, we have

$$\|u - U\|_{L^\infty(\partial\Omega)} \leq C \left\| \left(-\frac{1}{2}I + \mathcal{K}_\Omega\right)(u - U) \right\|_{L^\infty(\partial\Omega)} ,$$

where C depends only on the $\mathcal{C}^2$ character of Ω and therefore

$$\|u - U\|_{L^\infty(\partial\Omega)} \leq C \lim_{t\to 0^+} \sup_{x\in\partial\Omega} \left| \mathcal{D}_\Omega(u - U)(x + t\nu_x) \right| .$$

Using (2.71), we readily get

$$||u - U||_{L^\infty(\partial\Omega)} \leq C|k - 1| \sup_{x \in \partial\Omega} \left| \int_D \nabla_y \Gamma(x - y) \cdot \nabla u(y) \, dy \right|$$

$$\leq C|k - 1| \sup_{x \in \partial\Omega} \left(\int_D |\nabla_y \Gamma(x - y)|^2 \, dy \right)^{\frac{1}{2}} ||\nabla u||_{L^2(D)} \, .$$

Since

$$||\nabla u||_{L^2(D)} \leq C\epsilon^{d/2} ||g||_{L^2(\partial\Omega)}$$

by (2.82) and $\sup_{x \in \partial\Omega}(\int_D |\nabla_y \Gamma(x-y)|^2 \, dy)^{1/2}$ is bounded by $C\epsilon^{d/2}$, we obtain the desired result. $\qquad\square$

Next, the following estimates hold.

Proposition 5.6 (i) *If Ω is a Lipschitz domain, then*

$$||H - U||_{L^2(\partial\Omega)} \leq C||u - U||_{L^2(\partial\Omega)} \leq C|k - 1| \, ||g||_{L^2(\partial\Omega)} \epsilon^d \, .$$

(ii) *If Ω is of class C^2, then*

$$||H - U||_{L^\infty(\partial\Omega)} \leq C||u - U||_{L^\infty(\partial\Omega)} \leq C|k - 1| \, ||g||_{L^2(\partial\Omega)} \epsilon^d \, .$$

(iii) *If Ω is of class C^2, then*

$$||H - U||_{L^\infty(\overline{\Omega})} \leq C|k - 1| \, ||g||_{L^2(\partial\Omega)} \epsilon^d \, .$$

(iv) *If Ω is of class C^2, then*

$$||H - U||_{W^{1,2}(\Omega)} \leq C|k - 1|^{\frac{1}{2}} \, ||g||_{L^2(\partial\Omega)} \epsilon^{\frac{3d}{4}} \, .$$

(v) *If Ω and $D \subset\subset \Omega$ are Lipschitz domains, then*

$$||\nabla H - \nabla U||_{L^\infty(\overline{D})} \leq C||u - U||_{L^2(\partial\Omega)} \leq C|k - 1| \, ||g||_{L^2(\partial\Omega)} \epsilon^d \, ,$$

where C depends on $dist(\partial\Omega, D)$.

Proof. Parts (i) and (ii) follow from the fact that

$$H - U = (\frac{1}{2}I + \mathcal{K}_\Omega)(u - U) \quad \text{on } \partial\Omega$$

together with the facts that

$$||\mathcal{K}_\Omega v||_{L^2(\partial\Omega)} \leq C||v||_{L^2(\partial\Omega)} \quad \text{if } \Omega \text{ is a Lipschitz domain,}$$
$$||\mathcal{K}_\Omega v||_{L^\infty(\partial\Omega)} \leq C'||v||_{L^\infty(\partial\Omega)} \quad \text{if } \Omega \text{ is of class } C^2 \, ,$$

where the constants C and C' depend only on the Lipschitz and C^2 characters of Ω, respectively. Part (iii) is a direct application of the maximum principle to the harmonic function $H - U$ and (ii).

To prove (iv) we write

$$\|\nabla(H-U)\|^2_{L^2(\Omega)} = \int_{\partial\Omega} \frac{\partial}{\partial\nu}(H-U)(H-U)$$

$$\leq \|H-U\|_{L^2(\partial\Omega)}\|\frac{\partial}{\partial\nu}(H-U)\|_{L^2(\partial\Omega)} \ .$$

Since, by using the fact from Theorem 2.24 that $K_\Omega : W^2_1(\partial\Omega) \to W^2_1(\partial\Omega)$ is a bounded operator together with Lemma 5.4, we have

$$\|\frac{\partial}{\partial\nu}(H-U)\|_{L^2(\partial\Omega)} \leq C\|H-U\|_{W^2_1(\partial\Omega)} \leq C\|u-U\|_{W^2_1(\partial\Omega)} \leq C\epsilon^{\frac{d}{2}}\|g\|_{L^2(\partial\Omega)} \ .$$

Therefore we get

$$\|\nabla(H-U)\|^2_{L^2(\Omega)} \leq C|k-1|\|g\|^2_{L^2(\partial\Omega)}\epsilon^{\frac{3d}{2}} \ .$$

Now, since $\nabla(H-U) = \nabla\mathcal{D}_\Omega(u-U)$, we obtain

$$\|\nabla H - \nabla U\|_{L^\infty(\overline{D})} \leq \sup_{x\in\overline{D}}\int_{\partial\Omega}|\nabla_x\Gamma(x-y)|^2\,d\sigma(y)\,\|u-U\|_{L^2(\partial\Omega)} \ ,$$

and consequently (v) holds, where the constant C depends on $\mathrm{dist}(\partial\Omega, D)$. This finishes the proof of the proposition.　　　　□

5.2 Asymptotic Expansion

As stated in the above theorem, we restrict our derivation to the case of a single inclusion ($m = 1$). We only give the details when considering the difference between the fields corresponding to one and zero inclusions. In order to further simplify notation we assume that the single inclusion D has the form $D = \epsilon B + z$, where $z \in \Omega$ and B is a bounded Lipschitz domain in $\mathbb{R}^d$ containing the origin. Here and throughout this book, ϵB denotes the set $\{\epsilon x | x \in B\}$. Suppose that the conductivity of D is a positive constant $k \neq 1$. Let $\lambda := (k+1)/(2(k-1))$ as before. Then by (2.73) and (2.65), the solution u of (2.61) takes the form

$$u(x) = U(x) - N_D(\lambda I - \mathcal{K}^*_D)^{-1}\left(\frac{\partial H}{\partial\nu}\bigg|_{\partial D}\right)(x) \ , \quad x \in \partial\Omega \ ,$$

where U is the background potential given in (2.62).

Define

$$H_n(x) := \sum_{|i|=0}^{n}\frac{1}{i!}(\partial^i H)(z)(x-z)^i.$$

Here we use the multi-index notation $i = (i_1,\ldots,i_d) \in \mathbb{N}^d$. Then we have from (2.66) that

$$\left\| \frac{\partial H}{\partial \nu} - \frac{\partial H_n}{\partial \nu} \right\|_{L^2(\partial D)} \leq \sup_{x \in \partial D} |\nabla H(x) - \nabla H_n(x)| |\partial D|^{1/2}$$

$$\leq \|H\|_{\mathcal{C}^{n+1}(\overline{D})} |x - z|^n |\partial D|^{1/2}$$

$$\leq C \|g\|_{L^2(\partial \Omega)} \epsilon^n |\partial D|^{1/2} \, .$$

Note that

$$\text{if } \int_{\partial D} h \, d\sigma = 0 \, , \text{ then } \int_{\partial D} (\lambda I - \mathcal{K}_D^*)^{-1} h \, d\sigma = 0 \, . \tag{5.10}$$

If $\int_{\partial D} h \, d\sigma = 0$, then we have for $x \in \partial \Omega$ that

$$\left| N_D (\lambda I - \mathcal{K}_D^*)^{-1} h(x) \right| = \left| \int_{\partial D} \left[N(x, y) - N(x, z) \right] (\lambda I - \mathcal{K}_D^*)^{-1} h(y) \, d\sigma(y) \right|$$

$$\leq C\epsilon |\partial D|^{1/2} \|h\|_{L^2(\partial D)} \, .$$

Since $\Delta H = \Delta H_n = 0$ in D, it then follows that

$$\sup_{x \in \partial \Omega} \left| N_D (\lambda I - \mathcal{K}_D^*)^{-1} \left(\left. \frac{\partial H}{\partial \nu} \right|_{\partial D} - \left. \frac{\partial H_n}{\partial \nu} \right|_{\partial D} \right)(x) \right|$$

$$\leq C\epsilon |\partial D|^{1/2} \left\| \frac{\partial H}{\partial \nu} - \frac{\partial H_n}{\partial \nu} \right\|_{L^2(\partial D)} \leq C \|g\|_{L^2(\partial \Omega)} \epsilon^{d+n} \, .$$

Therefore, we have

$$u(x) = U(x) - N_D (\lambda I - \mathcal{K}_D^*)^{-1} \left(\left. \frac{\partial H_n}{\partial \nu} \right|_{\partial D} \right)(x) + O(\epsilon^{d+n}), \quad x \in \partial \Omega \, , \tag{5.11}$$

where the $O(\epsilon^{d+n})$ term is dominated by $C\|g\|_{L^2(\partial \Omega)} \epsilon^{d+n}$ for some C depending only on c_0. Note that

$$(\lambda I - \mathcal{K}_D^*)^{-1} \left(\left. \frac{\partial H_n}{\partial \nu} \right|_{\partial D} \right)(x) = \sum_{|i|=1}^{n} (\partial^i H)(z)(\lambda I - \mathcal{K}_D^*)^{-1} \left(\frac{1}{i!} \nu_x \cdot \nabla (x-z)^i \right)(x) \, .$$

Since $D = \epsilon B + z$, one can prove by using the change of variables $y = (x - z)/\epsilon$ and the expression of $\mathcal{K}_D^*$ defined by (2.29) that

$$(\lambda I - \mathcal{K}_D^*)^{-1} \left(\nu_x \cdot \nabla (x-z)^i \right)(x) = \epsilon^{|i|-1} (\lambda I - \mathcal{K}_B^*)^{-1} \left(\nu_y \cdot \nabla y^i \right) \left(\frac{1}{\epsilon}(x - z) \right) \, .$$

Put

$$\phi_i(x) := (\lambda I - \mathcal{K}_B^*)^{-1} \left(\nu_y \cdot \nabla y^i \right)(x), \quad x \in \partial B \, . \tag{5.12}$$

Then we get

$$N_D(\lambda I - \mathcal{K}_D^*)^{-1}\left(\left.\frac{\partial H_n}{\partial \nu}\right|_{\partial D}\right)(x) \tag{5.13}$$

$$= \sum_{|i|=1}^{n} \frac{1}{i!}(\partial^i H)(z)\epsilon^{|i|-1}\int_{\partial D} N(x,y)\phi_i(\epsilon^{-1}(y-z))\,d\sigma(y)$$

$$= \sum_{|i|=1}^{n} \frac{1}{i!}(\partial^i H)(z)\epsilon^{|i|+d-2}\int_{\partial B} N(x,\epsilon y + z)\phi_i(y)\,d\sigma(y)\,.$$

We now have from (2.56) and (5.13)

$$N_D(\lambda I - \mathcal{K}_D^*)^{-1}\left(\left.\frac{\partial H_n}{\partial \nu}\right|_{\partial D}\right)(x)$$

$$= \sum_{|i|=1}^{n} \frac{1}{i!}(\partial^i H)(z)\epsilon^{|i|+d-2}\sum_{|j|=0}^{+\infty}\frac{1}{j!}\epsilon^{|j|}\partial_z^j N(x,z)\int_{\partial B} y^j \phi_i(y)d\sigma(y)\,.$$

Observe that since H is a harmonic function in Ω we may compute

$$\sum_{|i|=l}\frac{1}{i!}(\partial^i H)(z)\Delta(y^i) = \Delta_y\left(\sum_{|i|=l}\frac{1}{i!}(\partial^i H)(z)y^i\right) = 0\,,$$

and therefore, by Green's formula, it follows that

$$\int_{\partial B}\sum_{|i|=l}\frac{1}{i!}(\partial^i H)(z)\nabla(y^i)\cdot\nu_y\,d\sigma(y) = 0\,.$$

Thus, in view of (5.10) and (5.12), the following identity holds:

$$\sum_{|i|=l}\frac{1}{i!}(\partial^i H)(z)\int_{\partial B}\phi_i(y)d\sigma(y) = 0 \quad \forall\, l \geq 1\,.$$

Recalling now from Lemma 2.30 the fact that

$$\epsilon^{d-2}N(x,\epsilon y + z) = \epsilon^{d-2}\sum_{|j|=0}^{n-|i|+1}\frac{1}{j!}\epsilon^{|j|}\partial_z^j N(x,z)y^j + O(\epsilon^{d+n-|i|})$$

for all $i, 1 \leq |i| \leq n$, and the definition of GPTs, we obtain the following pointwise asymptotic formula. For $x \in \partial\Omega$,

$$u(x) = U(x) - \epsilon^{d-2}\sum_{|i|=1}^{n}\sum_{|j|=1}^{n-|i|+1}\frac{\epsilon^{|i|+|j|}}{i!j!}(\partial^i H)(z)M_{ij}\partial_z^j N(x,z)$$

$$+\, O(\epsilon^{d+n})\,. \tag{5.14}$$

Observing that the formula (5.14) still contains $\partial^i H$ factors, we see that the remaining task is to convert (5.14) to a formula given solely by U and its derivatives.

As a simplest case, let us now take $n = 1$ to find the leading-order term in the asymptotic expansion of $u|_{\partial\Omega}$ as $\epsilon \to 0$. According to (v) in Proposition 5.6 we have

$$|\nabla H(z) - \nabla U(z)| \leq C\epsilon^d \|g\|_{L^2(\partial\Omega)} , \qquad (5.15)$$

and therefore, we deduce from (5.14) that

$$u(x) = U(x) - \epsilon^d \sum_{|i|=1,|j|=1} (\partial^i U)(z) M_{ij} \partial^j N(x, z) + O(\epsilon^{d+1}) , \qquad x \in \partial\Omega ,$$

which is, in view of (4.10), exactly the formula derived in [132] and [84] when D has a $\mathcal{C}^{1+\alpha}$-boundary for some $\alpha > 0$.

We now return to (5.14). Recalling that by Green's formula $U = -\mathcal{S}_\Omega(g) + \mathcal{D}_\Omega(U|_{\partial\Omega})$ in Ω, substitution of (5.14) into (2.64) immediately yields that, for any $x \in \Omega$,

$$H(x) = U(x)$$
$$-\epsilon^{d-2} \sum_{|i|=1}^{n} \sum_{|j|=1}^{n-|i|+1} \frac{\epsilon^{|i|+|j|}}{i!j!} (\partial^i H)(z) M_{ij} \mathcal{D}_\Omega(\partial_z^j N(\cdot, z))(x) + O(\epsilon^{d+n}) . \qquad (5.16)$$

In (5.16) the remainder $O(\epsilon^{d+n})$ is uniform in the $\mathcal{C}^n$-norm on any compact subset of Ω for any n, and therefore

$$(\partial^l H)(z) + \sum_{|i|=1}^{n} \epsilon^{d-2} \sum_{|j|=1}^{n-|i|+1} \epsilon^{|i|+|j|} (\partial^i H)(z) P_{ijl} = (\partial^l U)(z) + O(\epsilon^{d+n}) \qquad (5.17)$$

for all $l \in \mathbb{N}^d$ with $|l| \leq n$, where

$$P_{ijl} = \frac{1}{i!j!} M_{ij} \partial_x^l \mathcal{D}_\Omega(\partial_z^j N(\cdot, z)) \Big|_{x=z} .$$

Define the operator

$$\mathcal{P}_\epsilon : (v_l)_{l \in \mathbb{N}^d, |l| \leq n} \mapsto \left(v_l + \epsilon^{d-2} \sum_{|i|=1}^{n} \sum_{|j|=1}^{n-|i|+1} \epsilon^{|i|+|j|} v_i P_{ijl} \right)_{l \in \mathbb{N}^d, |l| \leq n} .$$

Observe that

$$\mathcal{P}_\epsilon = I + \epsilon^d \mathcal{R}_1 + \cdots + \epsilon^{n+d-1} \mathcal{R}_{n-1} .$$

Defining the matrices $\mathcal{Q}_p, p = 1, \ldots, n-1$, by

$$(I + \epsilon^d \mathcal{R}_1 + \cdots + \epsilon^{n+d-1} \mathcal{R}_{n-1})^{-1} = I + \epsilon^d \mathcal{Q}_1 + \cdots + \epsilon^{n+d-1} \mathcal{Q}_{n-1}$$
$$+ O(\epsilon^{n+d}) \qquad (5.18)$$

for small ϵ, we finally obtain that

$$((\partial^i H)(z))_{i\in\mathbb{N}^d,|i|\leq n} = \left(I + \sum_{p=1}^{n} \epsilon^{d+p-1} \mathcal{Q}_p\right)((\partial^i U)(z))_{i\in\mathbb{N}^d,|i|\leq n} + O(\epsilon^{d+n})\,,$$

(5.19)

which yields the main result of this chapter stated in Theorem 5.1.

We also have a complete asymptotic expansion of the solutions of the Dirichlet problem.

Theorem 5.7 *Suppose that the inclusion consists of a single component, and let v be the solution of (5.1) with the Neumann condition replaced by the Dirichlet condition $v|_{\partial\Omega} = f$. Let V be the solution of $\Delta V = 0$ in Ω with $V|_{\partial\Omega} = f$. The following pointwise asymptotic expansion on $\partial\Omega$ holds for $d = 2,3$:*

$$\frac{\partial v}{\partial \nu}(x) = \frac{\partial V}{\partial \nu}(x) - \epsilon^{d-2} \sum_{\substack{|i|=1}}^{n} \sum_{\substack{|j|=1}}^{n-|i|+1} \frac{\epsilon^{|i|+|j|}}{i!j!}$$

$$\times \left[\left(\left(I + \sum_{p=1}^{n+2-|i|-|j|-d} \epsilon^{d+p-1} \mathcal{Q}_p\right)(\partial^l V(z))\right)_i M_{ij}\partial_z^j \frac{\partial}{\partial\nu_x}G(x,z)\right]$$

$$+ O(\epsilon^{d+n})\,,$$

(5.20)

where the remainder $O(\epsilon^{d+n})$ is dominated by $C\epsilon^{d+n}\|f\|_{W^2_{\frac{1}{2}}(\partial\Omega)}$ for some C independent of $x \in \partial\Omega$. Here $G(x,z)$ is the Dirichlet Green's function; M_{ij}, $i,j \in \mathbb{N}^d$, are the GPTs; and $\mathcal{Q}_p$ is the operator defined in (5.18), where $\mathcal{P}_{ijl}$ is defined, in this case, by

$$P_{ijl} = \frac{1}{i!j!}M_{ij}\partial_x^l \mathcal{S}_\Omega\left(\partial_z^j\left(\frac{\partial}{\partial\nu_x}G\right)(\cdot,z)\right)\bigg|_{x=z}.$$

Theorem 5.7 can be proved in exactly the same manner as Theorem 5.1. We begin with Theorem 2.34. Then the same arguments give us

$$v(x) = V(x) - \epsilon^{d-2} \sum_{\substack{|i|=1}}^{n} \sum_{\substack{|j|=1}}^{n-|i|+1} \frac{\epsilon^{|i|+|j|}}{i!j!}(\partial^i H)(z)M_{ij}\partial_z^j G(x,z) + O(\epsilon^{d+n})\,.$$

From this we can get (5.20) as before.

Before concluding this section, we shall make a remark. The following formulae (5.21) and (5.22) are not exactly asymptotic formulae since the function H still depends on ϵ. However, since these formulae are simple and useful for solving the inverse problem in Chapter 7, we make a record of them as a theorem.

Theorem 5.8 *We have*

$$
u(x) = H(x) + \epsilon^{d-2} \sum_{|i|=1}^{n} \sum_{|j|=1}^{n-|i|+1} \frac{\epsilon^{|i|+|j|}}{i!j!} \partial^i H(z) M_{ij} \partial^j \Gamma(x - z)
$$
$$
+ O(\epsilon^{d+n}) ,
$$
(5.21)

where $x \in \partial\Omega$ and the $O(\epsilon^{d+n})$ term is dominated by $C\|g\|_{L^2(\partial\Omega)}\epsilon^{d+n}$ for some C depending only on c_0, and H is given in (2.64). Moreover,

$$
H(x) = - \sum_{|i|=1}^{n} \sum_{|j|=1}^{n-|i|+1} \frac{1}{i!j!} \epsilon^{|i|+|j|+d-2} \partial^i H(z) M_{ij} \partial^j \Gamma(x-z) + O(\epsilon^{d+n}) ,
$$
(5.22)

for all $x \in \mathbb{R}^d \setminus \overline{\Omega}$.

Proof. Beginning with the representation formula (2.63), one can show in the same way as in the derivation of (5.11) that

$$
u(x) = H(x) + \mathcal{S}_D(\lambda I - \mathcal{K}_D^*)^{-1}\left(\frac{\partial H_n}{\partial \nu}\bigg|_{\partial D}\right)(x) + O(\epsilon^{d+n}) , \quad x \in \partial\Omega ,
$$

for $x \in \partial\Omega$. Then the rest is parallel to the previous arguments.

The formula (5.22) can be derived using (2.67). $\qquad\square$

5.3 Derivation of the Asymptotic Formula for Closely Spaced Small Inclusions

An asymptotic formula similar to (5.2) was obtained for closely spaced inclusions in [29]. In this section we present the formula and its derivation in brief.

Let D denote a set of m closely spaced inclusions inside Ω:

$$
D = \cup_{s=1}^{m} D_s := \cup_{s=1}^{m}(\epsilon B_s + z) ,
$$

where $z \in \Omega$, $\epsilon > 0$ is small and B_s, for $s = 1,\ldots,m$, is a bounded Lipschitz domain in $\mathbb{R}^d$. We suppose in addition to (H1) and (H2) in Sect. 4.10 that the set D is well separated from the boundary $\partial\Omega$, i.e., $\mathrm{dist}(D,\partial\Omega) > c_0 > 0$.

Let $g \in L_0^2(\partial\Omega)$. The voltage potential in the presence of the set D of conductivity inclusions is denoted by u. It is the solution to

$$
\begin{cases}
\nabla\cdot\left(\chi(\Omega \setminus \bigcup_{s=1}^{m} \overline{D_s}) + \sum_{s=1}^{m} k_s\chi(D_s)\right)\nabla u = 0 \quad \text{in } \Omega , \\[2mm]
\dfrac{\partial u}{\partial \nu}\bigg|_{\partial\Omega} = g , \int_{\partial\Omega} u = 0 .
\end{cases}
$$
(5.23)

The background voltage potential is denoted by U as before.

Based on the arguments given in Theorem 2.31, the following theorem was proved in [207].

Theorem 5.9 *The solution u of the problem (5.23) can be represented as*

$$u(x) = H(x) + \sum_{s=1}^{m} \mathcal{S}_{D_s} \psi^{(s)}(x) , \quad x \in \Omega , \tag{5.24}$$

where the harmonic function H is given by

$$H(x) = -\mathcal{S}_{\Omega}(g)(x) + \mathcal{D}_{\Omega}(f)(x), \quad x \in \Omega, \quad f := u|_{\partial\Omega} ,$$

and $\psi^{(s)} \in L_0^2(\partial D_s)$, $s = 1, \cdots , m$, satisfies the integral equation

$$(\lambda_s I - \mathcal{K}_{D_s}^*)\psi^{(s)} - \sum_{l \neq s} \frac{\partial(\mathcal{S}_{D_l}\psi^{(l)})}{\partial\nu^{(s)}}\Big|_{\partial D_s} = \frac{\partial H}{\partial\nu^{(s)}}\Big|_{\partial D_s} \quad \text{on } \partial D_s .$$

Moreover, $\forall\, n \in \mathbb{N}$, a constant $C_n = C(n, \Omega, \mathrm{dist}(D, \partial\Omega))$ exists independent of $|D|$ and the conductivities $k_s, s = 1, \dots, m$, such that

$$\|H\|_{\mathcal{C}^n(\overline{D})} \leq C_n \|g\|_{L^2(\partial\Omega)} .$$

One can also prove the following theorem.

Theorem 5.10 *The solution u to (5.23) can be represented as*

$$u(x) = U(x) - \sum_{s=1}^{m} N_{D_s} \psi^{(s)}(x) , \quad x \in \partial\Omega ,$$

where $\psi^{(s)}$, $s = 1, \dots, m$, is defined by (2.65).

Following the arguments presented in Sect. 5.2, we only outline the derivation of an asymptotic expansion of u leaving the details to the reader.

For $x \in \partial\Omega$, by using the change of variables $y = (x - z)/\epsilon$, we may write

$$\sum_{s=1}^{m} N_{D_s} \psi^{(s)}(x) = \epsilon^{d-1} \sum_{s=1}^{m} \int_{\partial B_s} N(x, \epsilon y + z)\psi^{(s)}(\epsilon y + z)\, d\sigma(y) . \tag{5.25}$$

We expand the Neumann function N as in (2.56)

$$N(x, \epsilon y + z) = \sum_{|j|=0}^{+\infty} \frac{1}{j!}\epsilon^{|j|}\partial_z^j N(x, z) y^j . \tag{5.26}$$

We then use the uniqueness of the solution to the integral equation (4.59) and the expansion of the harmonic function H,

$$H(x) := H(z) + \sum_{|i|=1}^{+\infty} \frac{1}{i!}(\partial^i H)(z)(x - z)^i, \quad x \in \overline{D} ,$$

to show that

$$\psi^{(s)}(\epsilon y + z) = \sum_{|i|=1}^{+\infty} \frac{\epsilon^{|i|-1}}{i!}(\partial^i H)(z)\phi_i^{(s)}(y) , \quad y \in \partial B_s , \qquad (5.27)$$

where $\phi_i^{(s)}$ is the solution to (4.59).

Substituting (5.26) and (5.27) into (5.25), we obtain

$$\sum_{s=1}^{m} N_{D_s}\psi^{(s)}(x) = \sum_{|i|=1}^{+\infty}\sum_{|j|=0}^{+\infty} \frac{\epsilon^{|i|+|j|+d-2}}{i!j!}(\partial^i H)(z)\partial_z^j N(x,z)$$
$$\times \sum_{s=1}^{m} \int_{\partial B_s} y^j \phi_i^{(s)}(y)\, d\sigma(y) .$$

If $j = 0$, then $\int_{\partial B_s} y^j \phi_i^{(s)}(y)\, d\sigma(y) = 0$ for $s = 1,\ldots,m$, and hence, we get

$$\sum_{s=1}^{m} N_{D_s}\psi^{(s)}(x) = \sum_{|i|=1}^{+\infty}\sum_{|j|=1}^{+\infty} \frac{\epsilon^{|i|+|j|+d-2}}{i!j!}(\partial^i H)(z)\partial_z^j N(x,z)M_{ij} , \qquad (5.28)$$

where M_{ij} is the generalized polarization tensor defined in (4.60).

We now convert the formula (5.28) to one given solely by U and its derivatives, without H. Using formula (5.17), we can show analogously to (v) in Proposition 5.6 that

$$|\partial^i H(z) - \partial^i U(z)| \le C\epsilon^d \|g\|_{L^2(\partial\Omega)} \quad \text{for } i \in \mathbb{N}^d ,$$

where C is independent of ϵ and g, and obtain the following theorem.

Theorem 5.11 *The following pointwise asymptotic expansion holds uniformly in $x \in \partial\Omega$ for $d = 2$ or 3:*

$$u(x) = U(x) - \sum_{|i|=1}^{d}\sum_{|j|=1}^{d} \frac{\epsilon^{|i|+|j|+d-2}}{i!j!}(\partial^i U)(z)\partial_z^j N(x,z)M_{ij} + O(\epsilon^{2d}) ,$$

where the remainder $O(\epsilon^{2d})$ is dominated by $C\epsilon^{2d}\|g\|_{L^2(\partial\Omega)}$ for some constant C independent of $x \in \partial\Omega$.

5.4 Derivation of the Asymptotic Formula for Anisotropic Inclusions

In this section, we use the same notation as above. For a given $g \in L_0^2(\partial\Omega)$, let u be the solution to the Neumann problem

$$\begin{cases} \nabla \cdot \gamma_\Omega(x)\nabla u = 0 \quad \text{in } \Omega \,, \\[2mm] \nu \cdot A\nabla u\Big|_{\partial\Omega} = g \,, \\[2mm] \displaystyle\int_{\partial\Omega} u(x)\,d\sigma(x) = 0 \,, \end{cases} \tag{5.29}$$

where the conductivity distribution $\gamma_\Omega = \chi(\Omega \setminus \overline{D})A + \chi(D)\widetilde{A}$ and $D = \epsilon B + z$.

The background potential U is the steady-state voltage potential in the absence of the conductivity inclusion, i.e., the solution to

$$\begin{cases} \nabla \cdot A\nabla U = 0 \quad \text{in } \Omega \,, \\[2mm] \nu \cdot A\nabla U\Big|_{\partial\Omega} = g \,, \\[2mm] \displaystyle\int_{\partial\Omega} U(x)\,d\sigma(x) = 0 \,. \end{cases} \tag{5.30}$$

Let $N^A(x,y)$, $x \in \partial\Omega$, $y \in \Omega$, be the Neumann function for $\nabla \cdot A\nabla$ on Ω; that is,

$$\begin{cases} \nabla \cdot A\nabla N^A(x,y) = -\delta_y \quad \text{in } \Omega \,, \\[2mm] \nu \cdot A\nabla N^A(x,y)\Big|_{\partial\Omega} = -\dfrac{1}{|\partial\Omega|} \,, \\[2mm] \displaystyle\int_{\partial\Omega} N^A(x,y)\,d\sigma(x) = 0 \,, \end{cases}$$

and $M_{ij}(A, \widetilde{A}, B)$ are the APTs. Following the same lines as in the derivation of (5.20), we can prove the following asymptotic expansion of the solution u to (5.29) on $\partial\Omega$; see [175].

Theorem 5.12 *For $x \in \partial\Omega$,*

$$u(x) = U(x) - \epsilon^d \sum_{|i|=1}^{d} \sum_{|j|=1}^{d-|i|+1} \frac{\epsilon^{|i|+|\beta|-2}}{i!j!} \partial^i U(z) M_{ij}(A, \widetilde{A}, B) \partial^j_z N^A(x,z) + O(\epsilon^{2d}) \,,$$

where the remainder $O(\epsilon^{2d})$ is dominated by $C\epsilon^{2d}$ for some constant C independent of $x \in \partial\Omega$ and z.

5.5 Further Results and Open Problems

First-order asymptotic formulae for eigenvalues of the Laplacian in domains with a small circular inclusion that is either perfectly conducting or perfectly insulating were derived in [259] and [260]. In [35], inclusions of arbitrary shape and of arbitrary conductivity contrast are considered. Note that letting the conductivity contrast of the inclusion tend to zero or infinity in our asymptotic expansion in [35] we do not arrive at Ozawa's formulae. This is an effect of non-commuting limits. The main reason behind this phenomenon is that the problem is a singularly perturbed one.

Following the integral approach developed in this chapter, full asymptotic expansions of solutions to Helmholtz and wave equations can be derived [25] as well as the heat equation $\partial_t u - \nabla \cdot (1 + (k-1)\chi(D))\nabla u = 0$. See [18].

The leading-order term in the asymptotic formula for the Helmholtz equation has been derived by Vogelius and Volkov in [299] (see also [39] where the second-order term in the asymptotic expansions of solutions to the Helmholtz equation is obtained). Their (variational) proof is radically different from the one presented here. Results similar to those presented in this chapter have been obtained in the context of the full (time-harmonic) Maxwell's equations in [45].

Finally, we mention that, in their interesting paper [60], Ben Hassen and Bonnetier considered a composite medium made of a periodic array of inclusions embedded in a homogeneous background material and compared the potential in this medium with the potential in a perturbed medium where a few inclusions have been misplaced. Away from the periodicity defect, they proved that the correction at first order of the perturbed potential can be expressed via a polarization tensor, which generalizes the one introduced in this book to periodic background media. These results could be useful in numerical analysis of the inverse conductivity problem in a highly heterogeneous medium.

6

Near-Boundary Conductivity Inclusions

Introduction

The voltage potentials change significantly when a conductivity inclusion D inside a conductor Ω is brought close to the boundary $\partial\Omega$. As shown in the previous chapter, if the inclusion D is small, then it can be modeled by a dipole. This approximation is valid when the field within the inclusion is nearly constant and the inclusion is not too close to the boundary. However, on decreasing the inclusion–boundary separation, the assumption that the field within the inclusion is nearly constant begins to fail because the inclusion–boundary interaction becomes significant.

The purpose of this chapter is to have a clearer picture of the inclusion–boundary interaction to making a reasonable extrapolation from the dipole approximation of a small inclusion inside a conductor to its signature when it is brought close to the boundary of the conductor.

This problem is of practical interest in many areas such as surface defect detection in the semiconductor industry and optical particle sizing. Many theoretical models have been developed, and many experimental measurements have been carried out in recent years, see [312].

We shall rigorously establish a new approximation that is valid when the inclusion is small and at a distance comparable with its diameter apart from the boundary of the conductor. Since the formula carries information about the location, the conductivity, and the volume of the inclusion, it can be efficiently exploited for imaging inclusions close to the boundary of the background conductor. In fact, since the boundary perturbation amplitude has a relative peak near the inclusion, the peak clearly manifests the presence of the inclusion. However, it is not trivial how this peak depends on the inclusion shape and its depth.

The outline of the chapter is as follows. The first section sets out optimal gradient estimates for solutions to the isotropic conductivity problem in the following two situations: when two circular conductivity inclusions are very close but not touching and when a circular inclusion is very close to the boundary of the domain where the inclusion is contained. These estimates imply that the gradient of the voltage potential stays bounded, and an asymptotic expansion of the solution can be derived when a small inclusion is brought close to the boundary of the conductor. The second section establishes an asymptotic expansion of the steady-state voltage potentials in the presence of a diametrically small conductivity inclusion that is nearly touching the boundary. The asymptotic formula extends those already derived in Chapter 5 for a small inclusion far away from the boundary of the background conductor and is expected to lead to very effective algorithms, which are aimed at determining the location and certain properties of the shape of a small inclusion that is nearly touching the boundary based on boundary measurements. Viability of the asymptotic formula is documented by a numerical example. Throughout this chapter, we follow the notation of Chapter 2.

6.1 Optimal Gradient Estimates

Suppose that Ω, which is a disk of radius ρ, contains an inclusion B, which is a disk of radius r. Suppose that the conductivity of Ω is 1 and that of B is $k \neq 1$. For a given $g \in C^\alpha(\partial\Omega)$, $\alpha > 0$, let u be the solution to the transmission problem (2.61).

The first question we consider is whether ∇u can be arbitrarily large as the inclusion B get closer to the boundary $\partial\Omega$. We are especially interested in the case of extreme conductivities $k = +\infty$ (a perfect conductor) or $k = 0$ (an insulated inclusion). This difficult question arises in the study of composite media; see [51].

If $0 < C_1 < k < C_2 < +\infty$ for some constants C_1 and C_2, a uniform upper bound on the gradient of u in a much more general setting has been derived by Li and Vogelius in [218]. Here we provide very precise estimates for $\|\nabla u\|_{L^\infty(\Omega)}$ for arbitrary conductivities.

According to Theorem 4.20, the solution u to (2.61) for a given Neumann data g can be represented as

$$u(x) = \mathcal{D}_\Omega(f)(x) - \mathcal{S}_\Omega(g)(x) + \mathcal{S}_B(\phi)(x), \quad x \in \Omega, \quad f := u\big|_{\partial\Omega}, \quad (6.1)$$

where $\phi \in L_0^2(\partial B)$ satisfies the integral equation

$$(\lambda I - \mathcal{K}_B^*)\phi = \frac{\partial}{\partial\nu}\left(\mathcal{D}_\Omega(f) - \mathcal{S}_\Omega(g)\right) \quad \text{on } \partial B,$$

with $\lambda = (k+1)/(2(k-1))$. Since B is a disk, it follows from (2.21) that $\mathcal{K}_B^*\phi = 0$ on ∂B and hence

$$\lambda\phi = \frac{\partial}{\partial\nu}\left(\mathcal{D}_\Omega(f) - \mathcal{S}_\Omega(g)\right) \quad \text{on } \partial B. \quad (6.2)$$

On the other hand, since $f = u|_{\partial\Omega}$, $\mathcal{D}_\Omega(f)|_- = (\frac{1}{2}I + \mathcal{K}_\Omega)f$ and Ω is a disk, we have

$$\frac{1}{2}f = -\mathcal{S}_\Omega(g) + \mathcal{S}_B(\phi) \quad \text{on } \partial\Omega . \tag{6.3}$$

It then follows from (6.2) and (6.3) that f and ϕ are the solutions of the following system of integral equations:

$$\begin{cases} \dfrac{1}{2}f - \mathcal{S}_B\phi = \mathcal{S}_\Omega g \quad \text{on } \partial\Omega , \\[2ex] \lambda\phi + \dfrac{\partial(\mathcal{D}_\Omega f)}{\partial\nu_B} = -\dfrac{\partial(\mathcal{S}_\Omega g)}{\partial\nu_B} \quad \text{on } \partial B . \end{cases}$$

Let x_1 be the point on ∂B closest to $\partial\Omega$ and x_2 be the point on $\partial\Omega$ closest to ∂B, and let R_B and R_Ω be reflections with respect to ∂B and $\partial\Omega$, respectively. One can easily see that $R_B R_\Omega$ and $R_\Omega R_B$ have unique fixed points in $\mathbb{R}^2 \setminus \overline{\Omega}$ and in B, respectively. Let us denote them by p_1 and p_2. Let J_1 be the line segment between p_1 and x_1 and J_2 that between p_2 and x_2.

The functions f and ϕ are given by explicit series analogous to those in Corollary 4.27, which converge absolutely and uniformly. Precise estimates of these explicit series lead us to the following theorem [31].

Theorem 6.1 *Let*

$$\epsilon := dist(B, \partial\Omega), \quad r^* := \sqrt{\frac{\rho - r}{\rho r}}, \quad \sigma := \frac{k-1}{k+1}\left(= \frac{1}{2\lambda}\right) ,$$

and let u be the solution to (2.61).

(i) *If $k < 1$, then a constant C_1 exists independent of k, r, ϵ, and g such that for ϵ small enough,*

$$\frac{C_1 \displaystyle\inf_{x \in J_1} |\langle \nabla\mathcal{S}_\Omega(g)(x), T_B(x_1)\rangle|}{1 + \sigma + 4r^*\sqrt{\epsilon}} \leq |\nabla u|_+(x_1)| ,$$

and

$$\frac{C_1 \displaystyle\inf_{x \in J_2} |\langle \nabla\mathcal{S}_\Omega(g)(x), T_\Omega(x_2)\rangle|}{1 + \sigma + 4r^*\sqrt{\epsilon}} \leq |\nabla u|_-(x_2)| .$$

Here T_B and T_Ω denote the positively oriented unit tangent vector fields on ∂B and $\partial\Omega$, respectively.

(ii) *For any $k \neq 1$, a constant C_2 exists independent of k, r, and ϵ such that for ϵ small enough,*

$$\|\nabla u\|_{L^\infty(\Omega)} \leq \frac{C_2\|g\|_{C^\alpha(\partial\Omega)}}{1 - |\sigma| + r^*\sqrt{\epsilon}} .$$

If z is the center of Ω and if $g(x) := a \cdot \nu_x$ on $\partial\Omega$ for some constant vector a, then $\mathcal{S}_\Omega(g) = -\frac{1}{2}a \cdot x + \text{constant}$, and hence we can achieve

$$\langle \nabla \mathcal{S}_\Omega(g)(x), T_B(x_1) \rangle \neq 0 \text{ and } \langle \nabla \mathcal{S}_\Omega(f)(x), T_\Omega(x_2) \rangle \neq 0 \quad \text{for any } x ,$$

by choosing a appropriately.

Theorem 6.1 shows that, in the case of the Neumann problem, if the inclusion is insulated ($k = 0$ and hence $\sigma = -1$), then

$$\frac{C_1'}{r^* \sqrt{\epsilon}} \leq \|\nabla u\|_{L^\infty(\Omega)} \leq \frac{C_2'}{r^* \sqrt{\epsilon}} ,$$

for some constants C_1' and C_2'. Thus ∇u blows up at the rate of $1/\sqrt{\epsilon}$ as long as the magnitude of r is much larger than that of ϵ. It also shows that the gradient blows up at the points x_1 and x_2. If r is of the same order as ϵ, then $r^* \approx 1/\sqrt{\epsilon}$ and hence ∇u does not blow up. In fact, it stays bounded and an asymptotic expansion of the solution as $\epsilon \to 0$ will be derived in the next section.

Note that for the Dirichlet problem the situation is reversed: ∇u blows up for a perfect conductor ($k = +\infty$); see [31].

Another interesting situation is when two circular conductivity inclusions are very close but not touching. To describe this second situation, let B_1 and B_2 be two circular inclusions contained in a matrix, which we assume to be the free space $\mathbb{R}^2$. For $s = 1, 2$, we suppose that the conductivity k_s of the inclusion B_s is a constant different from the constant conductivity of the matrix, which is assumed to be 1 for convenience. The conductivity k_s of the inclusion may be 0 or $+\infty$. The conductivity problem considered in this case is the following transmission problem for a given entire harmonic function H:

$$\begin{cases} \nabla \cdot \left(1 + \sum_{s=1,2} (k_s - 1)\chi(B_s)\right) \nabla u = 0 \quad \text{in } \mathbb{R}^2 , \\ u(x) - H(x) = O(|x|^{-1}) \quad \text{as } |x| \to +\infty . \end{cases} \tag{6.4}$$

The gradient ∇u of the solution u to (6.4) represents the perturbation of the field ∇H in the presence of inclusions B_1 and B_2. We are interested in the behavior of the gradient of the solution to the equation (6.4) as the distance between B_1 and B_2 goes to zero. Optimal bounds on ∇u can be proved. To state them, let us recall the notation used in Sect. 4.11. For $s = 1, 2$, let $B_s = B_{r_s}(z_s)$, the disk centered at z_s and of radius r_s. Let R_s, $s = 1, 2$, be the reflection with respect to ∂B_s; i.e.,

$$R_s(x) := \frac{r_s^2(x - z_s)}{|x - z_s|^2} + z_s, \quad s = 1, 2 .$$

It is easy to see that the combined reflections $R_1 R_2$ and $R_2 R_1$ have unique fixed points. Let I be the line segment between these two fixed points. Let x_s, $s = 1, 2$, be the point on ∂B_s closest to the other disk.

We also let

$$r_{\min} := \min(r_1, r_2), \quad r_{\max} := \max(r_1, r_2), \quad r_* := \sqrt{(2r_1 r_2)/(r_1 + r_2)} \,.$$

Finally let

$$\lambda_s := \frac{k_s + 1}{2(k_s - 1)} \,, \quad s = 1, 2, \quad \text{and} \quad \tau := \frac{1}{4\lambda_1 \lambda_2} \,.$$

Based on Corollary 4.27, the following result for the behavior of the gradient is obtained in [32, 31].

Theorem 6.2 *Let* $\epsilon := \mathrm{dist}(B_1, B_2)$, *and let* $\nu^{(s)}$ *and* $T^{(s)}$, $s = 1, 2$, *be the unit normal and tangential vector fields to* ∂B_s, *respectively. Let* u *be the solution of (6.4).*

(i) *If* ϵ *is sufficiently small, there is a constant* C_1 *independent of* k_1, k_2, r_1, r_2, *and* ϵ *such that*

$$\frac{C_1 \inf\limits_{x \in I} |\langle \nabla H(x), \nu^{(s)}(x_s) \rangle|}{1 - \tau + (r_*/r_{\min})\sqrt{\epsilon}} \leq |\nabla u|_+(x_s)|, \quad s = 1, 2\,, \tag{6.5}$$

provided that k_1, $k_2 > 1$, *and*

$$\frac{C_1 \inf\limits_{x \in I} |\langle \nabla H(x), T^{(s)}(x_s) \rangle|}{1 - \tau + (r_*/r_{\min})\sqrt{\epsilon}} \leq |\nabla u|_+(x_s)|, \quad s = 1, 2\,, \tag{6.6}$$

provided that k_1, $k_2 < 1$.

(ii) *Let* Ω *be a bounded set containing* B_1 *and* B_2. *Then there is a constant* C_2 *independent of* k_1, k_2, r_1, r_2, ϵ, *and* Ω *such that*

$$\|\nabla u\|_{L^\infty(\Omega)} \leq \frac{C_2 \|\nabla H\|_{L^\infty(\Omega)}}{1 - |\tau| + (r_*/r_{\max})\sqrt{\epsilon}} \,. \tag{6.7}$$

Note that, if $H(x) = a \cdot x$ for some constant vector a, which is the most interesting case, then

$$\langle \nabla H(x), \nu^{(s)}(x_s) \rangle = \langle a, \nu^{(s)}(x_s) \rangle \,,$$

and hence it does not vanish if we choose a appropriately.

Theorem 6.2 quantifies the behavior of ∇u in terms of the conductivities of the inclusions, their radii, and the distance between them. For example, if k_1 and k_2 degenerate to $+\infty$ or zero, then $\tau = 1$ and hence (6.5) and (6.7) read as follows:

$$\frac{C_1'}{(r_*/r_{\min})\sqrt{\epsilon}} \leq |\nabla u(x_s)|, \quad s = 1, 2, \quad \|\nabla u\|_{L^\infty(\Omega)} \leq \frac{C_2'}{(r_*/r_{\max})\sqrt{\epsilon}} \,, \tag{6.8}$$

for some constants C_1' and C_2', which shows that ∇u blows up at the rate of $1/\sqrt{\epsilon}$ as the inclusions get closer. It further shows that the gradient blows up at x_s which is the point on ∂B_s closest to the other disk.

The proofs of the above optimal estimates make use of quite explicit but non-trivial expansion formulae, which are analogous to those derived in Corollary 4.27. They are achieved by using a significantly different method from [69], [218], and [76].

6.2 Asymptotic Expansions

Suppose that $D = \epsilon B + z$, where $z \in \Omega$ is such that $\mathrm{dist}(z, \partial\Omega) = \delta\epsilon$. Here B is a bounded domain in $\mathbb{R}^2$ containing the origin with a connected $\mathcal{C}^2$-boundary and the constant $\delta > \max_{x \in \partial B} |x|$. Let u denote the voltage potential in the presence of the conductivity inclusion D, that is, the solution to (2.61). Recall that the background voltage potential U is the unique solution to (2.62).

In this case, a more complicated asymptotic formula first established in [13] should be used instead of (5.20). The dipole-type expansion (5.20) is valid only when the potential u within the inclusion D is nearly constant. On decreasing $\mathrm{dist}(D, \partial\Omega)$, this assumption begins to fail because the interaction between D and $\partial\Omega$ becomes significant. The approximation in [13], which is valid when the inclusion is at a distance comparable with its diameter apart from the boundary, provides some essential insight for understanding this interaction. Moreover, since it carries information about the location, the conductivity, and the volume of the inclusion, it can be efficiently exploited for imaging near-boundary inclusions.

6.2.1 Main Results

To mathematically set our expansion in this case, let z_0 be the normal projection of z onto $\partial\Omega$. With the notation of Chapter 4, the following asymptotic formula holds.

Theorem 6.3 *Suppose that $g \in \mathcal{C}^1(\partial\Omega)$ and Ω is of class $\mathcal{C}^2$. Then the following asymptotic expansion holds uniformly on $\partial\Omega$:*

$$(u - U)(x) = -\epsilon \nabla U(z_0) \cdot \left(\int_{\partial B} N(x, z + \epsilon y)(\lambda I - \mathcal{K}_B^*)^{-1}(\nu)\, d\sigma(y) \right)$$
$$+ O(\epsilon^{3/2})\,.$$

Moreover, if $|x - z_0| \gg O(\epsilon)$, then

$$(u - U)(x) = -\epsilon^2 \nabla U(z_0) \cdot M \nabla N(x, z_0)$$
$$+ O(\epsilon^{5/2})\,,$$

where $M = \int_{\partial B} y(\lambda I - \mathcal{K}_B^*)^{-1}(\nu)\, d\sigma(y)$ is the first-order polarization tensor.

Since $\int_{\partial B} N(x, z+\epsilon y)(\lambda I - \mathcal{K}_B^*)^{-1}(\nu)\, d\sigma(y) = O(1)$ for x near z_0, Theorem 6.3 shows that $(u - U)(x) = O(\epsilon)$ near z_0, whereas $(u - U)(x) = O(\epsilon^2)$ for x far away from z_0. Thus, $u - U$ has a relative peak near z_0.

6.2.2 Proof of Theorem 6.3

Since
$$\nabla H = \nabla U + \nabla \mathcal{D}_\Omega(u - U) \quad \text{in } \Omega\,,$$

we obtain from (2.73) that for $x \in \partial\Omega$,

$$(u - U)(x) + \int_{\partial D} N(x, y)(\lambda I - \mathcal{K}_D^*)^{-1}(\nu \cdot \nabla \mathcal{D}_\Omega(u - U))(y)\, d\sigma(y)$$
$$= -\int_{\partial D} N(x, y)(\lambda I - \mathcal{K}_D^*)^{-1}(\nu \cdot \nabla U)(y)\, d\sigma(y)\,. \tag{6.9}$$

This is a representation formula for the perturbations $u - U$ on $\partial\Omega$.

For $v \in L^\infty(\partial\Omega)$, let

$$Tv(x) := \int_{\partial D} N(x, y)(\lambda I - \mathcal{K}_D^*)^{-1}(\nu \cdot \nabla \mathcal{D}_\Omega v)(y)\, d\sigma(y), \quad x \in \partial\Omega\,. \tag{6.10}$$

Since $(\lambda I - \mathcal{K}_D^*)^{-1}(\nu \cdot \nabla \mathcal{D}_\Omega v)$ has mean value zero, we get

$$Tv(x) = \int_{\partial D} \frac{N(x, y) - N(x, z)}{\epsilon}(\lambda I - \mathcal{K}_D^*)^{-1}(\epsilon\nu \cdot \nabla \mathcal{D}_\Omega v)(y)\, d\sigma(y)\,. \tag{6.11}$$

We view (6.9) as an integral equation

$$(I + T)(u - U) = F \quad \text{on } \partial\Omega\,, \tag{6.12}$$

where the definition of F is obvious. We now investigate the invertibility of $I + T$ in $\mathcal{C}^0(\partial\Omega)$.

Lemma 6.4 *Suppose that $\partial\Omega$ is of class $\mathcal{C}^2$. Then there is a constant C independent of ϵ such that*

$$\|Tv\|_{L^\infty(\partial\Omega)} \leq C\|v\|_{L^\infty(\partial\Omega)}\,, \tag{6.13}$$

for any $v \in L^\infty(\partial\Omega)$.

Proof. Let $v \in L^\infty(\partial\Omega)$. Using (6.11), we get

$$|Tv(x)| \leq \frac{1}{\epsilon}\left(\int_{\partial D} |N(x, y) - N(x, z)|^p\, d\sigma(y)\right)^{1/p}$$
$$\times \|(\lambda I - \mathcal{K}_D^*)^{-1}(\epsilon\nu \cdot \nabla \mathcal{D}_\Omega v)\|_{L^q(\partial D)}\,,$$

where $1/p + 1/q = 1$, $p, q > 1$. We observe that for each $y \in \partial D$

$$|\nabla \mathcal{D}_\Omega v(y)| \leq C \frac{1}{\operatorname{dist}(y, \partial\Omega)} \|v\|_{L^\infty(\partial\Omega)} \,,$$

and hence

$$\|(\lambda I - \mathcal{K}_D^*)^{-1}(\epsilon \nu \cdot \nabla \mathcal{D}_\Omega v)\|_{L^q(\partial D)} \leq \|\epsilon \nu \cdot \nabla \mathcal{D}_\Omega v\|_{L^q(\partial D)}$$
$$\leq C \epsilon^{1/q} \|v\|_{L^\infty(\partial\Omega)} \,. \tag{6.14}$$

On the other hand, since Ω is a $\mathcal{C}^2$ domain, $-(1/2)\, I + \mathcal{K}_\Omega$ is invertible on $L^\infty(\partial\Omega)$, and hence on $L^q(\partial\Omega)$ for all $2 \leq q \leq +\infty$. Therefore we get from (2.53)

$$\frac{1}{\epsilon} \sup_{x \in \partial\Omega} \left(\int_{\partial D} |N(x,y) - N(x,z)|^p \, d\sigma(y) \right)^{1/p}$$
$$\leq \frac{C}{\epsilon} \sup_{x \in \partial\Omega} \left(\int_{\partial D} \left| \left(-\frac{1}{2} I + \mathcal{K}_\Omega \right) (N(\cdot, y) - N(\cdot, z))(x) \right|^p \, d\sigma(y) \right)^{1/p}$$
$$\leq \frac{C}{\epsilon} \sup_{x \in \partial\Omega} \left(\int_{\partial D} |\Gamma(x - y) - \Gamma(x - z)|^p \, d\sigma(y) \right)^{1/p} \,.$$

Thus we get

$$\frac{1}{\epsilon} \sup_{x \in \partial\Omega} \left(\int_{\partial D} |N(x,y) - N(x,z)|^p \, d\sigma(y) \right)^{1/p}$$
$$\leq \frac{C}{\epsilon} \sup_{x \in \partial\Omega} \left(\int_{\partial D} |y - z|^p |\nabla_y \Gamma(x - y^*)|^p \, d\sigma(y) \right)^{1/p} \leq C \epsilon^{-1 + 1/p} \,,$$

where y^* denotes some point between y and z. This together with (6.14) yields (6.13). $\qquad\square$

Lemma 6.5 *If $\partial\Omega$ is of class $\mathcal{C}^2$, then the operator $I + T$ is invertible on $\mathcal{C}^0(\partial\Omega)$.*

Proof. Since $\partial\Omega$ is of class $\mathcal{C}^2$, T is a compact operator on $\mathcal{C}^0(\partial\Omega)$. Thus by Fredholm's alternative it suffices to prove the injectivity of $I + T$.

Suppose that $(I + T)v = 0$ on $\partial\Omega$. Then

$$\left(-\frac{1}{2} I + \mathcal{K}_\Omega \right) v + \left(-\frac{1}{2} I + \mathcal{K}_\Omega \right) T v = 0 \quad \text{on } \partial\Omega \,.$$

It then follows from (2.53) and (2.28) that

$$-v(x) + \mathcal{D}_\Omega v(x) \Big|_- + \int_{\partial D} \Gamma(x-y)(\lambda I - \mathcal{K}_D^*)^{-1}(\nu \cdot \nabla \mathcal{D}_\Omega v)(y) \, d\sigma(y) = 0, \quad x \in \partial\Omega \,.$$

Let $H := \mathcal{D}_\Omega v$ in Ω. Then v on $\partial\Omega$ can be extended to Ω by

$$v(x) = H(x) + \mathcal{S}_D(\lambda I - \mathcal{K}_D^*)^{-1}(\nu \cdot \nabla H)(x), \quad x \in \Omega .$$

Hence v is a solution of the transmission problem $\nabla \cdot (1 + (k - 1)\chi_D)\nabla v = 0$. Then by (2.63) and the uniqueness of the representation (2.64), we get

$$H(x) = \mathcal{D}_\Omega(v)(x) - \mathcal{S}_\Omega(\frac{\partial v}{\partial \nu})(x), \quad x \in \Omega ,$$

which yields

$$\mathcal{S}_\Omega(\frac{\partial v}{\partial \nu})(x) = 0, \quad x \in \Omega .$$

Thus we get $\partial v / \partial \nu = 0$ on $\partial\Omega$ and hence $v = $ constant in Ω. Since $\int_{\partial\Omega} v\, d\sigma = -\int_{\partial\Omega} Tv\, d\sigma = 0$, we conclude that $v \equiv 0$. This completes the proof. $\square$

So far we have proved that

$$u(x) - U(x) = (I + T)^{-1}(F)(x), \quad x \in \partial\Omega . \tag{6.15}$$

To derive an asymptotic expansion of $u - U$ on $\partial\Omega$, we now investigate the asymptotic behavior of the operator T as $\epsilon \to 0$.

Lemma 6.6 *Suppose that $\partial\Omega$ is of class $\mathcal{C}^2$ and $D = \epsilon B + z$ as before. Let z_0 be the normal projection of z onto $\partial\Omega$. For $f \in \mathcal{C}^0(\partial\Omega)$, let*

$$s_f(\epsilon) := \sup_{|x - z_0| \leq \epsilon} |f(x) - f(z_0)| . \tag{6.16}$$

Then,

$$\sup_{x \in \partial D} |\epsilon \nabla \mathcal{D}_\Omega(f)(x)| \leq C(s_f(\sqrt{\epsilon}) + \sqrt{\epsilon})\|f\|_{L^\infty(\partial\Omega)} , \tag{6.17}$$

where C is independent of ϵ and f.

Proof. Without loss of generality we may assume that $\|f\|_{L^\infty(\partial\Omega)} = 1$. Taking the gradient of $\mathcal{D}_\Omega(f)$, we get

$$\begin{aligned}
\frac{\partial \mathcal{D}_\Omega(f)}{\partial x_1}(x) &= \frac{1}{2\pi} \int_{\partial\Omega} \Big[\frac{(x_1 - y_1)^2 - (x_2 - y_2)^2}{|x - y|^4}\nu_1(y) \\
&\quad + \frac{2(x_1 - y_1)(x_2 - y_2)}{|x - y|^4}\nu_2(y)\Big] f(y)d\sigma(y) \\
\frac{\partial \mathcal{D}_\Omega(f)}{\partial x_2}(x) &= \frac{1}{2\pi} \int_{\partial\Omega} \Big[\frac{(x_2 - y_2)^2 - (x_1 - y_1)^2}{|x - y|^4}\nu_2(y) \\
&\quad + \frac{2(x_1 - y_1)(x_2 - y_2)}{|x - y|^4}\nu_1(y)\Big] f(y)d\sigma(y) ,
\end{aligned}$$

for $x \in \partial D$. Thus (6.17) is a direct consequence of the following lemma.

Lemma 6.7 *Define*

$$w(x) := \frac{\epsilon}{2(z_0 - x) \cdot \nu_{z_0}}, \qquad x \in \partial D , \tag{6.18}$$

where ν_{z_0} is the outward normal to $\partial \Omega$ at z_0. Let $h \in C^0(\partial \Omega)$. Then for each $x \in \partial D$

$$\left| \frac{1}{\pi} \int_{\partial \Omega} \frac{\epsilon(x_j - y_j)^2}{|x-y|^4} h(y) d\sigma(y) - w(x)h(z_0) \right| \leq C(s_h(\sqrt{\epsilon}) + (\sqrt{\epsilon}))\|h\|_{L^\infty(\partial\Omega)} , \tag{6.19}$$

$j = 1, 2,$

$$\left| \frac{1}{\pi} \int_{\partial \Omega} \frac{\epsilon(x_1 - y_1)(x_2 - y_2)}{|x-y|^2} h(y) d\sigma(y) \right| \leq C(s_h(\sqrt{\epsilon}) + (\sqrt{\epsilon}))\|h\|_{L^\infty(\partial\Omega)} , \tag{6.20}$$

as $\epsilon \to 0$.

Proof. By rotation and translation if necessary, we may assume that $z_0 = 0$ and $\nu_{z_0} = (0, -1)$ so that $z = (0, \delta\epsilon)$. Then there is $\eta_0 > 0$ such that

$$\Omega \cap C_{\eta_0}(0) = \left\{ (x', x_d) \ : \ x_d > \varphi(x') \right\} \cap C_{\eta_0}(0) ,$$

where $C_{\eta_0}(0)$ is the cube centered at 0 with side length $2\eta_0$ and φ is a C^2 function near 0 such that $\varphi(0) = 0$ and $\nabla\varphi(0) = 0$. Choose $\eta = \sqrt{\epsilon} < \eta_0$, and let

$$\frac{1}{\pi} \int_{\partial \Omega} \frac{\epsilon(x_j - y_j)^2}{|x-y|^4} h(y) d\sigma(y) = \frac{1}{\pi} \int_{\partial\Omega \cap C_\eta(0)} + \frac{1}{\pi} \int_{\partial\Omega \setminus \overline{C}_\eta(0)} := I_1(x) + I_2(x) .$$

It is easy to see that

$$|I_2(x)| \leq C\frac{\epsilon}{\eta}\|h\|_{L^\infty(\partial\Omega)}, \qquad x \in \partial D . \tag{6.21}$$

Suppose $j = 1$. For $x \in \partial D$, write $x = z + \epsilon(v_1, v_2)$, where $|(v_1, v_2)| \leq C < \delta$. Then $I_1(x)$ takes the form

$$\epsilon I_1(x) = \frac{1}{\pi} \int_{|y'|\leq\delta} \frac{\epsilon|y' - \epsilon v_1|^2}{[|y' - \epsilon v_1|^2 + |\delta\epsilon + \epsilon v_2 - \varphi(y')|^2]^2} g(y') \, dy' ,$$

where $g(y') := h(\varphi(y'))\sqrt{1 + |\nabla\varphi(y')|^2}$. Since $|\varphi(y')| \leq C|y'|^2$ for some C, we get

$$\frac{1}{[|y' - \epsilon v_1|^2 + |\delta\epsilon + \epsilon v_2 - \varphi(y')|^2]^2}$$

$$= \frac{1}{(|y' - \epsilon v_1|^2 + (\delta\epsilon + \epsilon v_2)^2)^2 \left[1 + \frac{\varphi(y')^2 - 2(\delta\epsilon + \epsilon v_2)\varphi(y')}{|y' - \epsilon v_1|^2 + (\delta\epsilon + \epsilon v_2)^2}\right]^2}$$

$$= \frac{1}{[|y' - \epsilon v_1|^2 + (\delta\epsilon + \epsilon v_2)^2]^2} \left[1 + O(|y'|^2 + \epsilon)\right] .$$

It then follows that

$$\epsilon I_1(x) = \frac{1}{\pi} \int_{|y'| \leq \sqrt{\epsilon}} \frac{\epsilon |y' - \epsilon v_1|^2}{[|y' - \epsilon v_1|^2 + \epsilon^2(\delta + v_2)^2]^2} g(y') \, dy' + O(\epsilon) .$$

After a change of variables $y' - \epsilon v_1 = \epsilon(\delta + v_2)t$, $I_1(x)$ takes the form

$$\epsilon I_1(x) = \frac{1}{\delta + v_2} \frac{1}{\pi} \int_{|\epsilon(\delta + v_2)t + \epsilon v_1| \leq \sqrt{\epsilon}} \frac{t^2}{(|t|^2 + 1)^2} g(\epsilon(\delta + v_2)t + \epsilon v_1) \, dt + O(\epsilon) .$$

Since

$$\int_{-\infty}^{\infty} \frac{t^2}{(|t|^2 + 1)^2} dt = \frac{\pi}{2} ,$$

it is now easy to show that

$$\left| \epsilon I_1(x) - \frac{1}{2(\delta + v_2)} g(0) \right| \leq C \sup_{|t| \leq \eta} |g(t) - g(0)| . \tag{6.22}$$

Observe that

$$\frac{1}{2(\delta + v_2)} = \frac{\epsilon}{2(z_0 - x) \cdot \nu_{z_0}} = w(x)$$

in the original coordinates. By (6.21) and (6.22) with $\eta = \sqrt{\epsilon}$, we get (6.19) when $j = 1$.

Estimate (6.19) when $j = 2$ can proved in exactly the same way using the fact that $\int_{-\infty}^{\infty} 1/(|t|^2 + 1)^2 \, dt = \pi/2$. Estimate (6.20) can also be proved in the exactly same way using the identity $\int_{-\infty}^{\infty} t/(|t|^2 + 1)^2 \, dt = 0$. $\square$

Lemma 6.6 shows that for $f \in \mathcal{C}^0(\partial\Omega)$

$$\begin{aligned}
\|Tf\|_{L^\infty(\partial\Omega)} &\leq C\epsilon^{-1+1/p} \|\epsilon\nabla\mathcal{D}_\Omega f\|_{L^q(\partial D)} \\
&\leq C(s_f(\sqrt{\epsilon}) + \sqrt{\epsilon})\|f\|_{L^\infty(\partial\Omega)} ,
\end{aligned} \tag{6.23}$$

where $1/p + 1/q = 1$, $p, q > 1$.

Moreover, one can show in a similar way that, if x is far away from z_0, then

$$|Tf(x)| \leq C\epsilon(s_f(\sqrt{\epsilon}) + \sqrt{\epsilon})\|f\|_{L^\infty(\partial\Omega)} . \tag{6.24}$$

We now investigate the asymptotic behavior of F as $\epsilon \to 0$. We suppose from now on that $g \in \mathcal{C}^1(\partial\Omega)$ and Ω is of class $\mathcal{C}^2$ so that $U \in \mathcal{C}^2(\overline{\Omega})$. We first observe that

$$\|F\|_{L^\infty(\partial\Omega)} \le C\epsilon\|\nabla U\|_{L^\infty(\partial D)} \ .$$

This can be proved in a similar way as before.

Since $U \in \mathcal{C}^2(\overline{\Omega})$,

$$\nabla U|_{\partial D} = \nabla U(z_0) + O(\epsilon) \ ,$$

which gives after a change of variables

$$F(x) = -\epsilon\nabla U(z_0)\cdot\left(\int_{\partial B} N(x, z + \epsilon y)(\lambda I - \mathcal{K}_B^*)^{-1}(\nu)\,d\sigma(y)\right) + O(\epsilon^2) \ , \quad (6.25)$$

if x is close to z_0. Moreover, if x is far away from z_0 or $|x - z_0| \gg O(\epsilon)$, then

$$\int_{\partial B} N(x, z + \epsilon y)(\lambda I - \mathcal{K}_B^*)^{-1}(\nu)\,d\sigma(y)$$
$$= \int_{\partial B} [N(x, z + \epsilon y) - N(x, z)](\lambda I - \mathcal{K}_B^*)^{-1}(\nu)\,d\sigma(y)$$
$$= \epsilon\nabla N(x, z)M + O(\epsilon^2)$$
$$= \epsilon\nabla N(x, z_0)M + O(\epsilon^2) \ ,$$

where $M = \int_{\partial B} y(\lambda I - \mathcal{K}_B^*)^{-1}(\nu)\,d\sigma(y)$ is the polarization tensor. Thus, in this case, we obtain

$$F(x) = -\epsilon^2\nabla U(z_0) \cdot M\nabla N(x, z_0) + O(\epsilon^3) \quad \text{if } |x - z_0| \gg O(\epsilon) \ . \quad (6.26)$$

We claim that

$$s_F(\sqrt{\epsilon}) = O(\sqrt{\epsilon}) \ . \quad (6.27)$$

In fact, since Ω is a $\mathcal{C}^2$ domain, $|\nabla_x N(x, y)| \le C|x - y|^{-1}$ for $x \in \partial\Omega$ and $y \in \Omega$. Therefore,

$$|F(x) - F(z_0)| \le \int_{\partial D} |N(z_0, y) - N(x, y)|\left|(\lambda I - \mathcal{K}_D^*)^{-1}(\nu \cdot \nabla U)(y)\right|\,d\sigma(y)$$
$$\le \left(\int_{\partial D} |N(z_0, y) - N(x, y)|^p\,d\sigma(y)\right)^{1/p}\|(\lambda I - \mathcal{K}_D^*)^{-1}(\nu \cdot \nabla U)\|_{L^q(\partial D)}$$
$$\le C\epsilon^{-1+1/p}\|\nabla U\|_{L^q(\partial D)}$$
$$\le C\|\nabla U\|_{L^\infty(\partial D)}|x - z_0| \ .$$

We then obtain from (6.23) and (6.24) that

$$F(x) = \begin{cases} O(\epsilon^{3/2}) & \text{if } |x - z_0| = O(\epsilon) \ , \\ O(\epsilon^{5/2}) & \text{if } |x - z_0| \gg O(\epsilon) \ . \end{cases} \quad (6.28)$$

Combining (6.15), (6.25), (6.26), and (6.28), we finally obtain Theorem 6.3.

6.2.3 A Numerical Example

Let us now document the viability of our results in Theorem 6.3 by numerical examples. Consider a unit disk in $\mathbb{R}^2$ with background conductivity 1 containing a single disk-shaped imperfection of small radius ϵ and conductivity k. The imperfection is centered at $z = (1 - \delta\epsilon, 0)$ on the axis $y = 0$ at a distance $(\delta - 1)\epsilon$ from the boundary where the constant $\delta > 1$. Let $z_0 = (1, 0)$.

Since

$$\int_{\partial D} \nu_y \, d\sigma(y) = 0 \text{ and } \int_{\partial\Omega} N(x, y) \, d\sigma(x) = 0, \text{ for } y \in \Omega \,,$$

then using property (2.21) we have

$$(\lambda I - \mathcal{K}_D^*)^{-1}(\nu)(y) = \frac{1}{\lambda}\nu_y, \forall \, y \in \partial\Omega$$

and

$$N(x, y) = -2\Gamma(x - y) \text{ modulo constants}, \forall \, x \in \partial\Omega, y \in \Omega \,.$$

See formula (2.58).

From Theorem 6.3 it then follows that

(i)
$$(u - U)(x) \simeq -\frac{\epsilon}{\pi\lambda}\nabla U(z_0)\cdot\left(\int_{\partial B} \ln|x - z - \epsilon y|\nu_y \, d\sigma(y)\right) \,,$$

for $x \in \partial\Omega$.

(ii)
$$(u - U)(x) \simeq -\frac{4\epsilon^2}{\lambda}\nabla U(z_0) \cdot \frac{x - z_0}{|x - z_0|^2}$$

if $|x - z_0| \gg O(\epsilon)$.

(iii)
$$(u - U)(z_0) \simeq -\frac{\epsilon}{\pi\lambda}\nabla U(z_0)\cdot\left(\int_{\partial B} \ln|\delta\nu_{z_0} - y|\nu_y \, d\sigma(y)\right) \,.$$

We now present numerical simulations from [13] using these asymptotic expansions. In these experiments, we examine numerically the transmission problem (2.61) in cylindrical coordinates (r, θ) with Neumann boundary data $g(1, \theta) = \cos\theta + \sin\theta$. The analytical solution of the homogeneous problem (2.62) is then given by $U(r, \theta) = r(\cos\theta + \sin\theta)$. Therefore, $(u - U)(z_0)$ can be approximated as follows:

$$(u - U)(z_0)$$
$$\simeq -\frac{\epsilon(k - 1)}{\pi(k + 1)}\int_0^{2\pi} \ln\left((\delta - \cos\theta)^2 + \sin^2\theta\right)(\cos\theta + \sin\theta) \, d\theta \,. \tag{6.29}$$

The first set of computations (see Figure 6.1) shows the dependence of the perturbation of the boundary conductivity $(u - U)|_{\partial\Omega}$ as a function of the distance variable δ for different values of ϵ and for a fixed imperfection conductivity of $k = 2$. The next three figures (Figure 6.2) show the results for a larger value of the conductivity, $k = 10$.

We observe that the minimal value (near $\theta = 0$) is constant, and this is clearer as the distance δ decreases. We can conclude that the perturbation amplitude is asymptotically first order in ϵ.

We can also plot these same results for $k = 10$ fixed as a function of δ with $\epsilon = 0.1$; see Figure 6.3 (a). We clearly observe the dependence of the amplitude and sharpness of the peak as a function of the distance.

The results of the above computations are summarized in Tables 6.1 and 6.2 where the maximal value of $|u - U|$ on the boundary $\partial\Omega$ is given as a function of the three parameters k, δ, and ϵ.

To check the influence of the angular position of the perturbation, a computation with $z = (0.5, 0.5)$ was performed. In Figure 6.4 we observe that the perturbation is indeed centered at $\theta = \pi/4$. We conclude that the angular position of the imperfection corresponds to the position of the perturbation peak.

Next, we compare in Table 6.3 the values of $(u - U)(z_0)$ computed from the asymptotic formula (6.29) with those computed by a direct simulation as in Tables 6.1 and 6.2.

Finally, we consider a homogeneous disk with a perfectly conducting circular imperfection. The boundary condition on the perimeter of the imperfection is homogeneous Dirichlet, $u = 0$. The results as a function of δ are shown in Figure 6.3 (b). As in the cases above,

(i) the peak of the perturbation corresponds to the angular position of the imperfection;

(ii) as the imperfection approaches the boundary, the peak's amplitude tends to a finite limit.

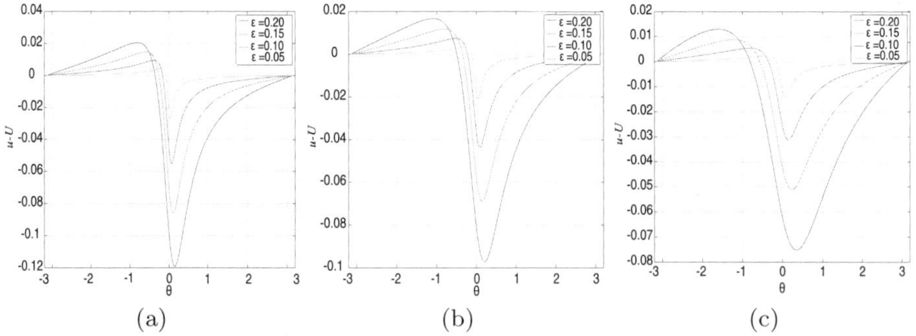

Fig. 6.1. $k = 2$ and ϵ varying with (a) $\delta = 1.5$, (b) $\delta = 2$, and (c) $\delta = 3$. Colors: blue $\epsilon = 0.2$; green $\epsilon = 0.15$; red $\epsilon = 0.1$; and cyan $\epsilon = 0.05$.

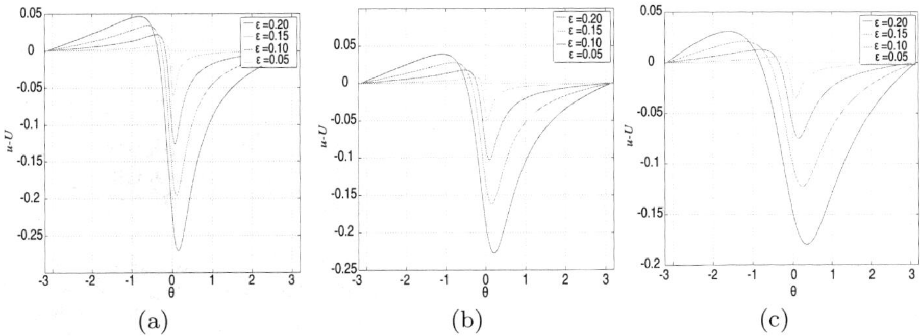

Fig. 6.2. $k = 10$ and ϵ varying with (a) $\delta = 1.5$, (b) $\delta = 2$, and (c) $\delta = 3$. Colors: blue $\epsilon = 0.2$; green $\epsilon = 0.15$; red $\epsilon = 0.1$; and cyan $\epsilon = 0.05$.

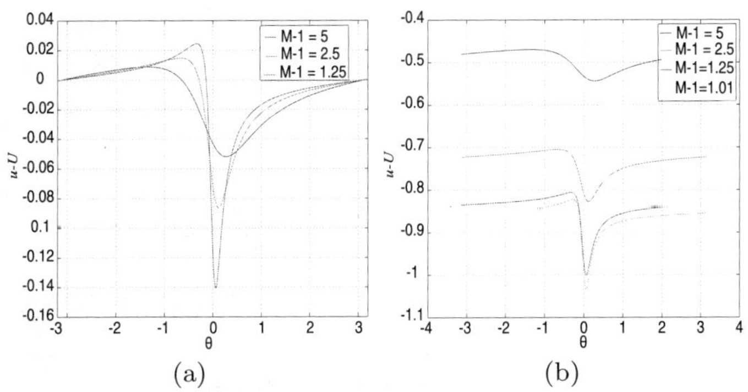

Fig. 6.3. $\epsilon = 0.1$ and varying distance δ with (a) $k = 10$, (b) $k = +\infty$. Colors: blue $\delta - 1 = 5$; green $\delta - 1 = 2.5$; red $\delta - 1 = 1.25$; and cyan $\delta - 1 = 1.01$.

	$\delta = 1.5$	$\delta = 2.0$	$\delta = 3.0$
$\epsilon = 0.20$	0.119 (**0.60**)	0.097 (**0.49**)	0.075 (**0.38**)
$\epsilon = 0.15$	0.086 (**0.57**)	0.069 (**0.46**)	0.051 (**0.34**)
$\epsilon = 0.10$	0.055 (**0.55**)	0.044 (**0.44**)	0.031 (**0.31**)
$\epsilon = 0.05$	0.027 (**0.54**)	0.021 (**0.42**)	0.014 (**0.28**)

Table 6.1. $\max_{\partial \Omega} |u - U|$ and $\max_{\partial \Omega} |u - U| / \epsilon$ (in bold) for $k = 2$.

	$\delta = 1.5$	$\delta = 2.0$	$\delta = 3.0$
$\epsilon = 0.20$	0.270 (**1.35**)	0.227 (**1.14**)	0.180 (**0.90**)
$\epsilon = 0.15$	0.196 (**1.30**)	0.162 (**1.07**)	0.123 (**0.82**)
$\epsilon = 0.10$	0.126 (**1.26**)	0.103 (**1.03**)	0.075 (**0.75**)
$\epsilon = 0.05$	0.061 (**1.22**)	0.049 (**1.00**)	0.035 (**0.69**)

Table 6.2. $\max_{\partial \Omega} |u - U|$ and $\max_{\partial \Omega} |u - U| / \epsilon$ (in bold) for $k = 10$.

	$\delta = 3.0$	$\delta = 4.0$	$\delta = 5.0$
$\epsilon = 0.05$	0.0118 (**0.236**)	0.0093 (**0.185**)	0.0076 (**0.152**)
	0.0116 (**0.232**)	0.0085 (**0.171**)	0.0068 (**0.135**)
$\epsilon = 0.02$	0.0046 (**0.228**)	0.0035 (**0.173**)	0.0028 (**0.140**)
	0.0046 (**0.232**)	0.0034 (**0.171**)	0.0027 (**0.135**)
$\epsilon = 0.01$	0.0023 (**0.230**)	0.0017 (**0.170**)	0.0014 (**0.135**)
	0.0023 (**0.232**)	0.0017 (**0.171**)	0.0014 (**0.135**)

Table 6.3. Comparison of $(u - U)(z_0)$ computed numerically (upper lines) and $(u - U)(z_0)$ computed from the asymptotic formula (6.29) (lower lines) for $k = 2$. Bold values are $(u - U)(z_0)/\epsilon$.

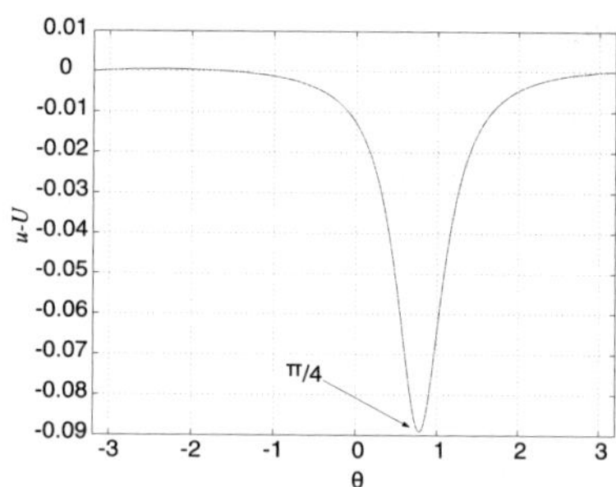

Fig. 6.4. Boundary perturbations for $z = (0.5, 0.5)$.

6.3 Further Results and Open Problems

One very interesting problem is to extend Theorem 6.2 to the three-dimensional case. We think that an estimate of the gradient of the voltage potential when two spheres of not necessary equal radii approaching one another can be obtained using a bispherical coordinate system that fits the given geometry. The bispherical coordinate system is a rotational system with two coordinate surfaces generated by rotating a complete circle and a circular arc, and a third one that describes a meridean plane. The surfaces of the two spheres are depicted from two different values of the coordinate variable describing the complete spheres, whereas the far field is limited to a small neighborhood of the origin within the parametric space of the second and third variables. See [239] and [86].

Impedance Imaging of Conductivity Inclusions

Introduction

Taking advantage of the smallness of the inclusions, Cedio-Fengya, Moskow, and Vogelius [84] used the leading-order term in the asymptotic expansion of u to find the locations z_s, $s = 1, \ldots, m$, of the inclusions and certain properties of the domains B_s, $s = 1, \ldots, m$ (relative size, orientation). The approach proposed in [84] is based on a least-squares algorithm. Ammari, Moskow, and Vogelius [42] also used this leading-order term to design a direct reconstruction method based on a variational formulation. The idea in [42] is to form the integral of the "measured boundary data" against harmonic test functions and choose the input current g so as to obtain an expression involving the inverse Fourier transform of distributions supported at the locations z_s, $s = 1, \ldots, m$. Applying a direct Fourier transform to this data then pins down the locations. This approach is similar to the method developed by Calderón [78] in his proof of uniqueness of the linearized conductivity problem and later by Sylvester and Uhlmann in their important work [285] on uniqueness in the three-dimensional inverse conductivity problem. The main disadvantage of this algorithm is the fact that it uses current sources of exponential type. This important practical issue, which we do not attempt to address, still needs to be resolved. A more realistic real-time algorithm for determining the locations of the inclusions has been developed by Kwon, Seo, and Yoon [208]. This fast, stable, and efficient algorithm is based on the observation of the pattern of a simple weighted combination of an input current g of the form $g = a \cdot \nu$ for some constant vector a and the corresponding output voltage. In all of these algorithms, the locations z_s, $s = 1, \ldots, m$, of the inclusions are determined with an error $O(\epsilon)$, and little about the domains B_s can be reconstructed. Furthermore, to practically implement these algorithms, one needs the magnitude of the inclusions to be very small.

In this chapter we apply the accurate asymptotic formula (5.2) for the purpose of identifying the location and certain properties of the shape of the conductivity inclusions. By improving the algorithm of Kwon, Seo, and

Yoon [208], we first design two real-time algorithms with good resolution and accuracy. We then describe the least-squares algorithm and the variational algorithm introduced in [42] and review the interesting approach proposed by Brühl, Hanke, and Vogelius [73]. Their method is in the spirit of the linear sampling method of Colton and Kirsch [100]. Furthermore, we present the simple pole method first developed in [52]. After that, we give Lipschitz-continuous dependence estimates for the reconstruction problem. These estimates, established by Friedman and Vogelius [132], bound the difference in the location and relative size of two sets of inclusions by the difference in the boundary voltage potentials corresponding to a fixed current distribution. We also provide upper and lower bounds on the moments of the unknown inclusions. We conclude the chapter by presenting efficient direct algorithms for reconstructing small anisotropic inclusions. We refer to [196, 200, 279, 283, 112, 284, 74, 71, 72, 156, 160, 161, 214, 227, 152, 70] for other numerical methods aimed at solving the inverse conductivity problem in different settings.

7.1 Preliminary

The methods of finding inclusions are based on the asymptotic expansion formula (5.4). However, the formula (5.4) is expressed in terms of the Neumann function $N(x, z)$, which depends on the domain Ω. There is a trick to overcoming this difficulty. For $g \in L_0^2(\partial\Omega)$, define the harmonic function $H[g](x)$, $x \in \mathbb{R}^d \setminus \overline{\Omega}$, by

$$H[g](x) := -\mathcal{S}_\Omega(g)(x) + \mathcal{D}_\Omega(u|_{\partial\Omega})(x) , \quad x \in \mathbb{R}^d \setminus \overline{\Omega} , \tag{7.1}$$

where u is the solution of (5.23). Since $-\mathcal{S}_\Omega(g)(x) + \mathcal{D}_\Omega(U|_{\partial\Omega})(x) = 0$ for $x \in \mathbb{R}^d \setminus \overline{\Omega}$, we have

$$H[g](x) = \mathcal{D}_\Omega(u|_{\partial\Omega} - U|_{\partial\Omega})(x) . \tag{7.2}$$

Then by substituting (5.4) into (7.2) and using a simple formula $\mathcal{D}_\Omega(N(\cdot - z))(x) = \Gamma(x - z)$ for $z \in \Omega$ and $x \in \mathbb{R}^d \setminus \overline{\Omega}$, which is a direct consequence of (2.53), we get

$$H[g](x) = -\sum_{s=1}^{m} \sum_{|i|=1}^{d} \sum_{|j|=1}^{d-|i|+1} \frac{\epsilon_s^{|i|+|j|+d-2}}{i!j!} \partial^i U(z_s) M_{ij}(k_s, B_s) \partial_z^j \Gamma(x - z_s)$$
$$+ O(\epsilon^{2d}) . \tag{7.3}$$

The first-order approximation, which will be mainly used for the reconstruction, takes a particularly simple form:

$$H[g](x) = -\sum_{s=1}^{m} \epsilon_s^d \nabla U(z_s) M(k_s, B_s) \nabla_z \Gamma(x - z_s) + O(\epsilon^{d+1}) \tag{7.4}$$

for all $x \in \mathbb{R}^d \setminus \overline{\Omega}$. Note that, if $|x| \to +\infty$, we have

$$H[g](x) = -\sum_{s=1}^{m} \epsilon_s^d \nabla U(z_s) M(k_s, B_s) \nabla_z \Gamma(x - z_s) + O\left(\frac{\epsilon^{d+1}}{|x|^d}\right). \tag{7.5}$$

Observe that $\nabla_z \Gamma(x - z_s) = O(|x|^{-d+1})$ as $|x| \to +\infty$.

If the inclusion has a symmetry, then the error term in (7.4) with $m = 1$ can be replaced with $O(\epsilon^{d+2})$, because the correction of order two is zero, as a consequence of Lemma 4.4. The following example illustrates this result.

Let $d = 2$, and consider a single inclusion $D = \epsilon B + z$ in $\Omega \subset \mathbb{R}^2$. We plot the quantity

$$\max_{x \in S} \ln \| H[g](x) + \epsilon^2 \nabla U(z) M \nabla_z \Gamma(x - z) \|$$

as a function of $\ln \epsilon$, where S is a $\mathcal{C}^2$-closed surface enclosing the domain Ω [46]. The graphics in Figure 7.2 demonstrate that the expression in (7.4) (with $d = 2$) is of order $O(\epsilon^4)$ for symmetric inclusions and of order $O(\epsilon^3)$ for non-symmetric ones.

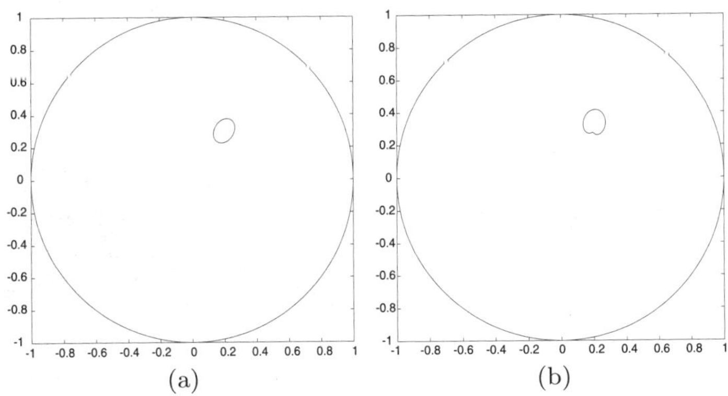

(a)   (b)

Fig. 7.1. Symmetric inclusion (a); non-symmetric inclusion (b).

7.2 Projection Algorithm — Reconstruction of a Single Inclusion

The projection algorithm was developed by Ammari and Seo in [43]. To bring out the main ideas of this algorithm, we only consider the case where D has one component of the form $\epsilon B + z$. Based on Theorem 5.1 and two more observations we rigorously reconstruct, with good resolution and accuracy, the location, the size, and the polarization tensors from the observation in the near field (x near $\partial\Omega$) and the far field (x far from $\partial\Omega$) of the pattern $H(x)$, which is computed directly from the current-voltage pairs.

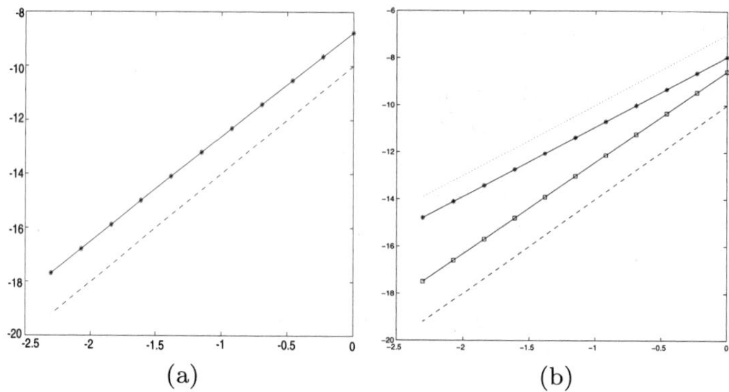

Fig. 7.2. Remainder of order $O(\epsilon^4)$ for (a); remainder of order $O(\epsilon^3)$ for (b).

The mathematical analysis provided in this section indicates that the projection algorithm has good resolution and accuracy.

As we said before, this algorithm makes use of constant current sources. For any unit vector $a \in \mathbb{R}^d$, $d = 2, 3$, let $H[a \cdot \nu]$ denote the function H in (2.64) corresponding to the Neumann data

$$g(y) = \frac{\partial}{\partial \nu}(a \cdot y) = a \cdot \nu_y , \quad y \in \partial\Omega .$$

The expression $D = \epsilon B + z$ requires some care because it can be expressed in infinitely many different ways. For a unique representation, we need to select a canonical domain B that is a representative domain of the set of all $D = \epsilon B + z$. Assume for the sake of simplicity that $k > 1$. Let $\mathcal{T}_\lambda$ be the set of all strictly star-shaped domains B satisfying

$$\int_B x\, dx = 0 , \quad |M(k, B)| = 1 ,$$

where $\det(M)$ is the determinant of the matrix M and $M(k, B)$ is the polarization tensor of Pólya–Szegö associated with the domain B and the conductivity $k = (2\lambda + 1)/(2\lambda - 1)$. Then, by using the essential fact from Chapter 4 that $M(k, B)$ is a symmetric positive-definite matrix and so, its determinant cannot vanish, it is not hard to see that, if $\epsilon_1 B_1 + z_1 = \epsilon_2 B_2 + z_2$, where B_1 and B_2 belong to $\mathcal{T}_\lambda$, then $z_1 = z_2, \epsilon_1 = \epsilon_2$, and $B_1 = B_2$. Note that if $0 < k < 1$ then $M(k, B)$ is a symmetric negative definite matrix. Throughout this chapter, we assume that $B \in \mathcal{T}_\lambda$.

The first step for the reconstruction procedure is to compute ϵ and $M(k, B)$ up to an error of order ϵ^d.

Theorem 7.1 (Size estimation) *Let S be a C^2 closed surface (or curve in $\mathbb{R}^2$) enclosing the domain Ω. Then for any vectors a and a^* we have*

$$\int_S \frac{\partial H[a \cdot \nu]}{\partial \nu}(x)\, a^* \cdot x\, d\sigma(x) - \int_S H[a \cdot \nu](x)\, a^* \cdot \nu_x\, d\sigma(x) \tag{7.6}$$

$$= -a^* \cdot (\epsilon^d M(k, B)a) + O(\epsilon^{2d}) \ .$$

Proof. Let Ω' denote the domain inside S; that is, $\partial\Omega' = S$. Since $S \subset \mathbb{R}^d \backslash \overline{\Omega}$, it follows from (2.67) that for any vector a, $H[a \cdot \nu] = -\mathcal{S}_D \phi$ on S, where

$$\phi = (\lambda I - \mathcal{K}_D^*)^{-1}\left(\frac{\partial H}{\partial \nu}\Big|_{\partial D}\right) \ .$$

Thus the left side of (7.6) is in fact equal to

$$-\int_S \frac{\partial}{\partial \nu}\left(\mathcal{S}_D\phi(x)\right)\, a^* \cdot x\, d\sigma(x) + \int_S \mathcal{S}_D\phi(x)\, a^* \cdot \nu_x\, d\sigma(x) \ . \tag{7.7}$$

Using the fact that $\Delta \mathcal{S}_D \phi = 0$ in $\mathbb{R}^d \setminus \partial D$ and the divergence theorem on $\Omega' \setminus \overline{D}$, we can see that the term in (7.7) equals

$$-\int_{\partial D} \frac{\partial(\mathcal{S}_D\phi(x))}{\partial \nu}\Big|_+ a^* \cdot x\, d\sigma(x) + \int_{\partial D} \mathcal{S}_D\phi(x)\, a^* \cdot \nu_x\, d\sigma(x) \ .$$

Then by the jump relation (2.27), it is equal to

$$-\int_{\partial D} a^* \cdot x\, \phi(x)\, d\sigma(x) \ .$$

Setting $\widetilde{h}(y) = \frac{\partial}{\partial \nu} H[a \cdot \nu](z + \epsilon y)$, we have by a change of variables

$$\int_{\partial D} a^* \cdot y\, \phi(y)\, d\sigma(y) = \epsilon^d \int_{\partial B} a^* \cdot y\, (\lambda I - \mathcal{K}_B^*)^{-1}\widetilde{h}(y)\, d\sigma(y) \ .$$

The estimate (v) in Proposition 5.6 provides the expansion

$$\int_{\partial B} a^* \cdot y\, (\lambda I - \mathcal{K}_B^*)^{-1}\widetilde{h}(y)\, d\sigma(y) = \int_{\partial B} a^* \cdot y\, (\lambda I - \mathcal{K}_B^*)^{-1}(\nu \cdot a)\, d\sigma(y) + O(\epsilon^d) \ ,$$

which leads us to the identity (7.6). $\square$

Now, let us explain how to compute ϵ and $M(k, B)$ up to an error of order ϵ^d using Theorem 7.1.

Let $\mathbb{A}$ be the $d \times d$ matrix defined by $\mathbb{A} = \sqrt{\mathbb{B}\mathbb{B}^T}$, where the pq-component of $\mathbb{B}$ is equal to

$$\int_S \frac{\partial H[e_p \cdot \nu]}{\partial \nu}(x)e_q \cdot x\, d\sigma(x) - \int_S H[e_p \cdot \nu](x)e_q \cdot \nu_x\, d\sigma(x) \ .$$

Here $\mathbb{B}^T$ is the transpose of the matrix $\mathbb{B}$ and $\{e_p\}_{p=1}^d$ is the standard basis of $\mathbb{R}^d$. Define

$$\epsilon^* = \sqrt[d^2]{|\mathbb{A}|}, \quad M^* := \frac{1}{(\epsilon^*)^d}\mathbb{A} \ .$$

According to Theorem 7.1, we immediately see that

$$\epsilon^* = \epsilon(1 + O(\epsilon^d)) \text{ and } M^* = M(k, B) + O(\epsilon^d) \ . \tag{7.8}$$

Note that slightly different size estimations can be obtained by making use of Lemma 4.14 and Theorem 4.16; see [82, 83]. It can be shown that

$$\frac{1}{k-1}a_{pp} \leq |D|(1 + O(|D|)) \leq \frac{k}{k-1}a_{pp} \ ,$$

where $(a_{pp})_{p=1,\dots,d}$ are the diagonal elements of $\mathbb{A}$, and

$$\frac{1}{d-1+\frac{1}{k}}\frac{\mathrm{Tr}(\mathbb{A})}{k-1} \leq |D|(1 + O(|D|)) \leq (d-1+k)\frac{(\mathrm{Tr}(\mathbb{A}^{-1}))^{-1}}{k-1} \ .$$

It can also be easily seen that all of these size estimations, even for moderate size volume, represent an improvement over the one given in Lemma 3.1.

Because of the normalization $|M(k, B)| = 1$, the knowledge of $M(k, B)$ does not determine k. Equivalently, it is not possible to determine ϵ and k simultaneously from the knowledge of the lowest-order term in the asymptotic expansion of the pattern H.

Observe that by construction the real matrix M^* is symmetric positive-definite. Let $0 < \kappa_1 \leq \dots \leq \kappa_{d-1} \leq \kappa_d$ be the eigenvalues of $M(k, B)$. Using once again the fact that $M(k, B)$ is a symmetric positive-definite matrix it follows that there is a constant C depending only on the Lipschitz character of B such that $C < \kappa_p < 1/C$, and therefore, for ϵ small enough, the eigenvalues $\{\kappa_*^{(p)}\}_{p=1}^d$ of M^* satisfy the same estimates.

Having recovered (approximately) the polarization tensor of Pólya–Szegö $M(k, B)$, we now compute an orthonormal basis of eigenvectors $a_*^{(1)}, \dots, a_*^{(d)}$ of M^*. We will use these eigenvectors for recovering the location z. Let Σ_p be a line parallel to $a_*^{(p)}$ such that

$$\mathrm{dist}\,(\partial\Omega, \Sigma_p) = O\left(\frac{1}{(\epsilon^*)^{d-1}}\right), \quad p = 1, \dots, d \ .$$

For any $x \in \Sigma_p$ it is readily seen from (5.22) and (7.8) that for background potentials U_p given by

$$U_p(x) = a_*^{(p)} \cdot x - \frac{1}{|\partial\Omega|}\int_{\partial\Omega} a_*^{(p)} \cdot y\, d\sigma(y) \ , \quad p = 1, \dots, d$$

(or equivalently for the currents $g = a_*^{(p)} \cdot \nu$), the following asymptotic expansion holds:

$$H[a_*^{(p)} \cdot \nu](x) = -\kappa_*^{(p)}\frac{(\epsilon^*)^d}{\omega_d|x-z|^d}(x-z) \cdot a_*^{(p)} + O\left(\frac{\epsilon^{2d}}{|x-z|^{d-1}}\right) \tag{7.9}$$

for all $x \in \Sigma_p$, where $\kappa_*^{(p)}$ is the eigenvalue of M^* associated with the eigenvector $a_*^{(p)}$.

In fact, this is the far-field expansion of the pattern $H[a_*^{(p)} \cdot \nu]$, from which we shall find the location z with an error of order $O(\epsilon^d)$. To get some insight, let us neglect the asymptotically small remainder $O(\epsilon^{2d})$ in the asymptotic expansion (7.9).

Our second important observation is that, since M^* is symmetric positive and the set of eigenvectors $(a_*^{(1)}, \ldots, a_*^{(d)})$ forms an orthonormal basis of $\mathbb{R}^d$, we will find exactly d points $z_*^p \in \Sigma_p, p = 1, \ldots, d$, so that $H[a_*^{(p)} \cdot \nu](z_*^p) = 0$. Finally, the point $z_* = \sum_{p=1}^d (z_*^p \cdot a_*^{(p)}) a_*^{(p)}$ is very close to z, namely $|z_* - z| = O(\epsilon^d)$.

Theorem 7.2 (Detection of the location) *Let $a_*^{(1)}, \ldots, a_*^{(d)}$ denote the mutually orthonormal eigenvectors of the symmetric matrix M^*. For any $p = 1, \cdots, d$, let $H[a_*^{(p)} \cdot \nu]$ be the function H in (2.64) corresponding to the Neumann data $g = a_*^{(p)} \cdot \nu$ and let Σ_p be a line with the direction $a_*^{(p)}$ so that $\mathrm{dist}\,(\partial\Omega, \Sigma_p) = O(1/(\epsilon^*)^{d-1})$. Then $z_*^p \in \Sigma_p$ exists so that $H[a_*^{(p)} \cdot \nu](z_*^p) = 0$. Moreover, the point $z_* = \sum_{p=1}^d (z_*^p \cdot a_*^{(p)})a_*^{(p)}$ satisfies the following estimate:*

$$|z_* - z| \leq C\epsilon^d , \tag{7.10}$$

where the constant C is independent of ϵ and z.

Proof. From (7.9) it follows that a positive constant C exists, independent of x, z, and ϵ such that

$$H[a_*^{(p)} \cdot \nu](x) \geq -\frac{\epsilon^d}{\omega_d |x - z|^{d-1}} \left(\kappa_*^{(p)} \frac{(x - z)}{|x - z|} \cdot a_*^{(p)} + C\epsilon^d \right) \text{ for all } x \in \Sigma_p ,$$

$$H[a_*^{(p)} \cdot \nu](x) \leq -\frac{\epsilon^d}{\omega_d |x - z|^{d-1}} \left(\kappa_*^{(p)} \frac{(x - z)}{|x - z|} \cdot a_*^{(p)} - C\epsilon^d \right) \text{ for all } x \in \Sigma_p .$$

For $x \in \Sigma_p$ satisfying

$$\frac{(x - z)}{|x - z|} \cdot a_*^{(p)} < -\frac{C}{\kappa_*^{(p)}} \epsilon^d ,$$

we have $H[a_*^{(p)} \cdot \nu](x) > 0$. On the other hand, for $x \in \Sigma_p$ satisfying

$$\frac{(x - z)}{|x - z|} \cdot a_*^{(p)} > \frac{C}{\kappa_*^{(p)}} \epsilon^d ,$$

we similarly have $H[a_*^{(p)} \cdot \nu](x) < 0$. Therefore, the zero point z_* satisfies

$$|(z_* - z) \cdot a_*^{(p)}| \leq C\epsilon^d, \text{ for } p = 1, \ldots, d ,$$

which implies that (7.10) holds, since $\{a_*^{(p)}\}_{p=1}^d$ forms an orthonormal basis of $\mathbb{R}^d$. $\square$

Finally, to find additional geometric features of the domain B and its conductivity k, we use higher order terms in the asymptotic expansion of H, which follows from a combination of the estimate (v) in Proposition 5.6 and the expansion (5.22):

$$H[a \cdot \nu](x) = - \sum_{|i|=1} \sum_{|j|=1}^{d} \frac{\epsilon^{|i|+|j|+d-2}}{j!} a \partial_z^j \Gamma(x-z) M_{ij} + O(\epsilon^{2d}) . \qquad (7.11)$$

Since z, ϵ, and the polarization tensor M are now recovered with an error $O(\epsilon^d)$, the reconstruction of the higher order polarization tensors M_{ij} for $|i| = 1$ and $2 \le |j| \le d$, could easily been done by inverting an appropriate linear system arising from (7.11). Then we could determine the conductivity k from the knowledge of M_{ij}, for $1 \le |i|, |j| \le d$.

The main results in this section are summarized in the following reconstruction procedure.

Projection Algorithm

For any unit vector a, let $H[a \cdot \nu]$ be the function H in (2.64) corresponding to the Neumann data $g(y) = a \cdot \nu_y, y \in \partial\Omega$. Let $\{e_p\}_{p=1}^d$ denote the standard orthonormal basis of $\mathbb{R}^d$. Let S be a C^2-closed surface (or curve in $\mathbb{R}^2$) enclosing the domain Ω.

Step 1 Compute $H[e_p \cdot \nu](x)$ for $x \in S$ to calculate the matrix $\mathbb{A} = \sqrt{\mathbb{B}\mathbb{B}^T}$, where the pq-component of $\mathbb{B}$ is equal to

$$\int_S \frac{\partial H[e_p \cdot \nu]}{\partial \nu}(x) e_q \cdot x \, d\sigma(x) - \int_S H[e_p \cdot \nu](x) e_q \cdot \nu_x \, d\sigma(x)$$

and $\mathbb{B}^T$ is the transpose of the matrix $\mathbb{B}$. Then

$$\epsilon^* = \sqrt[d^2]{|\mathbb{A}|} = \epsilon(1 + O(\epsilon^d)) \quad \text{and} \quad M^* := \frac{1}{(\epsilon^*)^d}\mathbb{A} = M(k, B) + O(\epsilon^d) .$$

Step 2 Compute an orthonormal basis $\{a_*^{(p)}\}_{p=1}^d$ of eigenvectors of the symmetric positive-definite matrix M^*.

Step 3 Consider Σ_p to be a line with the direction $a_*^{(p)}$ so that dist $(\partial\Omega, \Sigma_p) = O(1/(\epsilon^*)^{d-1})$ and $z_*^p \in \Sigma_p$ so that $H[a_*^{(p)} \cdot \nu](z_*^p) = 0$. Then the point $z_* = \sum_{p=1}^d (z_*^p \cdot a_*^{(p)})a_*^{(p)}$ satisfies the estimate $|z_* - z| = O(\epsilon^d)$.

Step 4 Recover the higher order polarization tensors M_{ij}, for $|i| = 1$ and $2 \le |j| \le d$, by solving an appropriate linear system arising from (7.11) and then determine the conductivity k from the knowledge of M_{ij}, for $1 \le |i|, |j| \le d$.

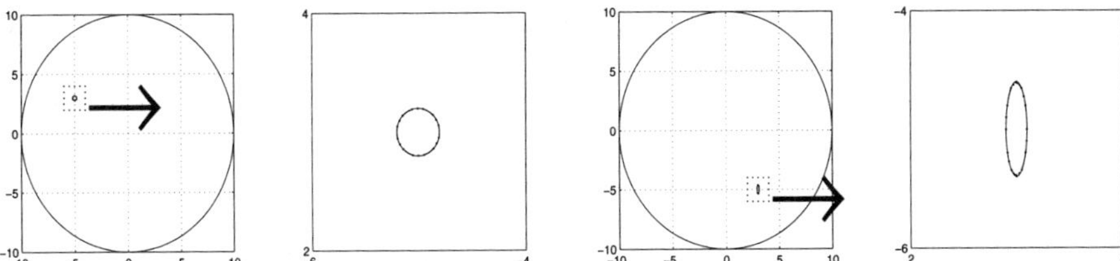

Fig. 7.3. Detection of the location and the polarization tensor of a small inclusion by the projection algorithm.

7.3 Quadratic Algorithm — Detection of Closely Spaced Inclusions

Recall that the projection algorithm uses only linear solutions. In this section, we design another algorithm using quadratic solutions. We apply this algorithm for the purpose of reconstructing the first-order polarization tensor and the center of closely spaced small inclusions from a finite number of boundary measurements.

Assume for the sake of simplicity that $d = 2$. Based on estimates (7.4) and (7.5), we have the following reconstruction procedure.

Quadratic Algorithm

Step 1 For $g_p = \partial x_p / \partial \nu$, $p = 1, 2$, measure $u|_{\partial\Omega}$.

Step 2 Compute the first-order polarization tensor $\epsilon^2 M = \epsilon^2 (m_{pq})^d_{p,q=1}$ for D by

$$\epsilon^2 m_{pq} = \lim_{t \to +\infty} 2\pi t H[g_p](te_q) .$$

Step 3 Compute $h_p = \lim_{t \to +\infty} 2\pi t H[g_3](te_p)$ for $g_3 = \frac{\partial(x_1 x_2)}{\partial \nu}, p = 1, 2$. Then the center is estimated by solving

$$z = (h_1, h_2)(\epsilon^2 M)^{-1} .$$

Step 4 Let the overall conductivity $\overline{k} = +\infty$ if the polarization tensor M is positive-definite. Otherwise assume $\overline{k} = 0$. Use results from Subsect. 4.11.1 to obtain the shape of the equivalent ellipse.

In order to collect data $u|_{\partial\Omega}$ in Step 1, we solve the direct problem (5.29) as follows. Using the formula (5.24) and the jump relations (2.27) and (2.28), we have, for $s = 1, \ldots, m$, the following equations:

$$\begin{cases} \dfrac{1}{2} u = \mathcal{K}_\Omega u - \mathcal{S}_\Omega g + \displaystyle\sum_{s=1}^{m} \mathcal{S}_{D_s} \psi^{(s)} & \text{on } \partial\Omega , \\[3ex] (\lambda_s I - \mathcal{K}^*_{D_s})\psi^{(s)} - \displaystyle\sum_{l \neq s} \dfrac{\partial(\mathcal{S}_{D_l}\psi^{(l)})}{\partial\nu^{(s)}}\Big|_{\partial D_s} = \dfrac{\partial H}{\partial\nu^{(s)}}\Big|_{\partial D_s} & \text{on } \partial D_s . \end{cases}$$

We solve the integral equation using the collocation method [204] and obtain $u|_{\partial\Omega}$ on $\partial\Omega$ for given data g.

A few words of explanation are required for Step 4. In order to determine the overall conductivity, it is necessary to know for every single inclusion both its individual conductivity k_s and size $|B_s|$, $s = 1, \ldots, m$. That is impossible; thus we assume *a priori* that $\overline{k}$ is either $+\infty$ or 0 depending on the sign of the detected polarization tensor. Therefore it is natural that the quadratic algorithm gives better information when the conductivity contrast between the background and the inclusions is high. We illustrate in Figure 7.4 the viability of this algorithm. Rigorous justification of its validity follows from the arguments we just went through for the projection algorithm.

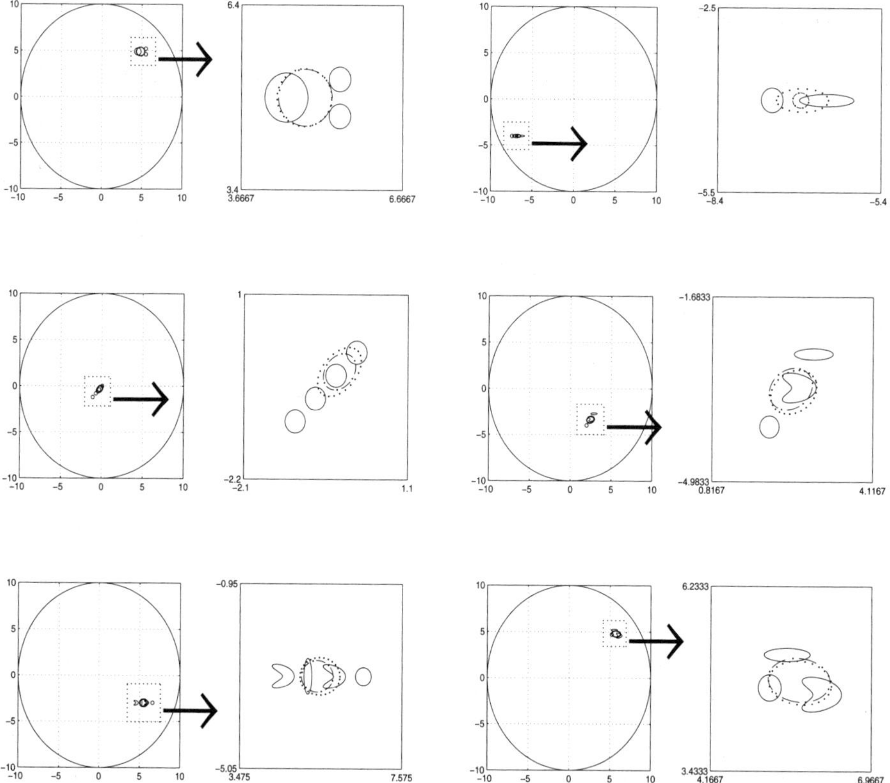

Fig. 7.4. Reconstruction of closely spaced small inclusions. The dashed line is the equivalent ellipse, and the dash-dot line is the detected ellipse. The numerical values are given in Table 7.1.

We conclude this section with a comment on stability. In general, the measured voltage potential contains unavoidable observation noise, so that

k_i	$a_0^i, a_1^i, a_2^i, b_0^i, b_1^i, b_2^i$	$\overline{k}$	$\overline{a}$	$\overline{b}$	$\overline{\theta}$	$\overline{z}$
		k	a	b	θ	z
100	5.5, 0.2, 0, 5.2, 0.2, 0	60.079	0.511	0.468	0.000	(4.838, 4.900)
100	5.5, 0.2, 0, 4.6, 0.2, 0	$+\infty$	0.502	0.461	0.000	(4.856, 4.899)
50	4.5, 0.4, 0, 4.9, 0.4, 0					
1.5	-7.4, 0.2, 0, -4, 0.2, 0	1.5	0.474	0.190	0.000	(-6.844, -4.000)
1.5	-6.4, 0.5, 0, -4, 0.1, 0	$+\infty$	0.146	0.123	0.000	(-6.875, -4.000)
100	0.1, 0.2, 0, 0, 0.2, 0					
100	-0.3, 0.2, 0, -0.4, 0.2, 0	3.88	0.511	0.315	0.785	(-0.236, -0.336)
1.5	-0.7, 0.2, 0, -0.8, 0.2, 0	$+\infty$	0.355	0.267	0.785	(-0.233, -0.333)
1.5	-1.1, 0.2, 0,-1.2, 0.2, 0					
5	2.9, 0.4, 0, -2.7, 0.1, 0	18.655	0.491	0.365	0.443	(2.494, -3.375)
100	2.5, 0.25, 0.2, -3.3, 0.25, 0.05	$+\infty$	0.458	0.351	0.443	(2.434, -3.321)
50	2.0, 0.2, 0, -4.0, 0.2, 0					
5	4.5, 0.15, 0.2, -3, 0.25, 0.05					
5	5.2, 0.1, 0, -3, 0.4, 0	5	0.507	0.419	-0.000	(5.502, -3.000)
5	5.8, 0.15, 0.2, -3, 0.25,0.05	$+\infty$	0.401	0.353	-0.000	(5.436, -3.000)
5	6.6, 0.2, 0, -3, 0.2, 0					
100	6.0, 0.25, 0.2, 4.6, 0.25, 0.05	100	0.549	0.331	-0.089	(5.728, 4.772)
100	5.5, 0.4, 0, 5.2, 0.1, 0	$+\infty$	0.540	0.329	-0.089	(5.712, 4.817)
100	5.2, 0.2, 0, 4.7, 0.2, 0					

Table 7.1. Table for Figure 7.4. Here $\overline{k}, \overline{z}$ are the overall conductivity and center defined by (4.84) and (4.85). $\overline{a}$, $\overline{b}$, and $\overline{\theta}$ are semi-axis lengths and the angle of orientation of the equivalent ellipse while a, b, and θ are those of detected ellipse assuming $k = +\infty$. The point z is the detected center.

we have to answer the stability question. Fortunately, the projection and quadratic algorithms are totally based on the observation of the pattern of H; thus, if

$$H^{\mathrm{meas}}[g](x) := -\mathcal{S}_\Omega(g)(x) + \mathcal{D}_\Omega(u^{\mathrm{meas}}) \quad \text{for } x \in \mathbb{R}^d \setminus \overline{\Omega} \,,$$

where u^{meas} is the measured voltage on the boundary, then we have the following stability estimate

$$|H^{\mathrm{meas}}[g](x) - H[g](x)| \leq \left| \int_{\partial\Omega} \frac{\partial \Gamma}{\partial \nu_y}(x - y)\left(u^{\mathrm{meas}} - u\right)(y)\, d\sigma(y) \right|$$

$$\leq C \, \|u^{\mathrm{meas}} - u\|_{L^2(\partial\Omega)} \,,$$

where C is a constant depending only on the distance from x to $\partial\Omega$. Thus we conclude that the projection and quadratic algorithms are not sensitive to the observation noise.

We now present another method using finitely many measurements, assuming that all inclusions are disks.

7.4 Simple Pole Method

This method is due to Kang and Lee [177]. It was first developed in [52]. Suppose that the inclusion is of the form $D = \cup_{s=1}^{m} D_s$ and each D_s is a disk, or $D_s = \epsilon_s B$, where B is a unit disk. In this case the polarization tensor $M^{(s)}$ associated with B is given by

$$M^{(s)}(= M(k_s, B)) = \pi \frac{2(k_s - 1)}{k_s + 1} I \,,$$

where I is the identity matrix. Therefore, in this case we obtain from (7.4) that

$$H[g](x) = \sum_{s=1}^{m} \frac{\epsilon_s^2(k_s - 1)}{k_s + 1} \frac{\nabla U(z_s) \cdot (x - z_s)}{|x - z_s|^2} + O(\epsilon^3), \quad x \in \mathbb{R}^2 \setminus \overline{\Omega} \,.$$

Thus, we get

$$H[\nu_1](x) + iH[\nu_2](x) = \sum_{s=1}^{m} \frac{\beta_s}{z - \alpha_s} + O(\epsilon^3), \quad z \in \mathbb{C} \setminus \overline{\Omega} \,,$$

where $\beta_s := \epsilon_s^2(k_s - 1)/(k_s + 1)$ and $\alpha_s = (z_s)_1 + i(z_s)_2$. Note that $H[\nu_2]$ is a harmonic conjugate of $H[\nu_1]$.

Therefore our inclusion detection problem reduces to the problem of finding the simple poles α_s and the residues β_s from the knowledge of a meromorphic function $f(z) = \sum_{s=1}^{m} \beta_s/(z - \alpha_s)$ on a circle $|z| = R$ enclosing all the poles.

It turns out that there is a nice way to locate the simple poles. By the Cauchy integral formula, we have

$$\frac{1}{2\pi i} \int_{|z|=R} z^n f(z) dz = \sum_{s=1}^{m} \beta_s \alpha_s^n \,.$$

The method of identification of simple poles is based on the following simple observations.

Lemma 7.3 *Suppose that the sequence $\{c_n\}$ takes the form $c_n = \sum_{s=1}^{m} \beta_s \alpha_s^n$, $n = 0, 1, \ldots$. If $l_1, \ldots, l_k$ satisfies the generating equation*

$$c_{n+m} + l_1 c_{n+m-1} + \cdots + l_m c_n = 0, \quad n = 0, 1, \ldots, m-1 \,, \tag{7.12}$$

then $\alpha_1, \alpha_2, \cdots, \alpha_m$ are solutions of

$$z^m + l_1 z^{m-1} + \cdots + l_m = 0 \,. \tag{7.13}$$

The converse is also true. Furthermore, if (7.12) holds, then it holds for all n.

Lemma 7.4 *Let c_n be as in the Lemma 7.3, and let*

$$D_n = \det \begin{pmatrix} c_0 & c_1 & \cdots & c_{n-1} \\ c_1 & c_2 & \cdots & c_n \\ \vdots & \vdots & & \vdots \\ c_{n-1} & c_n & \cdots & c_{2n-2} \end{pmatrix}.$$

Then

$$D_n = \begin{cases} \beta_1\beta_2\cdots\beta_m \prod_{i<j}(\alpha_i - \alpha_j)^2 & \text{if } n = m\,, \\ 0 & \text{if } n > m\,. \end{cases} \tag{7.14}$$

Lemmas 7.3 and 7.4 suggest that, if we know the number m of simple poles, then we first solve the system of equations (7.12) to find $l_1,\ldots,l_m$. We then solve the equation (7.13) to find the poles $\alpha_1,\ldots,\alpha_m$. Once we find $\alpha_1,\ldots,\alpha_m$, it is a simple matter to find $\beta_1,\ldots,\beta_m$. The most serious difficulty in finding poles comes from the fact that we do not know their number aforehand. In order to determine this number, we use the formula (7.14). That is, we start with a bound N of the number of poles and compute the determinants in (7.14) for $n = N, N-1, \ldots$, until it becomes non-zero. The first number for which the determinant is non-zero is the number of simple poles we seek to determine.

Of course, these computations are performed within a given tolerance. The result of a numerical test in a simple situation is given in [177].

We note that the problem of reconstructing multiple thin inclusions can be reduced to a problem of finding simple poles for which the simple pole method may be applied; see a recent paper by Ammari, Beretta, and Francini[14].

7.5 Least-Squares Algorithm

In this section we consider m inclusions $D_s, s = 1,\ldots,m$, each of the form $D_s = \epsilon_s B_s + z_s$ where each $B_s \in \mathcal{T}_{\lambda_s}$. Here $\lambda_s = (k_s + 1)/(2(k_s - 1))$. Let S be a $\mathcal{C}^2$-closed surface (or curve in $\mathbb{R}^2$) enclosing the domain Ω. The least-squares algorithm is based on the minimization of a discrete L^2-norm of the residual

$$H[g](x) + \sum_{s=1}^{m} \sum_{|i|=1}^{d} \sum_{|j|=1}^{d} \frac{\epsilon_s^{|i|+|j|+d-2}}{i!j!}(\partial^i U)(z_s)\partial_z^j \Gamma(x - z_s)M_{ij}^s$$

on S. Here $M_{ij}^s = M_{ij}(k_s, B_s)$. We select L equidistant points, $x_1,\ldots,x_L$, on S, and we seek to determine the unknown parameters of the inclusions D_s as the solution to the non-linear least-squares problem

$$\min \sum_{l=1}^{L} \left| H[g](x_l) + \sum_{s=1}^{m} \sum_{|i|=1}^{d} \sum_{|j|=1}^{d} \frac{\epsilon_s^{|i|+|j|+d-2}}{i!j!}(\partial^i U)(z_s)\partial_z^j \Gamma(x_l - z_s)M_{ij}^s \right|^2.$$

We minimize over $\{m, z_s, \epsilon_s, k_s, B_s\}$ when all parameters are unknown; however, there may be considerable non-uniqueness of the minimizer in this general case. If the inclusions are assumed to be of the form $z_s + \epsilon_s Q_s B$, for a common known domain B, but unknown locations z_s and rotations Q_s, then if ϵ_s and k_s are known, the least-squares algorithm can be applied to successfully determine the number m of inclusions, the locations z_s and the rotations Q_s, as demonstrated by numerical examples in [84].

7.6 Variational Algorithm

This algorithm is based on the original idea of Calderón [78], which was, by the way of a low amplitude perturbation formula, to reduce the reconstruction problem to the calculations of an inverse Fourier transform. It may require quite a number of boundary measurements, but if these are readily available, then the approach is simple and the implementation is fast.

For arbitrary $\eta \in \mathbb{R}^d$, one assumes that one is in possession of the boundary data for the voltage potential u, whose corresponding background potential is given by $U(y) = e^{i(\eta+i\eta^\perp)\cdot y}$ (boundary current $g_\eta(y) = i(\eta+i\eta^\perp)\cdot\nu_y e^{i(\eta+i\eta^\perp)\cdot y}$ on $\partial\Omega$), where $\eta^\perp \in \mathbb{R}^d$ is orthogonal to η with $|\eta| = |\eta^\perp|$.

If S is a $\mathcal{C}^2$-closed surface (or curve in $\mathbb{R}^2$) enclosing the domain Ω, then analogously to (7.6), one can easily prove that

$$
\begin{aligned}
\mathcal{E}(\eta) :=& \int_S \frac{\partial}{\partial\nu} H[g_\eta](y)\, e^{i(\eta-i\eta^\perp)\cdot y}\, d\sigma(y) \\
&- i \int_S H[g_\eta](y)\, \nu_y \cdot (\eta - i\eta^\perp)\, e^{i(\eta-i\eta^\perp)\cdot y}\, d\sigma(y) \\
=& \sum_{s=1}^{m} \epsilon_s^d(\eta + i\eta^\perp)\cdot M^s \cdot (\eta - i\eta^\perp)e^{2i\eta\cdot z_s} + O(\epsilon^{d+1})\,,
\end{aligned}
\tag{7.15}
$$

where $\epsilon = \sup_s \epsilon_s$ and $M^s = M(k_s, B_s)$.

Recall that the function $e^{2i\eta\cdot z_s}$ (up to a multiplicative constant) is exactly the Fourier transform of the Dirac function δ_{-2z_s} (a point mass located at $-2z_s$). Multiplication by powers of η in the Fourier space corresponds to differentiation of the Dirac function. The function $\mathcal{E}(\eta)$ is therefore (approximately) the Fourier transform of a linear combination of derivatives of point masses; i.e.,

$$
\check{\mathcal{E}} \simeq \sum_{s=1}^{m} \epsilon_s^d L_s \delta_{-2z_s}\,,
$$

where L_s is a second-order constant coefficient differential operator, whose coefficients depend on the polarization tensor of Pólya–Szegö M^s, and $\check{\mathcal{E}}$ represents the inverse Fourier transform of $\mathcal{E}(\eta)$.

The variational algorithm then consists in sampling the values of $\mathcal{E}(\eta)$ at some discrete set of points and then calculating the corresponding discrete inverse Fourier transform. After a re-scaling (by $-1/2$) the support of this inverse Fourier transform yields the location of the inclusions. Once the locations are known, one may calculate the polarization tensors of Pólya–Szegö by solving the appropriate linear system arising from (7.15).

To estimate the number of the sampling points needed for an accurate discrete Fourier inversion of $\mathcal{E}(\eta)$, we remind the reader of the main assertion of the so-called Shannon's sampling theorem [108]: A function f is completely specified (by a very explicit formula) by the sampled values $\{f(c_0 + \pi n/h)\}_{n=-\infty}^{+\infty}$ if and only if the support of the Fourier transform of f is contained inside $[-h, h]$. For the variational algorithm this suggests two things: (1) If the inclusions are contained inside a square of side $2h$, then we need to sample $\mathcal{E}(\eta)$ at a uniform, infinite, rectangular grid of mesh-size π/h to obtain an accurate reconstruction; (2) if we only sample the points in this grid for which the absolute values of the coordinates are less than K, then the resulting discrete inverse Fourier transform will recover the location of the inclusions with a resolution of $\delta = \pi/K$. In summary, we need (conservatively) of the order $(2h)^d/\delta^d$ sampled values of $\mathcal{E}(\eta)$ to reconstruct, with a resolution δ, a collection of inclusions that lie inside a square of side $2h$. The reader is referred to [301] for a review of the fundamental mechanism behind the FFT method for inverting the quantity in (7.15).

The following numerical examples from [42] clearly demonstrate the viability of the variational approach.

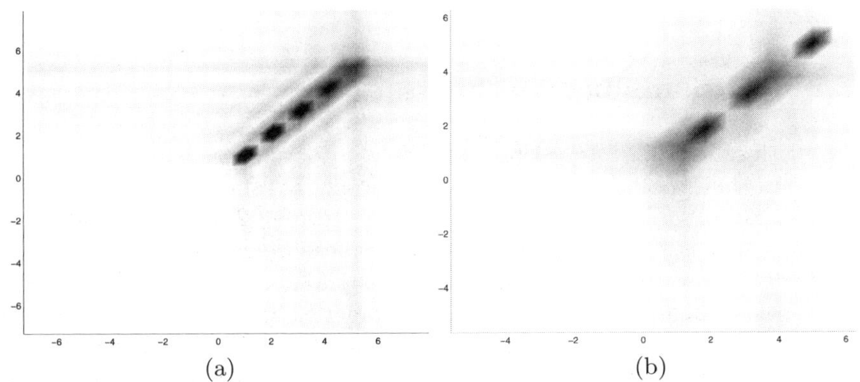

Fig. 7.5. Five inclusions: (a) 30×30 sample points, (b) 20×20 sample points.

We take the domain Ω to be the square $[-10, 10] \times [-10, 10]$, and we insert five inclusions in the shape of balls, with the sth-ball positioned at the point (s, s). We take each M^s to be $10 \times I$ and $\epsilon = 0.1$. We sample $\mathcal{E}(\eta)$ on the square $[-3, 3] \times [-3, 3]$ with a uniform 30×30 grid in (a) (900 sample points) and 20×20 grid in (b) (400 sample points). We are thus following the recipe from above, with $h = 10$ and $K = 3$. We should expect recovery of the locations of all inclusions, with a resolution $\delta = \pi/3$. The discrete inverse Fourier transform yields the gray-level (intensity) plot shown in Figure 7.5. In Figure 7.5(a) we can see that the five balls are still distinctly visible.

In order to simulate errors in the boundary measurements, as well as in the different approximations, we add on the order of 10% of random noise to the values of $\mathcal{E}(\eta)$. We see from Figure 7.6 that the reconstruction is quite stable.

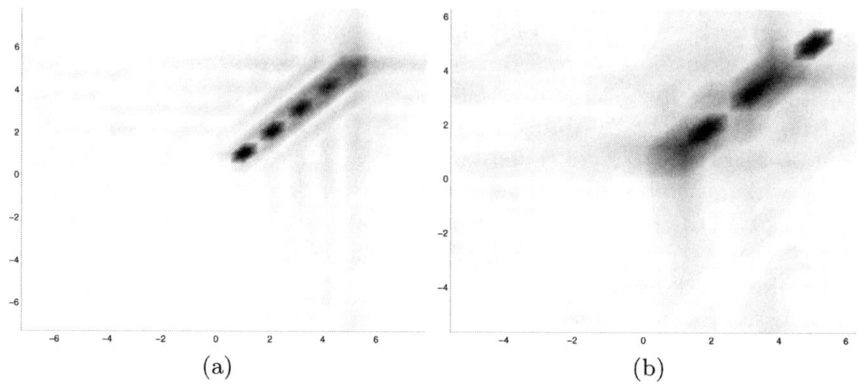

(a)	(b)

Fig. 7.6. Five inclusions with 10% noise (a) 30×30 sample points, (b) 20×20 sample points.

7.7 Linear Sampling Method

We now describe the interesting approach proposed by Brühl, Hanke, and Vogelius in their recent paper [73]. This approach is related to the linear sampling method of Colton and Kirsch [100] (see also [192] and [71]) and allows one to reconstruct small inclusions by taking measurements only on some portion of $\partial\Omega$. It also has some similarities to the MUltiple Signal Classification (MUSIC)-type algorithm developed by Devaney [110, 213] for estimating the locations of a number of point-like scatterers. We refer to Cheney [87] and Kirsch [193] for detailed discussions of the connection between the MUSIC algorithm and the linear sampling method.

Let $\partial\omega$ be a subset of $\partial\Omega$ with positive measure, and define $L_0^2(\partial\omega)$ to be the subspace of functions in $L^2(\partial\omega)$ with zero integral over $\partial\omega$. Let $D = \cup_{s=1}^{m}(\epsilon B_s + z_s)$ be a collection of small inclusions with conductivities $0 < k_s \neq 1 < +\infty, s = 1,\ldots,m$, and satisfying

$$|z_s - z_{s'}| \geq 2c_0 > 0 \quad \forall\, s \neq s' \quad \text{and} \quad \text{dist}(z_s,\partial\Omega) \geq 2c_0 > 0 \quad \forall\, s . \quad (7.16)$$

For a function $g \in L_0^2(\partial\omega)$, we can solve the problems

$$\begin{cases} \nabla \cdot \left(1 + (k-1)\chi(D)\right)\nabla u = 0 & \text{in } \Omega , \\[2mm] \dfrac{\partial u}{\partial \nu} = g & \text{on } \partial\omega , \\[2mm] \dfrac{\partial u}{\partial \nu} = 0 & \text{on } \partial\Omega \setminus \partial\omega , \\[2mm] \displaystyle\int_{\partial\omega} u(x)\,d\sigma(x) = 0 , \end{cases} \tag{7.17}$$

and

$$\begin{cases} \Delta U = 0 & \text{in } \Omega , \\[2mm] \dfrac{\partial U}{\partial \nu} = g & \text{on } \partial\omega , \\[2mm] \dfrac{\partial U}{\partial \nu} = 0 & \text{on } \partial\Omega \setminus \partial\omega , \\[2mm] \displaystyle\int_{\partial\omega} U(x)\,d\sigma(x) = 0 . \end{cases} \tag{7.18}$$

Define the partial Neumann-to-Dirichlet map on $L_0^2(\partial\omega)$ by $\Lambda_D(y) = u|_{\partial\omega}$. Let Λ_0 be the partial Neumann-to-Dirichlet map on $L_0^2(\partial\omega)$ for the case in which no conductivity inclusions are present. We seek to use $\Lambda_D - \Lambda_0$ to determine D. In this connection we first establish the following.

Lemma 7.5 *The operator* $\Lambda_D - \Lambda_0 : L_0^2(\partial\omega) \rightarrow L_0^2(\partial\omega)$ *is compact, self-adjoint, positive (respectively, negative) semi-definite, if* $0 < k_s < 1$ *(respectively* $1 < k_s < +\infty$) *for all* $s = 1, \ldots, m$.

Proof. Let $g \in L_0^2(\partial\omega)$, and let u and U denote the solutions of (7.17) and (7.18). An easy application of Green's formula gives

$$u(x) = \mathcal{D}_\Omega(u|_{\partial\Omega}) + (k-1)\int_D \nabla u(y) \cdot \nabla\Gamma(x-y)\,dy - \int_{\partial\omega} g(y)\Gamma(x-y)\,d\sigma(y)$$

and

$$U(x) = \mathcal{D}_\Omega(U|_{\partial\Omega}) - \int_{\partial\omega} g(y)\Gamma(x-y)\,d\sigma(y), \quad x \in \Omega .$$

Subtracting these two equations and letting x go to $\partial\Omega$ yields

$$(\tfrac{1}{2}I - \mathcal{K}_\Omega)(u - U) = (k-1)\int_D \nabla u(y) \cdot \nabla\Gamma(x-y)\,dy , \quad x \in \partial\Omega .$$

By using (2.28) and Lemma 2.29 together with the fact that

$$\int_{\partial\omega} (u - U)(y)\,d\sigma(y) = 0 ,$$

the above equation implies that

$$(\Lambda_D - \Lambda_0)g(x) = (1 - k)\int_D \nabla u(y) \cdot \nabla N(x,y)\, dy + C \quad \text{for } x \in \partial\omega\,,$$

where the constant C is given by

$$C = (k - 1)\int_{\partial\omega}\int_D \nabla u(y) \cdot \nabla N(x,y)\, dy\, d\sigma(x)\,.$$

By using (2.82) and (2.83), we can prove that

$$||u - U||_{L^2(\partial\omega)} \leq C||\nabla u||_{L^2(D)} \leq C'||g||_{L^2(\partial\omega)}\,,$$

for some positive constant C' independent of g, which indicates that $\Lambda_D - \Lambda_0$ is bounded. Indeed, from the smoothness of $\int_D \nabla u(y) \cdot \nabla N(x,y)\, dy|_{\partial\omega}$, we conclude that $\Lambda_D - \Lambda_0 : L_0^2(\partial\omega) \to L_0^2(\partial\omega)$ is compact. Thus, in order to prove that $\Lambda_D - \Lambda_0$ is self-adjoint, it suffices to show that it is symmetric. Consider $h \in L_0^2(\partial\omega)$ and v and V to be the solutions of (7.17) and (7.18), respectively, corresponding to the Neumann data h. Using integration by parts, we can establish the following identity:

$$\int_{\partial\omega}(\Lambda_D - \Lambda_0)(g)h = -\int_\Omega \nabla(u - U) \cdot \nabla(v - V) + \sum_{s=1}^m (1 - k_s)\int_{\epsilon B_s + z_s} \nabla u \cdot \nabla v$$

$$= \int_\Omega \left(1 + \sum_{s=1}^m (k_s - 1)\chi(\epsilon B_s + z_s)\right)\nabla(u - U) \cdot \nabla(v - V)$$

$$+ \sum_{s=1}^m (1 - k_s)\int_{\epsilon B_s + z_s} \nabla U \cdot \nabla V\,.$$

It results in, as desired, that $\Lambda_D - \Lambda_0 : L_0^2(\partial\omega) \to L_0^2(\partial\omega)$ is self-adjoint, positive (respectively, negative) semi-definite, if $0 < k_s < 1$ (respectively, $1 < k_s < +\infty$) for all $s = 1,\ldots,m$. $\qquad\square$

Next, let $\widetilde{N}$ be the solution to

$$\begin{cases} \Delta_x \widetilde{N}(x,z) = -\delta_z & \text{in } \Omega, \\[2mm] \dfrac{\partial \widetilde{N}}{\partial \nu_x}\Big|_{\partial\omega} = -\dfrac{1}{|\partial\omega|}\,, \\[2mm] \dfrac{\partial \widetilde{N}}{\partial \nu_x}\Big|_{\partial\Omega\backslash\partial\omega} = 0\,, \\[2mm] \displaystyle\int_{\partial\omega} \widetilde{N}(x,z)\, d\sigma(x) = 0 & \text{for } z \in \Omega\,. \end{cases} \tag{7.19}$$

Similarly to (5.4), we can prove without any new difficulties that

$$(\Lambda_D - \Lambda_0)(g)(x) = -\epsilon^d \sum_{s=1}^{m} \nabla U(z_s) M(k_s, B_s) \nabla_z \widetilde{N}(x, z_s) + O(\epsilon^{d+1}) \,,$$

uniformly on $\partial \omega$, where the remainder $O(\epsilon^{d+1})$ is bounded by $C\epsilon^{d+1}$ in the operator norm of $\mathcal{L}(L_0^2(\partial \omega), L_0^2(\partial \omega))$ and U is the background solution, that is, the solution of (7.18). Here $\mathcal{L}(L_0^2(\partial \omega), L_0^2(\partial \omega))$ is the set of linear bounded operators on $L_0^2(\partial \omega)$. Define the operator $T : L_0^2(\partial \omega) \to L_0^2(\partial \omega)$ by

$$T(g) = - \sum_{s=1}^{m} \nabla U(z_s) M(k_s, B_s) \nabla_z \widetilde{N}(\cdot, z_s) \,. \tag{7.20}$$

Since U depends linearly on g, T is linear. Corresponding to Lemma 7.5, the following result can be obtained.

Lemma 7.6 *The operator $T : L_0^2(\partial \omega) \to L_0^2(\partial \omega)$ is compact, self-adjoint, positive (respectively, negative) semi-definite, if $0 < k_s < 1$ (respectively, $1 < k_s < +\infty$) for all $s = 1, \ldots, m$.*

Proof. We first observe that T is a finite-dimensional operator, and hence, it is compact. Moreover, to prove that T is self-adjoint it suffices to show that it is symmetric. Let g and h be in $L_0^2(\partial \omega)$ and denote U and V as the background solutions corresponding, respectively, to g and h. We have

$$\int_{\partial \omega} T(g)h = - \sum_{s=1}^{m} \nabla U(z_s) M(k_s, B_s) \int_{\partial \omega} \nabla_z \widetilde{N}(x, z_s) \frac{\partial V}{\partial \nu}(x) \, d\sigma(x)$$

$$= - \sum_{s=1}^{m} \nabla U(z_s) M(k_s, B_s) \int_{\partial \Omega} \nabla_z \widetilde{N}(x, z_s) \frac{\partial V}{\partial \nu}(x) \, d\sigma(x) \,.$$

But since $\nabla_x \widetilde{N} = -\nabla_z \widetilde{N}$, we have $\Delta_x \nabla_z \widetilde{N} = \nabla_x \delta_{x=z}$ and therefore

$$\int_{\partial \Omega} \nabla_z \widetilde{N}(x, z_s) \frac{\partial V}{\partial \nu}(x) \, d\sigma(x) = \nabla V(z_s) \,.$$

Consequently,

$$\int_{\partial \omega} T(g)h = - \sum_{s=1}^{m} \nabla U(z_s) M(k_s, B_s) \nabla V(z_s) \,.$$

From the symmetry and the positive definiteness of the matrices $M(k_s, B_s)$ established in Theorem 4.11, we infer that T is self-adjoint, positive (respectively, negative) semi-definite, if $0 < k_s < 1$ (respectively, $1 < k_s < +\infty$) for all $s = 1, \ldots, m$. $\qquad\square$

Introduce now the linear operator $\mathcal{G} : L_0^2(\partial \omega) \to \mathbb{R}^{d \times m}$ defined by

$$\mathcal{G}g = (\nabla U(z_1), \ldots, \nabla U(z_m)) \,. \tag{7.21}$$

Endowing $\mathbb{R}^{d \times m}$ with the standard Euclidean inner product,

$$\langle a, b \rangle = \sum_{s=1}^{m} a_s \cdot b_s \quad \text{for } a = (a_1, \ldots, a_m), b = (b_1, \ldots, b_m), a_s, b_s \in \mathbb{R}^d ,$$

we then obtain

$$\langle \mathcal{G}g, a \rangle = \sum_{s=1}^{m} a_s \cdot \nabla U(z_s) = \int_{\partial\omega} \left(\sum_{s=1}^{m} a_s \cdot \nabla \widetilde{N}(x, z_s) \right) g(x) \, d\sigma(x) ,$$

for arbitrary $a = (a_1, \ldots, a_m) \in \mathbb{R}^{d \times m}$.

Therefore, the adjoint $\mathcal{G}^* : \mathbb{R}^{d \times m} \to L_0^2(\partial\omega)$ is given by

$$\mathcal{G}^* a = \sum_{s=1}^{m} a_s \cdot \nabla \widetilde{N}(\cdot, z_s) . \tag{7.22}$$

A characterization of the range of the operator T is obtained in the following lemma due to Brühl, Hanke, and Vogelius [73].

Lemma 7.7 (i) $\mathcal{G}^*$ *is injective;*
(ii) $\mathcal{G}$ *is surjective;*
(iii) $T = \mathcal{G}^* \mathcal{M} \mathcal{G}$, *where*

$$\mathcal{M}a = \left(M(k_1, B_1)a_1, \ldots, M(k_m, B_m)a_m \right), \quad a = (a_1, \ldots, a_m) \in \mathbb{R}^{d \times m} ;$$

(iv) $Range(T) = span \left\{ e_p \cdot \nabla \widetilde{N}(\cdot, z_s), \ p = 1, \ldots, d; \ s = 1, \ldots, m \right\}$, *where* $\{e_p\}_{p=1}^{d}$ *is the standard basis of* $\mathbb{R}^d$.

Proof. Suppose that $\mathcal{G}^* a = 0$; then the function $w(x) = \sum_{s=1}^{m} a_s \cdot \widetilde{N}(x, z_s)$ solves the Cauchy problem $\Delta w = 0$ in $\Omega \setminus \cup_{s=1}^{m} \{z_s\}, w = \partial w / \partial \nu = 0$ on $\partial\omega$, and from the uniqueness of the solution to this problem, we deduce that $w \equiv 0$. The dipole singularity of $\widetilde{N}(x, z_s)$ at z_s implies that $a_s = 0$, and thus, assertion (i) holds. Assertion (ii) follows from (i) and the well-known relation between the ranges and the null spaces of adjoint finite-dimensional operators: $Range(\mathcal{G}) = Ker(\mathcal{G}^*)^\perp$. Using (7.20), (7.21), and (7.22), it is easy to see that (iii) holds. Now according to (iii), we write $Range(T) = Range(\mathcal{G}^* \mathcal{M} \mathcal{G}) = Range(\mathcal{G}^*)$, since $\mathcal{M}$ and $\mathcal{G}$ are surjective. This yields (iv). $\qquad\square$

Now we present the main tool for the identification of the locations z_s. The following theorem is also due to Brühl, Hanke, and Vogelius [73].

Theorem 7.1. *Let* $e \in \mathbb{R}^d \setminus \{0\}$. *A point* $z \in \Omega$ *belongs to the set* $\{z_s : s = 1, \ldots, m\}$ *if and only if* $e \cdot \nabla_z \widetilde{N}(\cdot, z)\big|_{\partial\omega} \in Range\ (T)$.

Proof.   Assume that $g_{z,e} = e \cdot \nabla_z \widetilde{N}(\cdot, z)|_{\partial\omega} \in \text{Range}\,(T)$. As a consequence of (iv), $g_{z,e}$ may be represented as

$$g_{z,e}(x) = \sum_{s=1}^{m} a_s \cdot \nabla_z \widetilde{N}(x, z_s) \quad \text{for } x \in \partial\omega \ .$$

But then by the uniqueness of a solution to the Cauchy problem, it follows that

$$\sum_{s=1}^{m} a_s \cdot \nabla_z \widetilde{N}(x, z_s) = e \cdot \nabla_z \widetilde{N}(x, z) \quad \text{for all } x \in \Omega \setminus (\cup_{s=1}^{m}\{z_s\} \cup \{z\}) \ .$$

This is only possible if $z \in \{z_s : s = 1, \ldots, m\}$, and so we have established the necessity of this condition. The sufficiency follows immediately from (iv) in Lemma 7.7. $\qquad\square$

The finite-dimensional self-adjoint operator T can be decomposed as

$$T = \sum_{p=1}^{dm} \lambda_p v_p \, v_p^*, \quad ||v_p||_{L^2(\partial\omega)} = 1 \ ,$$

say with $|\lambda_1| \geq |\lambda_2| \geq \ldots \geq |\lambda_{dm}| > 0$. Let $P_p : L_0^2(\partial\omega) \rightarrow \text{span}\,\{v_1, \ldots, v_p\}$, $p = 1, \ldots, dm$, be the orthogonal projector $P_p = \sum_{q=1}^{p} v_q \, v_q^*$.
From Theorem 7.1 it follows that

$$z \in \{z_s : s = 1, \ldots, m\} \quad \text{iff} \quad (I - P_{dm})(e \cdot \nabla_z \widetilde{N}(\cdot, z)|_{\partial\omega}) = 0 \ ,$$

or equivalently, if we define the angle $\theta(z) \in [0, \pi/2)$ by

$$\cot \theta(z) = \frac{||P_{dm}(e \cdot \nabla_z \widetilde{N}(\cdot, z)|_{\partial\omega})||_{L^2(\partial\omega)}}{||(I - P_{dm})(e \cdot \nabla_z \widetilde{N}(\cdot, z)|_{\partial\omega})||_{L^2(\partial\omega)}} \ ,$$

then we have

$$z \in \{z_s : s = 1, \ldots, m\} \quad \text{iff} \quad \cot \theta(z) = +\infty \ .$$

On the other hand, since $\Lambda_D - \Lambda_0$ is a self-adjoint and compact operator on $L_0^2(\partial\omega)$, it admits, by the spectral theorem, the spectral decomposition

$$\Lambda_D - \Lambda_0 = \sum_{p=1}^{+\infty} \kappa_p^\epsilon v_p^\epsilon \, (v_p^\epsilon)^* \ , \quad ||v_p^\epsilon||_{L^2(\partial\omega)} = 1 \ ,$$

with $|\kappa_1^\epsilon| \geq |\kappa_2^\epsilon| \geq \ldots \geq |\kappa_{dm}^\epsilon| \geq \ldots \geq 0$. Let $P_p^\epsilon : L_0^2(\partial\omega) \rightarrow \text{span}\,\{v_1^\epsilon, \ldots, v_p^\epsilon\}$, $p = 1, 2, \ldots$, be the orthogonal projector $P_p^\epsilon = \sum_{q=1}^{p} v_q^\epsilon \, (v_q^\epsilon)^*$. Standard arguments from perturbation theory for linear operators [186] give (after appropriate enumeration of $\kappa_p^\epsilon, p = 1, \ldots, dm$)

$$\kappa_p^\epsilon = \epsilon^d \kappa_p + O(\epsilon^{d+1}) \quad \text{for } p = 1, 2, \ldots , \tag{7.23}$$

where we have set $\kappa_p = 0$ for $p > dm$, and

$$P_p^\epsilon = P_{dm} + O(\epsilon) \quad \text{for } p \geq dm , \tag{7.24}$$

provided that one makes appropriate choices of eigenvectors v_p^ϵ and $v_p, p = 1, \ldots, dm$.

Now in view of (7.23), the number m of inclusions may be estimated by looking for a gap in the set of eigenvalues of $\Lambda_D - \Lambda_0$. In order to recover the locations $z_s, s = 1, \ldots, m$, one can estimate, using (7.24), the $\cot \theta(z)$ by

$$\cot \theta_p(z) = \frac{||P_p^\epsilon (e \cdot \nabla_z \widetilde{N}(\cdot, z))|_{\partial \omega})||_{L^2(\partial \omega)}}{||(I - P_p^\epsilon)(e \cdot \nabla_z \widetilde{N}(\cdot, z)|_{\partial \omega})||_{L^2(\partial \omega)}} .$$

If one plots $\cot \theta_{dm}(z)$ as a function of z, we may see large values for z that are close to the positions z_s. The viability of this direct approach has been documented by several numerical examples in [73]. In particular, its ability to efficiently locate a high number of inclusions has been clearly demonstrated.

When comparing the different methods that have been designed for imaging small inclusions, it is fair to point out that the variational method and the sampling linear approach use "many boundary measurements." In contrast, the projection algorithm, the quadratic algorithm, and the least-squares algorithm only rely on "single measurements," and not surprisingly, they are more limited in their abilities to effectively locate a higher number of small inclusions.

7.8 Lipschitz-Continuous Dependence and Moment Estimations

7.8.1 Lipschitz-Continuous Dependence

We now prove a Lipschitz-continuous dependence of the location and relative size of two sets of inclusions on the difference in the boundary voltage potentials corresponding to a fixed current distribution. This explains the practical success of various numerical algorithms to detect the location and size of unknown small inclusions.

Consider two arbitrary collections of inclusions

$$D = \cup_{s=1}^m (\epsilon \rho_s B + z_s) \text{ and } D' = \cup_{s=1}^{m'} (\epsilon \rho_s' B + z_s') ,$$

which both satisfy (7.16). The parameter ϵ determines the common length scale of the inclusions and the parameters $\rho_s, 0 < c_0 \leq \rho_s \leq C_0$, for some constant C_0, determine their relative sizes. We suppose that all inclusions have the same known conductivity $0 < k \neq 1 < +\infty$. Let u and u' denote the corresponding voltage potentials [with fixed boundary current $g \in L_0^2(\partial\Omega)$]. It is crucial to assume that $\nabla U(x) \neq 0, \forall\, x \in \Omega$, where U is the background solution. Introduce $H[g] = -\mathcal{S}_\Omega g + \mathcal{D}_\Omega u$ and $H'[g] = -\mathcal{S}_\Omega g + \mathcal{D}_\Omega u'$.

By iterating the asymptotic formula (7.3), we arrive at the following expansions:

$$
\begin{aligned}
H[g](x) &= -\sum_{s=1}^{m}\sum_{|i|=1}^{d}\sum_{|j|=1}^{d}\frac{(\epsilon\rho_s)^{|i|+|j|+d-2}}{i!j!}(\partial^i U)(z_s)\partial_z^j\Gamma(x-z_s)M_{ij}(k,B) \\
&\quad + O(\epsilon^{2d})\,,
\end{aligned}
$$

$$
\begin{aligned}
H'[g](x) &= -\sum_{s=1}^{m'}\sum_{|i|=1}^{d}\sum_{|j|=1}^{d}\frac{(\epsilon\rho_s')^{|i|+|j|+d-2}}{i!j!}(\partial^i U)(z_s')\partial_z^j\Gamma(x-z_s')M_{ij}(k,B) \\
&\quad + O(\epsilon^{2d})\,.
\end{aligned}
$$
$$(7.25)$$

The following theorem, due to Friedman and Vogelius [132], shows that for small ϵ the locations of the inclusions z_s and their relative sizes ρ_s depend Lipschitz-continuously on $\epsilon^{-d}\|H[g] - H'[g]\|_{L^\infty(S)}$ for any $\mathcal{C}^2$-closed surface (or curve in $\mathbb{R}^2$) S enclosing the domain Ω.

Theorem 7.8 *Let S be a $\mathcal{C}^2$-closed surface (or curve in $\mathbb{R}^2$) enclosing the domain Ω. Constants $0 < \epsilon_0, \delta_0$, and C exist such that, if $\epsilon < \epsilon_0$ and $\epsilon^{-d}\|H[g] - H'[g]\|_{L^\infty(S)} < \delta_0$, then*

(i) $m = m'$, and, after appropriate reordering,

(ii) $|z_s - z_s'| + |\rho_s - \rho_s'| \leq C\left(\epsilon^{-d}\|H[g] - H'[g]\|_{L^\infty(S)} + \epsilon\right).$

The constants ϵ_0, δ_0 and C depend on $c_0, C_0, \Omega, S, B, k$ but are otherwise independent of the two sets of inclusions.

Proof. From (7.25) we get

$$
\begin{aligned}
\epsilon^{-d}\Big(H[g](x) - H'[g](x)\Big) &= \Bigg[\sum_{s=1}^{m'}(\rho_s')^d(\partial U)(z_s')\partial_z\Gamma(x-z_s')M(k,B) \\
&\quad - \sum_{s=1}^{m}(\rho_s)^d(\partial U)(z_s)\partial_z\Gamma(x-z_s)M(k,B)\Bigg] + O(\epsilon)\,,
\end{aligned}
$$

for all $x \in S$. Suppose now the assertion $m = m'$ is not true. Then a function of the form $F(x) = \sum_{s=1}^{m'}\partial_z\Gamma(x-z_s')\cdot\alpha_s' - \sum_{s=1}^{m}\partial_z\Gamma(x-z_s)\cdot\alpha_s$ exists, with $\alpha_s' \neq 0$ and $\alpha_s \neq 0$, such that $F(x) = 0$ for all $x \in S$. To see that α_s' as well as α_s are not zero, we use the fact that ∇U never vanishes and that the polarization tensor $M(k,B)$ is invertible. Let Ω' denote the region outside S. From the uniqueness of a solution to $\Delta F = 0$ in $\Omega', F = 0$ on $S, F(x) = O(|x|^{-d+1})$ as $|x| \to +\infty$, it follows that $\partial F/\partial\nu = 0$ on S. But F is also harmonic in $\mathbb{R}^d \setminus (\{z_s\} \cup \{z'_s\})$. From the uniqueness of a solution to the Cauchy problem for the Laplacian, we then conclude that $F \equiv 0$ in $\mathbb{R}^d$. This contradicts contradicts the fact that $m \neq m'$.

When it comes to proving (ii) assume for the sake of simplicity that $U(x) = x_1 - (1/|\partial|\Omega|) \int_{\partial\Omega} U$ (corresponding to the boundary current $g = \nu_1$). Then

$$
\epsilon^{-d}\left(H[g](x) - H'[g](x) \right) = \sum_{s=1}^{m} \Big[(\rho'_s)^d \partial_z \Gamma(x - z'_s)
$$
$$
- (\rho_s)^d \partial_z \Gamma(x - z_s) \Big] (M(k, B))_1 + O(\epsilon) \, ,
\tag{7.26}
$$

for all $x \in S$, where $(M(k, B))_1$ is the first column of the matrix $M(k, B)$. A simple calculation shows that, for some $\overline{\rho_s}$ and $\overline{z_s}$,

$$
\sum_{s=1}^{m} \Big[(\rho'_s)^d \partial_z \Gamma(x - z'_s) - (\rho_s)^d \partial_z \Gamma(x - z_s) \Big] (M(k, B))_1
$$
$$
= \sum_{s=1}^{m} \Big[d(\rho'_s - \rho_s)(\overline{\rho_s})^{d-1} \partial_z \Gamma(x - z'_s) + \rho_s^d (z'_s - z_s) \cdot \partial_z^2 \Gamma(x - \overline{z_s}) \Big] (M(k, B))_1
$$
$$
= \sum_{s=1}^{m} \left(|z_s - z'_s| + |\rho_s - \rho'_s| \right)
$$
$$
\times \sum_{s=1}^{m} \Big[d\, \partial\rho_s \, (\overline{\rho_s})^{d-1} \partial_z \Gamma(x - z'_s) + \rho_s^d \partial z_s \cdot \partial_z^2 \Gamma(x - \overline{z_s}) \Big] (M(k, B))_1 \, ,
$$

where

$$
\partial\rho_s = \frac{(\rho'_s - \rho_s)}{\sum_{s=1}^{m} \left(|z_s - z'_s| + |\rho_s - \rho'_s| \right)}
$$

and

$$
\partial z_s = \frac{(z'_s - z_s)}{\sum_{s=1}^{m} \left(|z_s - z'_s| + |\rho_s - \rho'_s| \right)} \, .
$$

Suppose the estimate (ii) is not true. Then perturbations $\partial\rho_s$ and ∂z_s exist with $\sum_{s=1}^{m} |\partial\rho_s| + |\partial z_s| = 1$, points $z_s \, (= z'_s = \overline{z_s})$, and parameters $\rho_s (= \rho'_s = \overline{\rho_s})$ so that

$$
G(x) = \sum_{s=1}^{m} \Big[d\, \partial\rho_s \, (\rho_s)^{d-1} \partial_z \Gamma(x - z_s) + \rho_s^d \partial z_s \cdot \partial_z^2 \Gamma(x - z_s) \Big] (M(k, B))_1 = 0
$$

for all $x \in S$. Just as was the case with F, the function G has a vanishing normal derivative on S and it is harmonic except at the points $\{z_s\}$ and $\{z'_s\}$. Therefore, by the unique continuation property of harmonic functions, $G \equiv 0$ and thus, $\partial\rho_s = \partial z_s = 0, s = 1, \ldots m$. This, however, would be a contradiction to the fact that $\sum_{s=1}^{m} |\partial \rho_s| + |\partial z_s| = 1$. We therefore conclude that the desired Lipschitz-continuous dependence estimate holds. $\qquad\square$

The factor ϵ^{-d} in front of $\|H[g] - H'[g]\|_{L^\infty(S)}$ is the best possible option; it follows immediately from (7.25) that even $|z_s - z'_s|$ and $|\rho_s - \rho'_s|$ are of order 1; then $\|H[g] - H'[g]\|_{L^\infty(S)}$ is of order ϵ^d. The use of the L^∞-norm of $H[g] - H'[g]$ on S is not essential; in fact other norms, such as the L^1-norm, can be used.

In the two-dimensional case, the results in Theorem 7.8 have some similarity to the results about the location of poles for meromorphic functions found in [233]. The idea is quite simple. Suppose $d = 2$; then (7.26) reads

$$\epsilon^{-2}\left(H[g](x) - H'[g](x) \right) = -\frac{1}{2\pi} \sum_{s=1}^{m'} (\rho'_s)^2 \frac{(x - z'_s)}{|x - z'_s|^2} (M(k, B))_1$$

$$+ \frac{1}{2\pi} \sum_{s=1}^{m} (\rho_s)^2 \frac{(x - z'_s)}{|x - z'_s|^2} (M(k, B))_1 + O(\epsilon) .$$

Identifying $\mathbb{R}^2$ with $\mathbb{C}$ as in the simple pole method yields

$$\epsilon^{-2}\left(H[g](x) - H'[g](x) \right) = \Re\left(\sum_{s=1}^{m'} \frac{\alpha'_s}{x - z'_s} - \sum_{s=1}^{m} \frac{\alpha_s}{x - z_s} \right) + O(\epsilon) ,$$

for all $x \in S$, where the constants $\alpha_s = -(1/2\pi)\rho_s^2((M(k, B))_{11} + i(M(k, B))_{12})$ and $\alpha'_s = -(1/2\pi)(\rho'_s)^2((M(k, B))_{11} + i(M(k, B))_{12})$ are of order 1. Therefore,

$$\sum_{s=1}^{m'} \frac{\alpha'_s}{x - z'_s} - \sum_{s=1}^{m} \frac{\alpha_s}{x - z_s} = \epsilon^{-2}\left(H[g](x) - H'[g](x) \right)$$

$$+ i\epsilon^{-2} \int_a^x \frac{\partial}{\partial \nu}\left(H[g](y) - H'[g](y) \right) d\sigma(y) + O(\epsilon) ,$$

for some complex constant $a \in S$.

Here

$$\int_a^x \frac{\partial}{\partial \nu}\left(H[g](y) - H'[g](y) \right) d\sigma(y)$$

is a harmonic conjugate to $H[g](x) - H'[g](x)$, and it satisfies

$$\left\| \int_a^x \frac{\partial}{\partial \nu}\left(H[g](y) - H'[g](y) \right) d\sigma(y) \right\|_{L^\infty(S)} \leq C \|H[g] - H'[g]\|_{L^\infty(S)} ,$$

for some constant C independent of ϵ. Since the poles $\{z_s\}$ and $\{z'_s\}$ are well separated and the pole residues $\{\rho_s\}$ and $\{\rho'_s\}$ are well bounded from zero, it follows from [233, Theorem 1] that parts (i) and (ii) in Theorem 7.8 hold.

7.8.2 Moment Estimations

Consider a collection of inclusions $D = \cup_{s=1}^{m}(\epsilon B_s + z_s)$, which satisfy (7.16). Our goal is to obtain upper and lower bounds on the moments of the unknown inclusions B_s. Observe that $\sum_{|i|=1}^{d} \partial^i U(z_s) x^i$ is a harmonic polynomial. Let S be a $\mathcal{C}^2$-closed surface (or curve in $\mathbb{R}^2$) enclosing the domain Ω. From

$$H[g](x) = -\sum_{s=1}^{m} \sum_{|i|=1}^{d} \sum_{|j|=1}^{d} \frac{\epsilon^{|i|+|j|+d-2}}{i!j!} (\partial^i U)(z_s) \partial_z^j \Gamma(x-z_s) M_{ij}^s + O(\epsilon^{2d}) \text{ on } S,$$

where $g = \partial U/\partial \nu$ and $M_{ij}^s = M_{ij}(k_s, B_s)$, we compute by Green's formula

$$\int_S \left(\frac{\partial}{\partial \nu} H[g]\, U - H[g]\, g \right) d\sigma$$

$$= -\sum_{s=1}^{m} \sum_{|i|=1}^{d} \sum_{|j|=1}^{d} \frac{\epsilon^{|i|+|j|+d-2}}{i!j!} \partial^i U(z_s) M_{ij}^s \partial^j U(z_s) + O(\epsilon^{2d}) \,.$$

Then, as a direct consequence of Theorem 4.13, the following moment estimations hold. Note that, in general, they are only meaningful if the conductivities $\{k_s\}_{s=1}^{m}$ and the locations $\{z_s\}_{s=1}^{m}$ are known.

Theorem 7.9 *We have*

$$\epsilon^{2-d} \left| \int_S \left(\frac{\partial}{\partial \nu} H[g]\, U - H[g]\, g \right) d\sigma \right| \leq \sum_{s=1}^{m} (k_s - 1) \int_{B_s} \left| \nabla \left(\sum_{|i|=1}^{d} \frac{\epsilon^{|i|}}{i!} \partial^i U(z_s) x^i \right) \right|^2 dx$$

and

$$\epsilon^{2-d} \left| \int_S \left(\frac{\partial}{\partial \nu} H[g]\, U - H[g]\, g \right) d\sigma \right| \geq \sum_{s=1}^{m} (1 - \frac{1}{k_s}) \int_{B_s} \left| \nabla \left(\sum_{|i|=1}^{d} \frac{\epsilon^{|i|}}{i!} \partial^i U(z_s) x^i \right) \right|^2 dx.$$

7.9 Detection of Anisotropic Inclusions

Efficient direct algorithms for reconstructing small anisotropic inclusions have been developed by Kang, Kim, and Kim in [175]. To bring out the main ideas of these algorithms we only consider the case where D has one component of the form $D = \epsilon B + z$. For a given $g \in L_0^2(\partial\Omega)$, let u be the solution to the Neumann problem (5.29). The background potential U is the steady-state voltage potential in the absence of the conductivity inclusion, i.e., the solution to (5.30). We now define a function $H^A[g]$ for $g \in L_0^2(\partial\Omega)$ by

$$H^A[g](x) = -\mathcal{S}_\Omega^A(g)(x) + \mathcal{D}_\Omega^A(u|_{\partial\Omega})(x), \quad x \in \mathbb{R}^d \setminus \overline{\Omega} \,. \tag{7.27}$$

By Theorem 5.12, the following asymptotic expansion of $H^A[g]$ outside Ω holds; see [175].

Theorem 7.10 *For $x \in \mathbb{R}^d \setminus \overline{\Omega}$,*

$$H^A[g](x) = -\epsilon^d \sum_{|i|=1}^{d} \sum_{|j|=1}^{d-|i|+1} \frac{\epsilon^{|i|+|j|-2}}{i!j!} \partial^i U(z) M_{ij} \partial_z^j \Gamma^A(x-z) + O(\frac{\epsilon^{2d}}{|x|^{d-1}}) .$$

$$(7.28)$$

Suppose now that $g = \nu \cdot Aa$ for a constant vector $a \in \mathbb{R}^d$. Therefore, $U(x) = a \cdot x$ and the formula (7.28) takes the form

$$H^A[g](x) = -\epsilon^d \sum_{|i|=1}^{d} \sum_{|j|=1}^{d} \frac{\epsilon^{|j|-1}}{j!} \partial^i U(z) M_{ij} \partial_z^j \Gamma^A(x-z) + O(\frac{\epsilon^{2d}}{|x|^{d-1}}) . \quad (7.29)$$

Then by explicitly computing $\partial_z^j \Gamma^A(x-z)$, we can show that

$$H^A[g](x) = \frac{1}{\omega_d} \langle a, \epsilon^d M A_* \frac{A_*(x-z)}{|A_*(x-z)|^d} \rangle + O(\frac{\epsilon^d}{|x|^d}) + O(\frac{\epsilon^{2d}}{|x|^{d-1}}) , \quad (7.30)$$

where $\omega_d = 2\pi$ if $d = 2$, and $\omega_d = 4\pi$ if $d = 3$, and $M = (M_{pq})$ is the first-order APT.

For a general Neumann data g, we have

$$H^A[g](x) = \frac{1}{\omega_d} \langle \nabla U(z), \epsilon^d M A_* \frac{A_*(x-z)}{|A_*(x-z)|^d} \rangle + O(\frac{\epsilon^d}{|x|^d}) + O(\frac{\epsilon^{d+1}}{|x|^{d-1}}) . \quad (7.31)$$

Since

$$\frac{A_*(x-z)}{|A_*(x-z)|^d} = \frac{A_*x}{|A_*x|^d} + O(|x|^{-d}) ,$$

we obtain from (7.30) and (7.31) the following far-field relations [175].

Theorem 7.11 *For $g \in L_0^2(\partial\Omega)$, let U be the solution of (5.30). Then, for $|x| = O(\epsilon^{-1})$,*

$$\omega_d |A_*x|^{d-1} H^A[g](x) = \langle \nabla U(z), \epsilon^d M A_* \frac{A_*x}{|A_*x|} \rangle + O(\epsilon^{d+1}) . \quad (7.32)$$

If $g = \nu \cdot Aa$, then for $|x| = O(\epsilon^{-d})$

$$\omega_d |A_*x|^{d-1} H^A[g](x) = \langle a, \epsilon^d M A_* \frac{A_*x}{|A_*x|} \rangle + O(\epsilon^{2d}) . \quad (7.33)$$

We note that (7.32) is a general far-field relation, whereas (7.33) is a formula with better precision.

Using (7.30), (7.32), and (7.33), we can detect the APT, the order of magnitude of D, and z.

Detection of APT: Now let $a = e_p$, or equivalently, $g = \nu \cdot Ae_p$, and choose $b_q = O(\epsilon^{-d})$ so that

$$A_* \frac{A_* b_q}{|A_* b_q|} = e_q, \quad p, q = 1, \ldots, d . \tag{7.34}$$

It then follows from (7.33) that

$$\epsilon^d M_{pq} = \omega_d |A_* b_q|^{d-1} H^A[g](b_q) + O(\epsilon^{2d}) . \tag{7.35}$$

Since ϵ is not known *a priori*, in actual computations we first find unit vectors b_q satisfying (7.34) and then compute $\omega_d |t A_* b_q|^{d-1} H^A[g](t b_q)$ as $t \to +\infty$. Since the first-order APT is invariant under translation as we can easily check, $\epsilon^d M$ is the first-order APT for the domain D.

Detection of Order of Magnitude: Having determined $\epsilon^d M$, we proceed to find the order of magnitude ϵ and the center z. Using Corollary 4.35, we can determine the order of magnitude of D. Let κ be the smallest (in absolute value) eigenvalue of $\epsilon^d M$. Then, $\epsilon^d |B| \approx |\kappa|$.

Detection of Center—Method 1: Let v_q, $q = 1, \cdots, d$, be orthonormal eigenvectors of the symmetric matrix $A_*(\epsilon^d M) A_*$ with the corresponding eigenvalue κ_q, and $a_q := A_* v_q$ and $g_q := \nu \cdot A a_q$. Let $x(t) := t a_q + O(\epsilon^{-1}) a_q^\perp$, where $a_q^\perp$ is a vector perpendicular to a_q. Then $|x(t)| = O(\epsilon^{-1})$ and hence, by (7.30), we get

$$H^A[g_q](x(t)) = \frac{\kappa_q}{\omega_d} \frac{|a_q|^2 t - a_q \cdot z}{|A_*(x(t) - z)|^d} + O(\epsilon^{2d}) . \tag{7.36}$$

Find the unique zero, and call it t_q, of $H^A[g_q](x(t))$ as a function of t for $q = 1, \cdots, d$. Let $\bar{z} = t_1 a_1 + \cdots + t_d a_d$. This $\bar{z}$ is the center. In fact, by the same argument as in [43], we can prove that $|\bar{z} - z| = O(\epsilon^d)$.

Detection of Center—Method 2: Let b_q, $q = 1, \cdots, d$, be the unit vector defined by (7.34). Then, from (7.32), we get

$$\omega_d |t A_* b_q|^{d-1} H^A[g](t b_q) = \langle \nabla U(z), \epsilon^d M e_q \rangle + O(\epsilon^{d+1}) . \tag{7.37}$$

Let $g = \nu \cdot A \nabla U$, where U is a second-order homogeneous harmonic polynomial. By computing $\omega_d |t A_* b_q|^{d-1} H^A[g](t b_q)$ as $t \to +\infty$, we recover $\langle \nabla U(z), \epsilon^d M e_q \rangle$, $q = 1, \cdots, d$. From this we now recover $\nabla U(z)$, and hence the center z modulo $O(\epsilon)$.

The precision of this method is $O(\epsilon)$, which is worse than Method 1. However, numerical experiments in the next section show that this method performs better when there is noise in the data.

Computational Experiments: We now present results of numerical experiments from [175]. In the following, Ω is assumed to be the disk centered at $(0, 0)$ with radius $r = 2$, and the background conductivity $A = I$. We also assume that $D = \epsilon B + z$, where B is the unit disk centered at $(0, 0)$. We note that, in the anisotropic case, D being a disk does not provide a special advantage. Moreover, in the process of solving the inverse problem, we do not use any *a priori* knowledge of D being a disk.

Let u be the solution of (5.29). In order to collect the data $u|_{\partial\Omega}$, we solve the direct problem (5.29) as follows: u is represented by

$$u(x) = \begin{cases} \mathcal{D}_\Omega^A u(x) - \mathcal{S}_\Omega^A g(x) + \mathcal{S}_D^A \phi(x) & \text{in } \Omega \setminus \overline{D}, \\ \mathcal{S}_D^{\tilde{A}} \psi(x) & \text{in } D, \end{cases}$$

where $u|_{\partial\Omega}$, ϕ, and ψ satisfy the following relations:

$$u = \mathcal{D}_\Omega^A u\big|_- - \mathcal{S}_\Omega^A g\big|_- + \mathcal{S}_D^A \phi \qquad \text{on } \partial\Omega,$$

$$\mathcal{D}_\Omega^A u - \mathcal{S}_\Omega^A g + \mathcal{S}_D^A \phi\big|_+ = \mathcal{S}_D^{\tilde{A}} \phi\big|_- \qquad \text{on } \partial D,$$

$$\frac{\partial}{\partial\nu}\mathcal{D}_\Omega^A u - \frac{\partial}{\partial\nu}\mathcal{S}_\Omega^A g + \frac{\partial}{\partial\nu}\mathcal{S}_D^A \phi\big|_+ = \frac{\partial}{\partial\tilde{\nu}}\mathcal{S}_D^{\tilde{A}} \phi\big|_- \qquad \text{on } \partial D.$$

We solve this integral equation using the collocation method [204] and obtain $u|_{\partial\Omega}$ on $\partial\Omega$ for given data g. We also add some noise to the computed data. Adding $p\%$ noise means that we have

$$u\left(1 + \frac{p}{100} \cdot \text{rand}(1)\right)$$

as the measured Dirichlet data. Here $\text{rand}(1)$ is the random number in $]-1, 1[$.

Reconstruction Algorithm 1:

Step 1 Obtain Dirichlet data u on $\partial\Omega$ for a given Neumann data $g_q = \nu \cdot A e_q$, $q = 1, 2$.

Step 2 For $p, q = 1, 2$, calculate $\lim_{t \to +\infty} w_2 t H^A[g_p](t e_q)$ to obtain the matrix $\epsilon^2 M$.

Step 3 Find orthonormal eigenvectors v_1, v_2 and corresponding eigenvalues κ_1, κ_2 of $\epsilon^2 M$. Let κ be the minimum of $|\kappa_1|, |\kappa_2|$. The order of magnitude of D is $\epsilon = \sqrt{\kappa |B|^{-1}}$.

Step 4 Let $g_j' = \nu \cdot A v_j$ and $x_q(t) = t v_q + \frac{1}{\epsilon} v_q^\perp$, $q = 1, 2$. Find the zero, say t_q, of $H^A[g_q'](x_q(t)) = v_q \cdot e_1 H^A[g](x_q(t)) + v_q \cdot e_2 H^A[g_2](x_q(t))$ as a function of t. We obtain the center $\overline{z} = t_1 v_1 + t_2 v_2$.

Reconstruction Algorithm 2: Step 4 in the above algorithm is replaced with

Step 4' For $g = \nu \cdot A\nabla(x_1 x_2)$, compute $h_q = \lim_{t \to +\infty} w_2 t H^A[g](t e_q)$, $q = 1, 2$. Then $(z_1, z_2) = (h_1, h_2) \begin{pmatrix} \epsilon^2 M_{12} & \epsilon^2 M_{22} \\ \epsilon^2 M_{11} & \epsilon^2 M_{12} \end{pmatrix}^{-1}$. We add the same amount of random noise in this step as well.

The following computational experiments from [175] clearly demonstrate the viability of the reconstruction algorithms. The first experiment is when $\widetilde{A} - A$ is positive-definite; the second one is when $\widetilde{A} - A$ is not positive-definite; the third one is to investigate the role of the condition number of $\widetilde{A} - A$ in the reconstruction process.

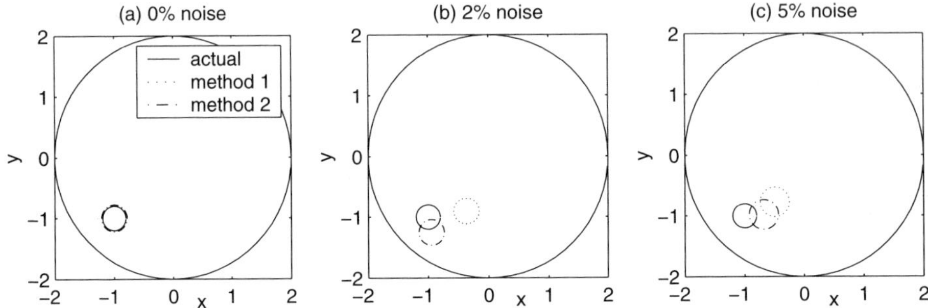

Fig. 7.7. First example.

z	r	noise(%)	$\overline{r}$	$\overline{z}_1$	$|z - \overline{z}_1|$
				$\overline{z}_2$	$|z - \overline{z}_2|$
		0	0.2204	$(-0.9994, -0.9994)$	8.1154e-004
				$(-0.9994, -0.9994)$	8.4362e-004
		2	0.2101	$(-0.3681, -0.9038)$	0.6391
$(-1, -1)$	0.2			$(-0.9445, -1.2519)$	0.2580
		5	0.2463	$(-0.4936, -0.7715)$	0.5556
				$(-0.6787, -0.9790)$	0.3220

Table 7.2. Results of the first example. Here r and $\overline{r}$ are the actual and computed radii, and z, $\overline{z}_1$ and $\overline{z}_2$ are the actual and the computed radii by Algorithms 1 and 2, respectively.

Experiment 1: Let $\widetilde{A} = \begin{pmatrix} 10 & 2 \\ 2 & 5 \end{pmatrix}$ and the actual inclusion, $D = (-1, -1) + 0.2B$. Note that $\widetilde{A} - A$ is positive-definite. Figure 7.7 shows the results when there is 0%, 2%, and 5% random noise. Figure 7.8 is the result when $\widetilde{A} = \begin{pmatrix} 10 & 1 \\ 1 & 2 \end{pmatrix}$ and $D = (0, 1) + 0.2B$.

These results show that both Algorithms 1 and 2 detect the order of magnitude of the inclusion fairly well even in the presence of noise. However, Algorithm 2 performs better than Algorithm 1 in detecting the center when

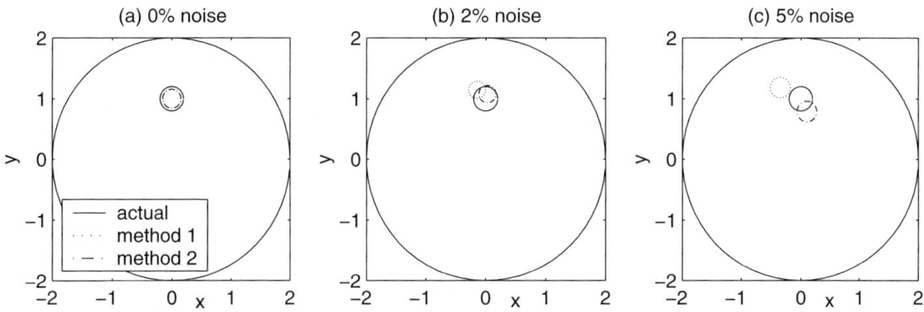

Fig. 7.8. Second example.

z	r	noise(%)	$\overline{r}$	$\overline{z}_1$	$|z - \overline{z}_1|$
				$\overline{z}_2$	$|z - \overline{z}_2|$
		0	0.1557	$(-0.0000, 0.9999)$	1.2316e-004
				$(-0.0000, 0.9998)$	1.6690e-004
		2	0.1417	$(-0.1421, 1.1468)$	0.2043
$(0, 1)$	0.2			$(0.0288, 1.0771)$	0.0823
		5	0.1689	$(-0.3499, 1.1841)$	0.3954
				$(0.1036, 0.7906)$	0.2336

Table 7.3. Results of the second example.

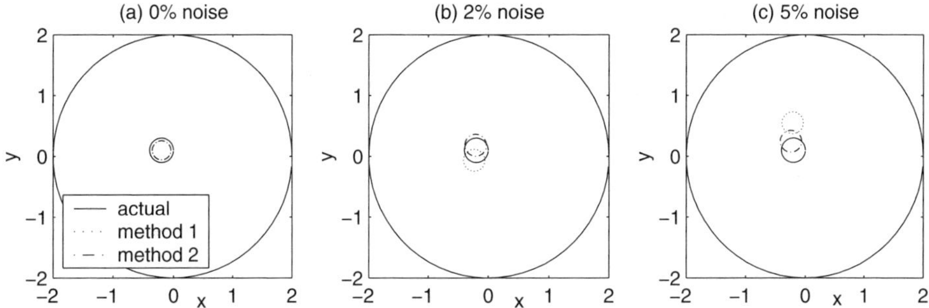

Fig. 7.9. Third example.

there is noise. A probable cause for this result is that the zeros of the functions in (7.36), which are already small in magnitude, are very sensitive to the noise.

Figure 7.9 shows that the location of the unknown inclusions does not affect the performance of the algorithms as long as they are away from $\partial\Omega$.

Experiment 2: This experiment is to see whether the algorithms work in the case where $\widetilde{A} - A$ is not positive- or negative-definite. Let $\widetilde{A} = \begin{pmatrix} 2 & 0 \\ 0 & \frac{1}{2} \end{pmatrix}$ and $D =$

z	r	noise(%)	$\overline{r}$	$\overline{z}_1$	$|z - \overline{z}_1|$
				$\overline{z}_2$	$|z - \overline{z}_2|$
		0	0.1559	$(-0.2000, 0.1000)$	1.2081e-005
				$(-0.2000, 0.1000)$	1.6354e-005
		2	0.1798	$(-0.2342, -0.0643)$	0.1678
$(-0.2, 0.1)$	0.2			$(-0.2108, 0.1830)$	0.0837
		5	0.1785	$(-0.2120, 0.5493)$	0.4495
				$(-0.2405, 0.2464)$	0.1519

Table 7.4. Results of the third example.

$(1,0)+0.2B$. Figure 7.10 shows the result. The algorithm seems to be working equally well for this case. It would be interesting to prove that the reconstruction formulae hold even when $\widetilde{A} - A$ is not positive- or negative-definite. In this example as well, Algorithm 2 performs better in detecting the center.

Experiment 3: This experiment tests how the condition number of $\widetilde{A} - A$ affects the precision of the algorithm. Suppose $A = I$. We first take $\widetilde{A} = \begin{pmatrix} \tau & 0 \\ 0 & 2 \end{pmatrix}$ and observe how the relative error $|z - \overline{z}|/\epsilon^2$ changes as τ increases. We then take $\widetilde{A} = \begin{pmatrix} \tau+1 & 0 \\ 0 & \tau \end{pmatrix}$ and make the same observations. Figure 7.11 compares changes of relative errors in these two cases where $\tau = 10, 10^2, 10^4, 10^5, 10^6$. It exhibits a clear difference: In the first case when the condition number of $\widetilde{A} - A$ increases as τ increases, the relative error is increasing, whereas in the second case when the condition number does not change, the error is stabilized. The second case is somewhat similar to the isotropic case and this kind of result is expected; see [181] or [23]. It is known that long and thin inclusions, or crack-like inclusions (inclusions of high Lipschitz character), are hard to detect; see, for example, [43]. This experiment suggests that in addition to this geometric obstruction, in the anisotropic case there is another obstruction of high condition number of $\widetilde{A} - A$.

Numerical results show that the second reconstruction algorithm performs better in the presence of noise. They also show that the reconstruction procedure works well even when $A - \widetilde{A}$ is not positive-or negative-definite, and that the error of reconstruction increases as the condition number of $A - \widetilde{A}$ increases. It would be interesting to investigate these points in a mathematically rigorous way.

7.10 Further Results and Open Problems

Following our approach throughout this chapter, we have designed efficient and robust algorithms for solving the inverse problem for the Helmholtz equation [19, 20]. We have developed two algorithms that use plane wave sources for identifying small electromagnetic or acoustic inclusions. The first algorithm, like the variational method in Sect. 7.6, reduces the reconstruction problem

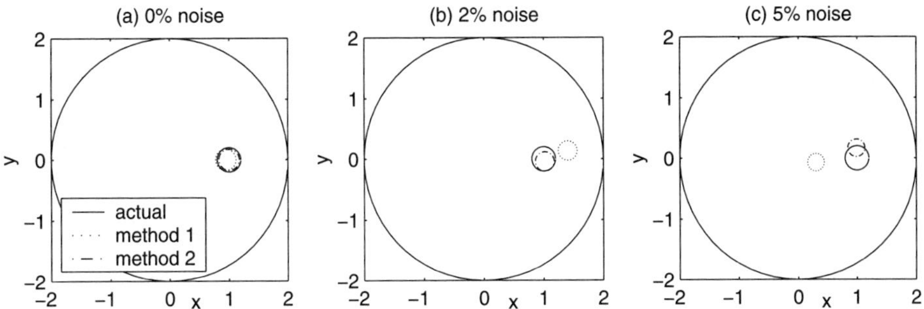

Fig. 7.10. Fourth example.

z	r	noise(%)	$\overline{r}$	$\overline{z}_1$	$\|z - \overline{z}_1\|$
				$\overline{z}_2$	$\|z - \overline{z}_2\|$
		0	0.1739	$(0.9447, -0.0000)$	0.0553
				$(1.0002, -0.0000)$	1.8443e-004
		2	0.1586	$(1.4031, 0.1347)$	0.4250
$(1,0)$	0.2			$(1.0186, -0.0427)$	0.0465
		5	0.1436	$(0.3048, -0.0702)$	0.6987
				$(0.9891, 0.1656)$	0.1660

Table 7.5. Results of the fourth example.

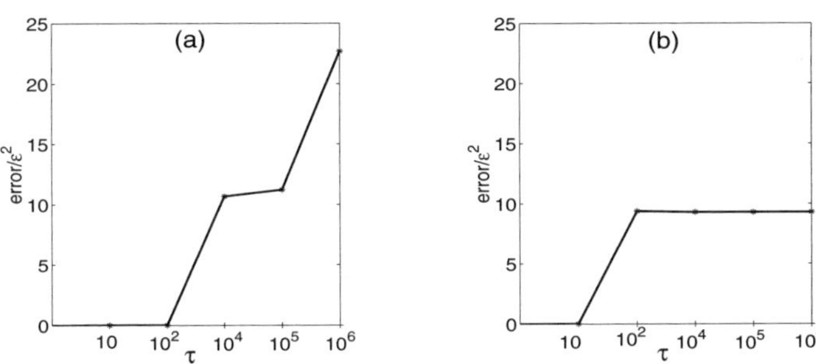

Fig. 7.11. The graphs show how the quantities $|z - \overline{z}|/\epsilon^2$ change as τ goes to $+\infty$. (a) The condition number of $\widetilde{A} - A$ is τ and the relative error increases. (b) The condition number of $\widetilde{A} - A$ is 1 and the relative error does not increase.

of the small inclusions to the calculation of an inverse Fourier transform. The second one is a MUSIC type of algorithm.

The methods presented in this chapter enable detection of the locations and the first-order polarization tensors from the boundary measurements. It is the detected polarization tensor that yields information about the size (and orientation) of the inclusion. However, the information from the first-order polarization tensor is a mixture of the conductivity and the volume. It is impossible to extract the conductivity from the first-order polarization tensor. A small inclusion with high conductivity and larger inclusion with lower conductivity can have the same first-order polarization tensor. It would be interesting and important to extract information about the material property, such as conductivity and anisotropy, of the inclusion from boundary measurements. It is likely that higher order polarization tensors yield such information.

Effective Properties of Electrical Composites

Introduction

The determination of the effective or macroscopic property of a two-phase medium is one of the classic problems in physics. Many distinguished scientists have extensively studied this question for generations, and they, no doubt, deserve for their contributions to be mentioned. The most famous scientists include Maxwell, Rayleigh, Lorentz, Debye, and Einstein, to name but a few.

To begin with, let us define rigorously what we understand by the concept of effective property. Consider $\Omega \subset \mathbb{R}^d$, a bounded domain with a connected Lipschitz boundary $\partial\Omega$, filled with some composite material that consists of a matrix of constant isotropic conductivity $\sigma_0 > 0$ and presents inside the following periodic spatial distribution: an array of periodically spaced cells, each of them wrapping a small isotropic conductivity inclusion that has constant conductivity $\sigma > 0$, of the form $\epsilon^{1+\beta}B$ for some $\beta > 0$. Here B denotes a bounded Lipschitz domain in $\mathbb{R}^d$ containing the origin, and $|B|$ is assumed to be equal to 1. The periodic array has period ϵ. For short, we refer to the material as a periodic dilute composite. As $\epsilon \to 0$, the volume fraction of the inclusions is $f = \epsilon^{d\beta}$.

Let $Y =]-1/2, 1/2[^d$ denote the unit cell and denote $\rho = \epsilon^\beta$. We set the periodic function

$$\gamma = \sigma_0 \chi(Y \setminus D) + \sigma \chi(D) \,,$$

where $D = \rho B$.

For a small parameter ϵ, $\gamma_\epsilon(x) := \gamma(x/\epsilon)$ makes a highly oscillating conductivity and represents the material property of the composite. Figure 8.1 shows a geometry of a composite.

Consider the conductivity problem

$$\nabla \cdot \gamma_\epsilon \nabla u_\epsilon = 0 \quad \text{in } \Omega \tag{8.1}$$

with an appropriate boundary condition on $\partial\Omega$. The theory of homogenization tells us that the solution u_ϵ converges weakly to a function u_0 in $W^{1,2}(\Omega)$

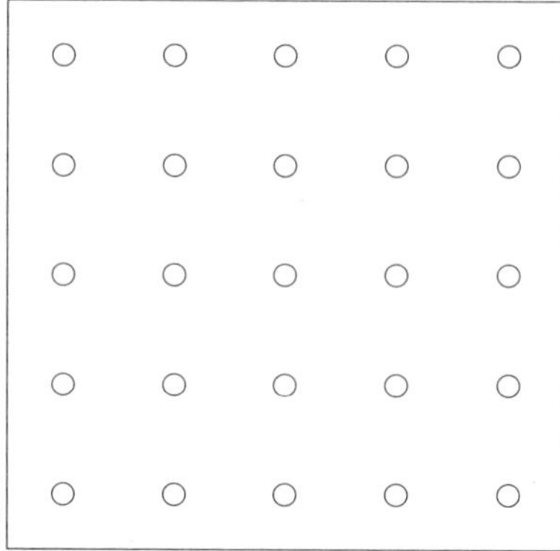

Fig. 8.1. Periodic composite material in $\mathbb{R}^2$. Inclusion $D = \rho B$, distance between inclusions ϵ, and the volume fraction $f = \rho^2$. Conductivity of inclusion equals σ, and conductivity of background equals σ_0.

and a constant (anisotropic) conductivity γ^* exists such that

$$\nabla \cdot \gamma^* \nabla u_0 = 0 \quad \text{in } \Omega . \tag{8.2}$$

The replacement of the original equation (8.1) by (8.2) is a valid approximation in a certain limit [61].

The coefficient γ^* is called an effective conductivity or a homogenized coefficient. It represents the overall macroscopic material property of the periodic composite material; see [173]. For a more intuitive approach, see [236]. See also [94] and [11] for applications to structural optimization.

In general, effective conductivities cannot be computed exactly except for a few configurations. We consider the problem of determining the effective property of the composite when the volume fraction $f = |D|$ goes to zero. In other words, the inclusions have much less volume than the matrix. This kind of material is called a dilute material. Many approximations for the effective properties of composites are based on the solution for dilute materials.

When the inclusion D is a disk or sphere, then the effective electrical conductivity, γ^*, of the composite medium is given by the well-known Maxwell–Garnett formula[1] [277]:

$$\gamma^* = \sigma_0 \left[1 + f \frac{d(\sigma - \sigma_0)}{(\sigma - \sigma_0) + d\sigma_0} + df^2 \frac{(\sigma - \sigma_0)^2}{((\sigma - \sigma_0) + d\sigma_0)^2} \right] I + o(f^2) , \tag{8.3}$$

where $d = 2, 3$ is the space dimension.

This formula has been generalized in many directions: to include higher power terms of the volume fraction f for spherical inclusions [171, 277, 311]; to include other shapes of the inclusion such as ellipses [310, 115, 134, 225, 114,

---

[1] Several different pairs of names are attached to this formula; see [236].

173, 140, 245, 81, 276, 215]; and to include the case when $f = O(1)$; see the book by Milton [236] and the one by Torquato [291] and the references therein.

This chapter begins with the derivation of an asymptotic expansion of the effective electrical conductivity of an isotropic composite medium for arbitrary shaped inclusions. The approach is valid for inclusions with Lipschitz boundaries and high contrast mixtures, and it enables us to compute higher-order terms in the asymptotic expansion of the effective conductivity. After that, with the help of the material developed in Chapter 2, we extend this derivation to anisotropic composites.

Our asymptotic expansions in this chapter have important implications for imaging composites. They show what information can be reconstructed from boundary measurements and how well. It is not surprising that the volume fractions and the GPTs form the only microstructural information that can be reconstructed from boundary measurements. The volume fraction is the simplest but most important piece of microstructural information. The GPTs involve microstructural information beyond that contained in the volume fractions (material contrast, inclusion shape, and orientation). Indeed, if arbitrary shaped inclusions orient according to a certain probability distribution, then our expansions show that only the moments of the orientational distribution functions of the inclusions can be recovered from (experimental) measurements of the effective conductivity of the composite. We refer to Hashin and Monteiro [147] and Torquato [292] for related interesting problems in imaging composites.

8.1 Computation of Effective Conductivity

In this section, we shall explain a scheme for deriving an asymptotic expansion of the effective property of the dilute composite material. This result is from [38]. Our approach can be viewed as a generalization of an elegant method that was first used for problems of the current form by Hasimoto [148, 261]. Hasimoto's method was designed to construct higher order terms in (8.3) when the inclusion is a sphere. It has been implemented numerically yielding results that are valid for fairly large volume fraction f [278].

The effective conductivity matrix $\gamma^* = (\gamma^*_{pq})_{p,q=1,\ldots,d}$ of Ω is defined by (see for instance [173, 236])

$$\gamma^*_{pq} := \int_Y (\sigma_0 \chi(Y \setminus D) + \sigma \chi(D)) \nabla u_p \cdot \nabla u_q \, ,$$

where u_p, for $p = 1, \ldots, d$, is the unique solution to the cell problem

$$\begin{cases} \nabla \cdot (\sigma_0 \chi(Y \setminus D) + \sigma \chi(D)) \nabla u_p = 0 \quad \text{in } Y \, , \\[2mm] u_p - x_p \ \text{periodic (in each direction) with period 1,} \\[2mm] \int_Y u_p = 0 \, . \end{cases} \tag{8.4}$$

Using Green's formula we can rewrite γ^* in the following form:

$$\gamma^*_{pq} = \sigma_0 \int_{\partial Y} u_q \frac{\partial u_p}{\partial \nu} . \tag{8.5}$$

The matrix γ^* depends on ϵ as a parameter and cannot be written explicitly. According to Theorem 2.41, the solution to (8.4) can be written as

$$u_p(x) = x_p + C_p + \mathcal{G}_D(\lambda I - \mathcal{B}_D^*)^{-1}(\nu_p)(x) \quad \text{in } Y, \quad p = 1, \ldots, d ,$$

where λ is given by

$$\lambda = \frac{\sigma + \sigma_0}{2(\sigma - \sigma_0)} . \tag{8.6}$$

For the sake of simplicity, we set for $p = 1, \ldots, d$,

$$\phi_p(y) = (\lambda I - \mathcal{B}_D^*)^{-1}(\nu_p)(y) \quad \text{for } y \in \partial D . \tag{8.7}$$

Thus we get from (8.5)

$$\gamma^*_{pq} = \sigma_0 \int_{\partial Y} (y_q + C + \mathcal{G}_D \phi_q(y)) \frac{\partial}{\partial \nu} (y_p + \mathcal{G}_D \phi_p(y)) \, d\sigma .$$

Because of the periodicity of $\mathcal{G}_D \phi_q$, we get

$$\int_{\partial Y} \frac{\partial}{\partial \nu} \mathcal{G}_D \phi_q \, d\sigma = \int_{\partial Y} \nu_q \mathcal{G}_D \phi_p \, d\sigma = \int_{\partial Y} \mathcal{G}_D \phi_q(y) \frac{\partial}{\partial \nu} \mathcal{G}_D \phi_p(y) \, d\sigma = 0 ,$$

and hence we have

$$\gamma^*_{pq} = \sigma_0 \left[\delta_{pq} + \int_{\partial Y} y_q \frac{\partial}{\partial \nu} \mathcal{G}_D \phi_p(y) \, d\sigma(y) \right] . \tag{8.8}$$

The periodicity of $\mathcal{G}_D \phi_p$ and the divergence theorem applied on $Y \setminus \overline{D}$ yield

$$\int_{\partial Y} y_q \frac{\partial}{\partial \nu} \mathcal{G}_D \phi_p(y) \, d\sigma = \int_{\partial D} y_q \frac{\partial}{\partial \nu} \mathcal{G}_D \phi_p \Big|_+ (y) \, d\sigma - \int_{\partial D} \nu_q \mathcal{G}_D \phi_p(y) \, d\sigma$$

$$= \int_{\partial D} y_q \phi_p(y) \, d\sigma + \int_{\partial D} y_q \frac{\partial}{\partial \nu} \mathcal{G}_D \phi_p \Big|_- (y) \, d\sigma$$

$$- \int_{\partial D} \nu_q \mathcal{G}_D \phi_p(y) \, d\sigma$$

$$= \int_{\partial D} y_q \phi_p(y) \, d\sigma .$$

Let

$$\psi_p(y) = \phi_p(\rho y) \quad \text{for } y \in \partial B .$$

Then by (8.8), we obtain

$$\gamma^* = \sigma_0 [I + f P] , \tag{8.9}$$

where $f = |D| = \rho^d$ is the volume fraction of D and $P := (P_{pq})$ is given by

$$P_{pq} := \int_{\partial B} y_q \psi_p(y)\, d\sigma(y), \quad p, q = 1, \ldots, d\,. \tag{8.10}$$

In order to derive an asymptotic expansion of γ^*, we now expand P in terms of ρ. In view of (2.94), the integral equation (8.7) can be rewritten as

$$(\lambda I - \mathcal{K}_D^*)\phi_p(x) - \int_{\partial D} \frac{\partial}{\partial \nu_x} R_d(x - y)\phi_p(y)\, d\sigma(y) = \nu_p(x), \quad x \in \partial D\,,$$

which, by an obvious change of variables, yields

$$(\lambda I - \mathcal{K}_B^*)\psi_p(x) - \rho^{d-1} \int_{\partial B} \frac{\partial}{\partial \nu_x} R_d(\rho(x - y))\psi_p(y)\, d\sigma(y) = \nu_p(x)\,, \tag{8.11}$$

for $x \in \partial B$.

By virtue of (2.95), we get

$$\nu \cdot \nabla R_d(\rho(x - y)) = -\frac{\rho}{d}\nu \cdot (x - y) + O(\rho^3)$$

uniformly in $x, y \in \partial B$. Since $\int_{\partial B} \psi_p(y)\, d\sigma(y) = 0$, we now have

$$(\lambda I - \mathcal{K}_B^*)\psi_p(x) - \frac{\rho^d}{d}\nu_x \cdot \int_{\partial B} y\psi_p(y)\, d\sigma(y) + O(\rho^{d+2}) = \nu_p(x), \quad x \in \partial B\,.$$

Therefore, we obtain

$$\psi_p = (\lambda I - \mathcal{K}_B^*)^{-1}(\nu_p) + \frac{\rho^d}{d} \sum_{l=1}^{d}(\lambda I - \mathcal{K}_B^*)^{-1}(\nu_l) \cdot \int_{\partial B} y_l \psi_p(y)\, d\sigma(y) \tag{8.12}$$

$$+ O(\rho^{d+2})\,.$$

Let $\widetilde{\psi}_p := (\lambda I - \mathcal{K}_B^*)^{-1}(\nu_p)$, $p = 1, \ldots, d$. Then $m_{pq} = \int_{\partial B} y_q \widetilde{\psi}_p(y)\, d\sigma(y)$, etc.

By iterating the formula (8.12), we get

$$\psi_p = \widetilde{\psi}_p + \frac{\rho^d}{d} \sum_{l=1}^{d} \widetilde{\psi}_l \int_{\partial B} y_l \widetilde{\psi}_p(y)\, d\sigma(y) + O(\rho^{d+2}) \quad \text{on } \partial B\,.$$

It then follows from the definition (8.10) of P that

$$P_{pq} = m_{pq} + \frac{\rho^d}{d} \sum_{l=1}^{d} m_{lq} m_{pl} + O(\rho^{d+2})\,,$$

and then we obtain from (8.9) the following theorem.

Theorem 8.1 *We have*

$$\gamma^* = \sigma_0 \left[I + f M (I - \frac{f}{d} M)^{-1} \right] + o(f^2) \,, \tag{8.13}$$

where M is the Pólya–Szegö polarization tensor associated with the scaled inclusion B and the conductivity $k = \sigma_0(2\lambda + 1)/(2\lambda - 1)$. Here λ is given by (8.6).

Formula (8.13) relates Theorem 4.16 with the theory of bounds in homogenization. See Milton [236] and Torquato [291] for detailed derivations of bounds in homogenization.

In the case of spherical inclusions, the Pólya–Szegö polarization tensor M is known exactly:

$$M = mI, m = \frac{d(\sigma - \sigma_0)}{\sigma - \sigma_0 + d\sigma_0} |B| \,, \tag{8.14}$$

and therefore, (8.13) yields the well-known Maxwell–Garnett formula (8.3).

Let $\mathcal{E}$ be an ellipse whose semi-axes are on the x_1- and x_2-axes and of length a and b, respectively. If $B = \frac{1}{|\mathcal{E}|} \mathcal{R}(\theta)\mathcal{E}$, where $\mathcal{R}(\theta) = \begin{pmatrix} \cos\theta & -\sin\theta \\ \sin\theta & \cos\theta \end{pmatrix}$, $\theta \in [0, \pi]$, and $|\mathcal{E}| = \pi ab$ is the volume of $\mathcal{E}$, then using Lemma 4.5 and Theorem 8.1, we obtain that the effective conductivity of the composite is given by

$$
\begin{aligned}
\gamma^* = \sigma_0 \Bigg[I + &(\frac{\sigma}{\sigma_0} - 1)\frac{f}{\pi ab} \\
\times \mathcal{R}(\theta) &\begin{pmatrix} \dfrac{a+b}{(a + \frac{\sigma}{\sigma_0}b) - \frac{f}{2}(\frac{\sigma}{\sigma_0} - 1)(a + b)} & 0 \\[2ex] 0 & \dfrac{a+b}{(\frac{\sigma}{\sigma_0}a + b) - \frac{f}{2}(\frac{\sigma}{\sigma_0} - 1)(a + b)} \end{pmatrix} \mathcal{R}^T(\theta) \Bigg] \\
&+ O(f^3) \,,
\end{aligned}
$$

where $\mathcal{R}^T$ denotes the transpose of $\mathcal{R}$.

This formula can be used to solve the inverse problem of determining the volume fraction f, the conductivity contrast σ/σ_0, the semi-lengths a and b, or the orientation θ of the inclusions from measurements of the effective conductivity of the composite. Indeed, if the elliptical inclusions orient according to a probability distribution $\Psi(\theta)$, then the effective conductivity

$$
\begin{aligned}
\gamma^* = \sigma_0 \Bigg[I + &(\frac{\sigma}{\sigma_0} - 1)\frac{f}{\pi ab} \times \int_0^{2\pi} \mathcal{R}(\theta) \\
\times &\begin{pmatrix} \dfrac{a+b}{(a + \frac{\sigma}{\sigma_0}b) - \frac{f}{2}(\frac{\sigma}{\sigma_0} - 1)(a + b)} & 0 \\[2ex] 0 & \dfrac{a+b}{(\frac{\sigma}{\sigma_0}a + b) - \frac{f}{2}(\frac{\sigma}{\sigma_0} - 1)(a + b)} \end{pmatrix} \\
&\times \mathcal{R}^T(\theta)\, \Psi(\theta)\, d\theta \Bigg] + O(f^3) \,,
\end{aligned}
$$

which shows that only the second moments of the orientational distribution functions of the inclusions $\Psi(\theta)$ can be recovered. See [307]. Using Lemma 4.5 and Theorem 8.1, this result can be trivially extended to arbitrary shaped inclusions.

The method presented above basically enables us to derive all the higher order terms of the asymptotic expansion of the effective conductivity. The construction of these terms depends only on the ability to continue the Taylor expansion (2.95).

For the sake of simplicity, we restrict ourselves to the two-dimensional case to derive in the same way the following theorem.

Theorem 8.2 *Suppose $d = 2$. The effective conductivity γ^* has an asymptotic expansion as the volume fraction $f \to 0$:*

$$\gamma^* = \sigma_0 \left[I + fM(I - \frac{f}{2}M)^{-1} + f^3 A \right] + O(f^4) , \tag{8.15}$$

where A is given by

$$A_{pq} = \sum_{\substack{|l|+|l'|=4 \\ |l|>0, |l'|>0}} c_{ll'} M_{lq} M_{pl'} , \quad p, q = 1, 2 .$$

Proof. Using the (higher-order) Taylor expansion

$$R_2(x) = R_2(0) - \frac{1}{4}(x_1^2 + x_2^2) + R_2^{(4)}(x) + O(|x|^6) \tag{8.16}$$

given in (2.98), we get

$$\nu \cdot \nabla R_2(\rho(x - y)) = -\frac{\rho}{2}\nu \cdot (x - y) + \rho^3 \nu \cdot \nabla_x R_2^{(4)}(x - y) + O(\rho^5) \tag{8.17}$$

uniformly in $x, y \in \partial B$. Write

$$R_2^{(4)}(x - y) = \sum_{|l|+|l'|=4} c_{ll'} x^l y^{l'} .$$

Then, for each fixed l', $\sum_l c_{ll'} x^l$ is harmonic since

$$\sum_l c_{ll'} x^l = \frac{1}{l'!} \partial_y^{l'} (R_2^{(4)}(x - y))\big|_{y=0} .$$

It follows from (8.11) that for $p = 1, 2$

$$(\lambda I - \mathcal{K}_B^*)\psi_p(x) - \frac{\rho^2}{2}\nu_x \cdot \int_{\partial B} y\psi_p(y)\, d\sigma(y)$$

$$-\rho^4 \sum_{|l|+|l'|=4} c_{ll'} (\nu \cdot \nabla x^l) \int_{\partial B} y^{l'} \psi_p(y)\, d\sigma(y) + O(\rho^6) = \nu_p(x), \quad x \in \partial B .$$

$$\tag{8.18}$$

Since $\int_{\partial B} \psi_p \, d\sigma = 0$ for $p = 1, 2$, we get

$$\psi_p = (\lambda I - \mathcal{K}_B^*)^{-1}(\nu_p) + \frac{\rho^2}{2} \sum_{l=1}^{2} (\lambda I - \mathcal{K}_B^*)^{-1}(\nu_l) \int_{\partial B} y_l \psi_p(y) \, d\sigma(y)$$

$$+\rho^4 \sum_{\substack{|l|+|l'|=4 \\ |l'|>0}} c_{ll'} (\lambda I - \mathcal{K}_B^*)^{-1}(\nu \cdot \nabla x^l) \int_{\partial B} y^{l'} \psi_p(y) \, d\sigma(y) + O(\rho^6) \, . \tag{8.19}$$

Let $\widetilde{\psi}^l := (\lambda I - \mathcal{K}_B^*)^{-1}(\nu \cdot \nabla x^l)$, and if $l = e_p$, let $\widetilde{\psi}_p := \widetilde{\psi}^l$, $p = 1, 2$. Then (8.19) takes the form

$$\psi_p = \widetilde{\psi}_p + \frac{\rho^2}{2} \sum_{l=1}^{2} \widetilde{\psi}_l \int_{\partial B} y_l \psi_p(y) \, d\sigma(y)$$

$$+\rho^4 \sum_{\substack{|l|+|l'|=4 \\ |l'|>0}} c_{ll'} \widetilde{\psi}^l \int_{\partial B} y^{l'} \psi_p(y) \, d\sigma(y) + O(\rho^6) \quad \text{on } \partial B \, . \tag{8.20}$$

In particular, we get

$$\psi_p = \widetilde{\psi}_p + O(\rho^2) \, . \tag{8.21}$$

Substituting (8.21) into (8.20), we obtain

$$\psi_p = \widetilde{\psi}_p + \frac{\rho^2}{2} \sum_{l=1}^{2} \widetilde{\psi}_l \int_{\partial B} y_l \psi_p(y) \, d\sigma(y)$$

$$+\rho^4 \sum_{\substack{|l|+|l'|=4 \\ |l'|>0}} c_{ll'} \widetilde{\psi}^l \int_{\partial B} y^{l'} \widetilde{\psi}_p(y) \, d\sigma(y) + O(\rho^6) \quad \text{on } \partial B \, .$$

It then follows from the definitions (8.10) of P and (4.4) of the generalized polarization tensors that

$$P_{pq} = m_{pq} + \frac{\rho^2}{2} \sum_{l=1}^{2} P_{pl} m_{lq} + \rho^4 \sum_{\substack{|l|+|l'|=4 \\ |l|>0,|l'|>0}} c_{ll'} M_{lq} M_{pl'} + O(\rho^6) \, .$$

Let A be the 2×2 matrix defined by

$$A_{pq} = \sum_{\substack{|l|+|l'|=4 \\ |l|>0,|l'|>0}} c_{ll'} M_{lq} M_{pl'}, \quad p, q = 1, 2 \, . \tag{8.22}$$

We then get

$$P = M + \frac{\rho^2}{2} PM + \rho^4 A + O(\rho^6) \, ,$$

and hence

$$P = M(I - \frac{\rho^2}{2}M)^{-1} + \rho^4 A + O(\rho^6) \, ,$$

which proves the theorem. $\square$

Let us consider a special but interesting case: the case where B is a disk. If we fix l' so that $|l'| = 1$ or 2, then $\sum_{|l|=4-|l'|} c_{ll'} y^l$ is a harmonic polynomial of degree 2 or 3, and hence we get from Proposition 4.7 that

$$\sum_{|l| \geq 2} c_{ll'} M_{lp} = 0 \, .$$

Therefore

$$A = \sum_{|l|=1} M_{lq} \sum_{|l'|=3} c_{ll'} M_{pl'} \, .$$

By Proposition 4.7 again, we can show that $A = 0$. Therefore, we get

$$\gamma^* = \sigma_0 \left[I + \rho^2 (I - \frac{\rho^2}{2}M)^{-1}M \right] + O(\rho^8) \, . \tag{8.23}$$

If B is a disk, we can even go further to obtain the full asymptotic expansion for the effective conductivity. Given an integer m, let $R^{(2s)}$ be the polynomial defined in (2.98). Write

$$\sum_{s=2}^{m} R_2^{(2s)}(x - y) = \sum_{s=2}^{m} \sum_{|l|+|l'|=2s} c_{ll'} x^l y^{l'} \, .$$

Then for each fixed l', $\sum_{|l|=2s-|l'|} c_{ll'} x^l$ is harmonic.

The same argument as before and (8.11) yield that, for $p = 1, 2$,

$$(\lambda I - \mathcal{K}_B^*)\psi_p(x) - \frac{\rho^2}{2} \nu_x \cdot \int_{\partial B} y \psi_p(y) \, d\sigma(y)$$

$$- \sum_{s=2}^{m} \rho^{2s} \sum_{|l|+|l'|=2s} c_{ll'} (\nu \cdot \nabla x^l) \int_{\partial B} y^{l'} \psi_p(y) \, d\sigma(y) + O(\rho^{2(m+1)}) = \nu_p(x) \, ,$$

and hence

$$\psi_p = \widetilde{\psi}_p + \frac{\rho^2}{2} \sum_{l=1}^{2} \widetilde{\psi}_l \int_{\partial B} y_l \psi_p(y) \, d\sigma(y)$$

$$+ \sum_{s=2}^{m} \rho^{2s} \sum_{|l|+|l'|=2s} c_{ll'} \widetilde{\psi}^l \int_{\partial B} y^{l'} \psi_p(y) \, d\sigma(y) + O(\rho^{2(m+1)}) \, . \tag{8.24}$$

Let $P_{pl} := \int_{\partial B} y^l \psi_p(y) \, d\sigma(y)$. We then get from (8.24)

$$\psi_p = \widetilde{\psi}_p + \frac{\rho^2}{2} \sum_{l=1}^{2} P_{pl}\widetilde{\psi}_l + \sum_{s=2}^{m} \rho^{2s} \sum_{\substack{|l|=2s-1 \\ |l'|=1}} c_{ll'} P_{pl'}\widetilde{\psi}^l$$

$$+ \sum_{s=2}^{m} \rho^{2s} \sum_{\substack{|l|+|l'|=2s \\ |l'|>1}} c_{ll'}\widetilde{\psi}^l \int_{\partial B} y^{l'} \psi_p(y)\, d\sigma(y) + O(\rho^{2(m+1)}) \,. \tag{8.25}$$

In particular,

$$\psi_p = \widetilde{\psi}_p + \frac{\rho^2}{2} \sum_{l=1}^{2} P_{pl}\widetilde{\psi}_l + \sum_{s=2}^{m} \rho^{2s} \sum_{\substack{|l|=2s-1 \\ |l'|=1}} c_{ll'} P_{pl'}\widetilde{\psi}^l + O(\rho^4) \,. \tag{8.26}$$

Since $\int_{\partial B} y^{l'} \widetilde{\psi}^l(y)\, d\sigma(y) = 0$ if $|l| = 1$ and $|l'| > 1$ by Proposition 4.7, we obtain by substituting (8.26) into (8.25)

$$\psi_p = \widetilde{\psi}_p + \frac{\rho^2}{2} \sum_{l=1}^{2} P_{pl}\widetilde{\psi}_l + \sum_{s=2}^{m} \rho^{2s} \sum_{\substack{|l|=2s-1 \\ |l'|=1}} c_{ll'} P_{pl'}\widetilde{\psi}^l + O(\rho^8) \,.$$

By iterating this argument we see that

$$\psi_p = \widetilde{\psi}_p + \frac{\rho^2}{2} \sum_{l=1}^{2} P_{pl}\widetilde{\psi}_l + \sum_{s=2}^{m} \rho^{2s} \sum_{\substack{|l|=2s-1 \\ |l'|=1}} c_{ll'} P_{pl'}\widetilde{\psi}^l + O(\rho^{2(m+1)}) \,.$$

It then follows from the definitions (8.10) of P and (4.4) of the generalized polarization tensors that

$$P_{pq} = m_{pq} + \frac{\rho^2}{2} \sum_{l=1}^{2} P_{pl}m_{lq} + \sum_{s=2}^{m} \rho^{2s} \sum_{\substack{|l|=2s-1 \\ |l'|=1}} c_{ll'} P_{pl'} \int_{\partial B} x_q \widetilde{\psi}^l(x)\, d\sigma(x)$$

$$+ O(\rho^{2(m+1)}) \,.$$

Observe that, since $\sum_{|l|=2s-1} c_{ll'}y^l$ is harmonic,

$$\sum_{|l|=2s-1} c_{ll'} \int_{\partial B} x_q \widetilde{\psi}^l(x)\, d\sigma(x) = \sum_{|l|=2s-1} c_{ll'} m_{lq} = 0 \,.$$

Therefore we finally have

$$P_{pq} = m_{pq} + \frac{\rho^2}{2} \sum_{l=1}^{2} P_{pl}m_{lq} + O(\rho^{2(m+1)}) \,,$$

or equivalently,

$$P = M(I - \frac{\rho^2}{2}M)^{-1} + O(\rho^{2(m+1)}) \,.$$

In conclusion, we get the following theorem.

Theorem 8.1. *If B is a disk, then the effective conductivity γ^* has an asymptotic expansion as $\rho \to 0$: For any integer m,*

$$\gamma^* = \sigma_0 \left[I + \rho^2 M (I - \frac{\rho^2}{2} M)^{-1} \right] + O((\rho^2)^{m+1}) , \qquad (8.27)$$

where M is the polarization tensor.

Using (8.14) we can rewrite (8.27) as

$$\gamma^* = \sigma_0 \left[1 + \frac{2f \frac{\sigma - \sigma_0}{\sigma + \sigma_0}}{1 - f \frac{\sigma - \sigma_0}{\sigma + \sigma_0}} \right] I + O(f^{m+1}) , \qquad (8.28)$$

for any m where $f = \rho^2$.

8.2 Anisotropic Composites

The asymptotic expansion formula (8.15) has been generalized in [28] to include anisotropic materials but only in the two-dimensional case. Suppose $d = 2$, and let the periodic anisotropic conductivity in the unit cell Y be defined by

$$\gamma = A\chi(Y \setminus D) + \widetilde{A}\chi(D) ,$$

where A and $\widetilde{A}$ are constant 2×2 positive-definite symmetric matrices with $A \neq \widetilde{A}$. Here Y and D are defined similarly to the isotropic case.

For a small parameter ϵ, we consider the problem of determining the effective anisotropic properties of the composite with anisotropic conductivity $\gamma(x/\epsilon)$ as $\epsilon \to 0$.

Write

$$A = \begin{pmatrix} a & b \\ b & c \end{pmatrix} , \quad a, c > 0 \text{ and } ac - b^2 > 0 .$$

The following result is proved in [28].

Theorem 8.3 *Suupose $d = 2$. Let K be the matrix defined by (2.111). Then we have an asymptotic formula for the effective conductivity*

$$\gamma^* = A + fM\left(I - 2fKM\right)^{-1} + O(f^3) , \qquad (8.29)$$

where $M = (m_{pq})_{1 \leq p,q \leq 2}$ is the first-order APT corresponding to the conductivity distribution $\gamma_B = A\chi(\mathbb{R}^2 \setminus B) + \widetilde{A}\chi(B)$.

To prove Theorem 8.3, we first note that the effective conductivity $\gamma^* = (\gamma^*_{pq})_{p,q=1,2}$ can be written as

$$\gamma_{pq}^* = \int_{\partial Y} u_p \nu \cdot A \nabla u_p \, d\sigma$$

$$= \int_{\partial Y} (y_q + c_q + \mathcal{G}_D^A g_q) \nu \cdot A \nabla (y_p + \mathcal{G}_D^A g_p) \, d\sigma$$

$$= \int_{\partial Y} y_q \nu \cdot A \nabla y_p \, d\sigma + \int_{\partial Y} y_q \nu \cdot A \nabla \mathcal{G}_D^A g_p \, d\sigma \; . \tag{8.30}$$

The last equality in the above holds because of the periodicity of $\mathcal{G}_D^A g_p$. After that, we prove the following lemma.

Lemma 8.4 *If $D = \rho B$, then for $p, q = 1, 2$,*

$$\int_{\partial Y} y_q \nu \cdot A \nabla \mathcal{G}_D^A g_p \, d\sigma = \rho^2 \int_{\partial B} y_q \psi_p(y) \, d\sigma \; , \tag{8.31}$$

where $\psi_p(y) = g_p(\rho y)$, $y \in B$.

Proof. By Green's formula

$$\int_{\partial (Y \setminus \overline{D})} \left[y_q \nu \cdot A \nabla \mathcal{G}_D^A g_p(y) - \mathcal{G}_D^A g_p(y) \nu \cdot A \nabla y_q \right] d\sigma = 0 \; ,$$

and hence we get from the jump relation (2.128) and the change of variable $y \to \rho y$,

$$\int_{\partial Y} y_q \nu \cdot A \nabla \mathcal{G}_D^A g_p \, d\sigma = \int_{\partial D} y_q \nu \cdot A \nabla \mathcal{G}_D^A g_p|_+ \, d\sigma - \int_{\partial D} \nu \cdot A \nabla y_q \mathcal{G}_D^A g_p \, d\sigma$$

$$= \int_{\partial D} y_q \left(g_p + \nu \cdot A \nabla \mathcal{G}_D^A g_p|_- \right) d\sigma - \int_{\partial D} y_q \nu \cdot A \nabla \mathcal{G}_D^A g_p|_- \, d\sigma$$

$$= \int_{\partial D} y_q g_p(y) \, d\sigma(y)$$

$$= \rho^2 \int_{\partial B} y_q g_p(\rho y) \, d\sigma(y) \; .$$

This completes the proof. $\qquad\qquad\qquad\qquad\qquad\qquad\qquad\qquad\qquad\qquad\qquad\square$

With the help of the above lemma and (8.30), we now prove Theorem 8.3. By (8.31), (8.30) now takes the form

$$\gamma^* = A + \rho^2 H \; , \tag{8.32}$$

where

$$H_{pq} = \int_{\partial B} y_q \psi_p(y) \, d\sigma(y), \quad p, q = 1, 2 \; . \tag{8.33}$$

Thanks to (2.126), (2.133) becomes

$$\begin{cases} \mathcal{S}_D^{\widetilde{A}} f_p - \mathcal{S}_D^A g_p - \mathcal{R}_D^A g_p = x_p \\ \nu \cdot \widetilde{A} \nabla \mathcal{S}_D^{\widetilde{A}} f_p|_- - \nu \cdot A \nabla \mathcal{S}_D^A g_p|_+ - \nu \cdot A \nabla \mathcal{R}_D^A g_p = \nu \cdot A \nabla x_p \end{cases} \quad \text{on } \partial D .$$
(8.34)

Making the change of variables $y \to \rho y$ and letting $\phi_p(y) = f_p(\rho y)$ and $\psi_p(y) = g_p(\rho y)$, the system of equations above becomes

$$\begin{cases} \mathcal{S}_B^{\widetilde{A}} \phi_p - \mathcal{S}_B^A \psi_p - \displaystyle\int_{\partial B} R^A(\rho(x-y))\psi_p(y)\, d\sigma(y) = x_p \\ \nu \cdot \widetilde{A} \nabla \mathcal{S}_B^{\widetilde{A}} \phi_p|_- - \nu \cdot A \nabla \mathcal{S}_B^A \psi_p|_+ \\ \qquad - \rho \displaystyle\int_{\partial B} \nu_x \cdot A \nabla_x R^A(\rho(x-y))\psi_p(y)\, d\sigma(y) = \nu \cdot A \nabla x_p \end{cases} \quad \text{on } \partial B .$$
(8.35)

Since R^A is smooth, we get from the Taylor expansion for a given $m \in \mathbb{N}$,

$$R^A(x) = R^A(0) + R_m^A(x) + E_m^A(x) ,$$
(8.36)

where

$$R_m^A(x) - \sum_{2 \le |i| \le 2m} r_i x^i \quad \text{and} \quad E_m^A(x) = O(|x|^{2(m+1)}) .$$

Moreover, since $\nabla \cdot A \nabla E_m^A = 0$ in Y by Lemma 2.42, a constant C independent of x and m exists such that

$$|E_m^A(x)| \le \frac{C|x|^{2m+2}}{(2m+2)! r^{2m+3}} \quad \text{for all } x \in \overline{D} ,$$
(8.37)

where $r = \text{dist}(D, \partial Y)$. Notice that the terms of odd degrees vanish because of the periodicity of $G_\sharp^A(x)$. Suppose that

$$R_m^A(x-y) = \sum_{|i|+|j| \le 2m} a_{ij} x^i y^j .$$
(8.38)

Here we use i, j for multi-indices. Since $\int_{\partial B} \psi_p \, d\sigma = 0$, we get

$$\int_{\partial B} R^A(\rho(x-y))\psi_p(y)\, d\sigma(y)$$
$$= \sum_{l=1}^{m} \rho^{2l} \sum_{\substack{|i|+|j|=2l \\ |i|,|j|>0}} a_{ij} x^i \int_{\partial B} y^j \psi_p \, d\sigma + C + O(\rho^{2(m+1)}) ,$$

where the constant C is

$$C = \sum_{l=1}^{m} \rho^{2l} \sum_{|i|=2l} a_{ij} \int_{\partial B} y^j \psi_p \, d\sigma .$$

We also get

$$\rho \int_{\partial B} \nu_x \cdot A\nabla_x R^A(\rho(x-y))\psi_p(y)\, d\sigma(y)$$

$$= \sum_{l=1}^{m} \rho^{2l} \sum_{\substack{|i|+|j|=2l \\ |i|,|j|>0}} a_{ij}(\nu \cdot A\nabla x^i) \int_{\partial B} y^j \psi_p \, d\sigma + O(\rho^{2(m+1)})\,.$$

Observe from (8.37) that the $O(\rho^{2(m+1)})$ term is bounded by

$$\frac{C\rho^{2(m+1)}\delta^{2m+2}}{(2m+2)!\, r^{2m+3}} \tag{8.39}$$

for some constant C where δ is the diameter of B. Let

$$H_{iq} := \int_{\partial B} y^i \psi_p \, d\sigma\,. \tag{8.40}$$

Define $T : L^2(\partial B) \times L^2(\partial B) \to W_1^2(\partial B) \times L^2(\partial B)$ by

$$T\begin{pmatrix} f \\ g \end{pmatrix} = \begin{pmatrix} \mathcal{S}_B^{\tilde{A}} f - \mathcal{S}_B^A g \\ \nu \cdot \tilde{A}\nabla \mathcal{S}_B^{\tilde{A}} f|_- - \nu \cdot A\nabla \mathcal{S}_B^A g|_+ \end{pmatrix}\,.$$

It then follows from (8.35) that

$$T\begin{pmatrix} \phi_p \\ \psi_p \end{pmatrix} - \sum_{l=1}^{m} \rho^{2l} \sum_{\substack{|i|+|j|=2l \\ |i|,|j|>0}} a_{ij} H_{pj} \begin{pmatrix} x^i \\ \nu \cdot A\nabla x^i \end{pmatrix}$$

$$- \begin{pmatrix} C \\ 0 \end{pmatrix} + O(\rho^{2(m+1)}) = \begin{pmatrix} x_p \\ \nu \cdot A\nabla x_p \end{pmatrix}\,,$$

and hence

$$\begin{pmatrix} \phi_p \\ \psi_p \end{pmatrix} = T^{-1}\begin{pmatrix} x_p \\ \nu \cdot A\nabla x_p \end{pmatrix}$$

$$+ \sum_{l=1}^{m} \rho^{2l} \sum_{\substack{|i|+|j|=2l \\ |i|,|j|>0}} a_{ij} H_{pj} T^{-1}\begin{pmatrix} x^i \\ \nu \cdot \nabla x^i \end{pmatrix} + T^{-1}\begin{pmatrix} C \\ 0 \end{pmatrix} + O(\rho^{2(m+1)})\,.$$

Notice that we use the fact that the second entry of $T^{-1}\begin{pmatrix} C \\ 0 \end{pmatrix}$ is zero, which was proved in Lemma 2.37. Let

$$\begin{pmatrix} \tilde{\phi}_i \\ \tilde{\psi}_i \end{pmatrix} = T^{-1}\begin{pmatrix} x^i \\ \nu \cdot A\nabla x^i \end{pmatrix}\,.$$

Then we have

$$\psi_p = \widetilde{\psi}_p + \sum_{l=1}^{m} \rho^{2l} \sum_{\substack{|i|+|j|=2l \\ |i|,|j|>0}} a_{ij} H_{pj} \widetilde{\psi}_i + O(\rho^{2(m+1)}) \, . \tag{8.41}$$

Since T^{-1} is bounded, the $O(\rho^{2(m+1)})$ term in (8.41) is also bounded by the quantity in (8.39) with a different constant C. Observe that $(\widetilde{\phi}_i, \widetilde{\psi}_i)$ is the solution to (4.86), and hence, anistropic polarization tensor (APT) M_{ij} is given by

$$M_{ij} = \int_{\partial B} x^j \psi_i \, d\sigma \, .$$

Substituting (8.41) in (8.33) yields

$$H_{pq} = m_{pq} + \sum_{l=1}^{m} \rho^{2l} \sum_{\substack{|i|+|j|=2l \\ |i|,|j|>0}} a_{ij} H_{pj} M_{iq} + O(\rho^{2(m+1)}) \, , \tag{8.42}$$

where $O(\rho^{2(m+1)})$ is bounded by the quantity in (8.39) with a different constant C. Notice that this formula includes H_{pj} in its expression.

In order to remove H_{pj} in (8.42), we can use the following formula:

$$H_{pj} = M_{pj} + \sum_{l=1}^{m} \rho^{2l} \sum_{\substack{|i|+|s|=2l \\ |i|,|s|>0}} a_{is} H_{ps} M_{ij} + O(\rho^{2(m+1)}), \quad 1 \leq |j| \leq 2m - 1 \, ,$$
$$\tag{8.43}$$

which can be obtained by substituting (8.41) in (8.40). Since ρ is small, one can solve (8.43) for H_{pj} in terms of M_{ij} and by (8.42) H_{pq} can be expressed solely by M_{ij}.

Suppose that $m = 1$ and let $f := \rho^2 = |D|$, the volume fraction of the inclusion. According to (2.110), $R_1(x) = -x \cdot Kx$. Hence

$$R_1(x - y) = -x \cdot Kx + 2x \cdot Ky - y \cdot Ky \, .$$

Therefore, in this case, (8.42) reads as follows:

$$H_{pq} = m_{pq} + f \sum_{s,l=1}^{2} a_{sl} H_{pl} m_{sq} + O(f^2) \, ,$$

where $2K = (a_{sl})$. In other words,

$$H = M + 2fHKM + O(f^2) \, ,$$

and hence

$$H = M\Big(I - 2fKM\Big)^{-1} + O(f^2) \, , \tag{8.44}$$

which yields the desired result. $\qquad\square$

In particular, if A is diagonal, then K is given by (2.123) and hence we obtain

$$\gamma^* = A + fM\left(I - \frac{f}{2}A^{-1}(I + c(A)E)M\right)^{-1} + O(f^3), \qquad (8.45)$$

where $c(A)$ is the number defined by (2.124) and $E = \begin{pmatrix} 1 & 0 \\ 0 & -1 \end{pmatrix}$. If A is isotropic, or $A = \sigma I$, then $c(A) = 0$ and the above formula becomes (8.15).

Note that, if A is diagonal, then we obtain

$$\gamma^* = A + fM\left(I - \frac{f}{2}A^{-1}(I + c(A)E)M\right)^{-1} + O(f^3) \,,$$

where $c(A)$ is the number defined by

$$c(A) := \frac{4\pi}{\sqrt{\det(A)}}\left(\frac{a}{24} + a\theta\left(i\sqrt{\frac{a}{c}}\right) - \frac{c}{24} - c\theta\left(i\sqrt{\frac{c}{a}}\right)\right),$$

and $E = \begin{pmatrix} 1 & 0 \\ 0 & -1 \end{pmatrix}$. If A is isotropic, or $A = \sigma_0 I$, then $c(A) = 0$ and the above formula becomes

$$\gamma^* = \sigma_0 I + fM\left(I - \frac{f}{2\sigma_0}M\right)^{-1} + O(f^3) \,,$$

and coincides with (8.13) since the first-order APT is equal to $\sigma_0 \times$ the first-order GPT.

8.3 Further Results and Open Problems

Since the construction of a full asymptotic expansion of the effective conductivity depends on the ability to continue the Taylor expansion of the periodic Green's function, it would be interesting to find an accurate way for doing this.

The formulae (8.15) and (8.29) will be extended to elastic composites. A general scheme to derive accurate asymptotic expansions of the elastic effective properties of dilute composite materials in terms of the elastic moment tensor and the volume fraction occupied by the elastic inclusions will be presented in Chapter 13. The formula is valid for general shaped Lipschitz inclusions with arbitrary phase moduli. Moreover, it exhibits an interesting feature of the effective elasticity tensor of composite materials: the presence of a distortion factor. The derivation of this formula is much more difficult than the one presented here for the effective conductivity because of the tensorial nature of the periodic Green's functions of the Lamé system.

Transmission Problem for Elastostatics

Introduction

In the preceding chapters, we considered isotropic and anisotropic conductivity problems. Now we turn to the system of elastostatics. After reviewing some well-known results on the solvability and layer potentials for the Lamé system, mostly from [104] and [121], we proceed to prove a representation formula for solutions of the Lamé system, which will be our main tool in later chapters. Next, we derive a complex representation of displacement fields. In the final section of this chapter, we construct a periodic Green's function for the Lamé system in the two-dimensional case and study the periodic transmission problem. We will use the results in this final section when we consider the effective properties of composite elastic materials.

9.1 Layer Potentials for the Lamé System

Let D be a bounded Lipschitz domain in $\mathbb{R}^d$, $d = 2, 3$, and (λ, μ) be the Lamé constants for D satisfying

$$\mu > 0 \quad \text{and} \quad d\lambda + 2\mu > 0 \, .$$

See Kupradze [206]. The elastostatic system corresponding to the Lamé constants λ, μ is defined by

$$\mathcal{L}_{\lambda,\mu}\mathbf{u} := \mu\Delta\mathbf{u} + (\lambda + \mu)\nabla\nabla \cdot \mathbf{u} \, .$$

The corresponding conormal derivative $\partial\mathbf{u}/\partial\nu$ on ∂D is defined to be

$$\frac{\partial\mathbf{u}}{\partial\nu} := \lambda(\nabla \cdot \mathbf{u})N + \mu(\nabla\mathbf{u} + \nabla\mathbf{u}^T)N \quad \text{on } \partial D \, , \tag{9.1}$$

where N is the outward unit normal to ∂D and the superscript T denotes the transpose of a matrix.

Notice that the conormal derivative has a direct physical meaning:

$$\frac{\partial \mathbf{u}}{\partial \nu} = \text{traction on } \partial D .$$

The vector $\mathbf{u}$ is the displacement field of the elastic medium having the Lamé coefficients λ and μ, and $(\nabla \mathbf{u} + \nabla \mathbf{u}^T)/2$ is the strain tensor.

Let us state a simple, but important, relation. The identity (9.2) is referred to as the divergence theorem.

Lemma 9.1 *If $\mathbf{u} \in W^{1,2}(D)$ and $\mathcal{L}_{\lambda,\mu}\mathbf{u} = 0$ in D, then for all $\mathbf{v} \in W^{1,2}(D)$,*

$$\int_{\partial D} \mathbf{v} \cdot \frac{\partial \mathbf{u}}{\partial \nu}\, d\sigma = \int_D \lambda(\nabla \cdot \mathbf{u})(\nabla \cdot \mathbf{v}) + \frac{\mu}{2}(\nabla \mathbf{u} + \nabla \mathbf{u}^T) \cdot (\nabla \mathbf{v} + \nabla \mathbf{v}^T)\, dx , \quad (9.2)$$

where for $d \times d$ matrices $a = (a_{ij})$ and $b = (b_{ij})$, $a \cdot b = \sum_{ij} a_{ij} b_{ij}$.

Proof. By the definition (9.1) of the conormal derivative, we get

$$\int_{\partial D} \mathbf{v} \cdot \frac{\partial \mathbf{u}}{\partial \nu}\, d\sigma = \int_{\partial D} \lambda(\nabla \cdot \mathbf{u})\mathbf{v} \cdot N + \mu \mathbf{v} \cdot (\nabla \mathbf{u} + \nabla \mathbf{u}^T)N\, d\sigma$$

$$= \int_D \lambda \nabla \cdot ((\nabla \cdot \mathbf{u})\mathbf{v}) + \mu \nabla \cdot ((\nabla \mathbf{u} + \nabla \mathbf{u}^T)\mathbf{v})\, dx .$$

Since

$$\nabla \cdot \left((\nabla \mathbf{u} + \nabla \mathbf{u}^T)\mathbf{v} \right) = \nabla(\nabla \cdot \mathbf{u}) \cdot \mathbf{v} + \Delta \mathbf{u} \cdot \mathbf{v} + \frac{1}{2}(\nabla \mathbf{u} + \nabla \mathbf{u}^T) \cdot (\nabla \mathbf{v} + \nabla \mathbf{v}^T) ,$$

we obtain (9.2) and the proof is complete. $\qquad\square$

We give now a fundamental solution to the Lamé system $\mathcal{L}_{\lambda,\mu}$ in $\mathbb{R}^d$.

Lemma 9.2 *A fundamental solution $\mathbf{\Gamma} = (\Gamma_{ij})_{i,j=1}^d$ to the Lamé system $\mathcal{L}_{\lambda,\mu}$ is given by*

$$\Gamma_{ij}(x) := \begin{cases} -\dfrac{A}{4\pi}\dfrac{\delta_{ij}}{|x|} - \dfrac{B}{4\pi}\dfrac{x_i x_j}{|x|^3} & \text{if } d = 3 , \\[2mm] \dfrac{A}{2\pi}\delta_{ij}\ln|x| - \dfrac{B}{2\pi}\dfrac{x_i x_j}{|x|^2} & \text{if } d = 2 , \end{cases} \qquad x \neq 0 ,$$

where

$$A = \frac{1}{2}\left(\frac{1}{\mu} + \frac{1}{2\mu + \lambda}\right) \quad and \quad B = \frac{1}{2}\left(\frac{1}{\mu} - \frac{1}{2\mu + \lambda}\right) . \qquad (9.3)$$

The function $\mathbf{\Gamma}$ is known as the Kelvin matrix of fundamental solutions.

Proof. We seek a solution $\mathbf{\Gamma} = (\Gamma_{ij})_{i,j=1}^d$ of

$$\mu \Delta \mathbf{\Gamma} + (\lambda + \mu)\nabla\nabla \cdot \mathbf{\Gamma} = \delta_0 I_d \quad \text{in } \mathbb{R}^d , \qquad (9.4)$$

where I_d is the $d \times d$ identity matrix and δ_0 is the Dirac mass at 0.

Taking the divergence of (9.4), we have

$$(\lambda + 2\mu)\Delta(\nabla \cdot \mathbf{\Gamma}) = \nabla\delta_0 \ .$$

Thus by Lemma 2.11

$$\nabla \cdot \mathbf{\Gamma} = \frac{1}{\lambda + 2\mu}\nabla\Gamma \ ,$$

where Γ is given by (2.8). Inserting this equation into (9.4) gives

$$\mu\Delta\mathbf{\Gamma} = \delta_0 \, I_d - \frac{\lambda + \mu}{\lambda + 2\mu}\nabla\nabla\Gamma \ .$$

Hence, it follows that

$$\Gamma_{ij}(x) := \begin{cases} -\dfrac{A}{4\pi}\dfrac{\delta_{ij}}{|x|} - \dfrac{B}{4\pi}\dfrac{x_i x_j}{|x|^3} & \text{if } d = 3 \ , \\[2ex] \dfrac{A}{2\pi}\delta_{ij}\ln|x| - \dfrac{B}{2\pi}\dfrac{x_i x_j}{|x|^2} & \text{if } d = 2 \ , \end{cases} \qquad x \neq 0 \ ,$$

modulo constants, where A and B are given by (9.3). $\square$

The single and double layer potentials of the density function φ on D associated with the Lamé parameters (λ, μ) are defined by

$$\mathcal{S}_D\varphi(x) := \int_{\partial D} \mathbf{\Gamma}(x - y)\varphi(y)\, d\sigma(y) \ , \quad x \in \mathbb{R}^d \ , \tag{9.5}$$

$$\mathcal{D}_D\varphi(x) := \int_{\partial D} \frac{\partial}{\partial\nu_y}\mathbf{\Gamma}(x - y)\varphi(y)\, d\sigma(y) \ , \quad x \in \mathbb{R}^d \setminus \partial D \ , \tag{9.6}$$

where $\partial/\partial\nu$ denotes the conormal derivative defined in (9.1). Thus, for $m = 1, \ldots, d$,

$$(\mathcal{D}_D\varphi(x))_m = \int_{\partial D} \lambda\frac{\partial\Gamma_{mi}}{\partial y_i}(x - y)\varphi(y) \cdot N(y)$$
$$+ \mu\left(\frac{\partial\Gamma_{mi}}{\partial y_j} + \frac{\partial\Gamma_{mj}}{\partial y_i}\right)(x - y)N_i(y)\varphi_j(y)\, d\sigma(y) \ .$$

Here we used the Einstein convention for the summation notation. As an immediate consequence of (9.2), we obtain the following lemma, which can be proved in the same way as the Green's representation (2.11) of harmonic functions.

Lemma 9.3 *If* $\mathbf{u} \in W^{1,2}(D)$ *and* $\mathcal{L}_{\lambda,\mu}\mathbf{u} = 0$ *in* D, *then*

$$\mathbf{u}(x) = \mathcal{D}_D(\mathbf{u}|_{\partial D})(x) - \mathcal{S}_D\left(\frac{\partial\mathbf{u}}{\partial\nu}\bigg|_{\partial D}\right)(x) \ , \quad x \in D \ , \tag{9.7}$$

and

$$\mathcal{D}_D(\mathbf{u}|_{\partial D})(x) - \mathcal{S}_D\left(\frac{\partial\mathbf{u}}{\partial\nu}\bigg|_{\partial D}\right)(x) = 0 \ , \quad x \in \mathbb{R}^d \setminus \overline{D} \ . \tag{9.8}$$

As before, let $\mathbf{u}|_+$ and $\mathbf{u}|_-$ denote the limits from outside D and inside D, respectively.

The following theorems are from Dahlberg, Kenig, and Verchota [104].

Theorem 9.4 (Jump formula, [104]) *Let D be a bounded Lipschitz domain in $\mathbb{R}^d, d = 2$ or 3. For $\varphi \in L^2(\partial D)$,*

$$\mathcal{D}_D\varphi|_\pm = (\mp\frac{1}{2}I + \mathcal{K}_D)\varphi \quad a.e. \text{ on } \partial D\,, \tag{9.9}$$

$$\frac{\partial}{\partial\nu}\mathcal{S}_D\varphi\Big|_\pm = (\pm\frac{1}{2}I + \mathcal{K}_D^*)\varphi \quad a.e. \text{ on } \partial D\,, \tag{9.10}$$

where $\mathcal{K}_D$ is defined by

$$\mathcal{K}_D\varphi(x) := p.v. \int_{\partial D} \frac{\partial}{\partial\nu_y}\mathbf{\Gamma}(x - y)\varphi(y)\, d\sigma(y) \quad a.e.\ x \in \partial D$$

and $\mathcal{K}_D^*$ is the adjoint operator of $\mathcal{K}_D$ on $L^2(\partial D)$; that is,

$$\mathcal{K}_D^*\varphi(x) := p.v. \int_{\partial D} \frac{\partial}{\partial\nu_x}\mathbf{\Gamma}(x - y)\varphi(y)\, d\sigma(y) \quad a.e.\ x \in \partial D\,.$$

It must be emphasized that, in contrast with the corresponding singular integral operators defined in (2.29) and (2.30) that arise when studying Laplace's equation (see Lemma 2.13), the singular integral operator $\mathcal{K}_D$ is not compact, even on bounded $\mathcal{C}^\infty$-domains [104].

Let Ψ be the vector space of all linear solutions of the equation $\mathcal{L}_{\lambda,\mu}\mathbf{u} = 0$ and $\partial\mathbf{u}/\partial\nu = 0$ on ∂D, or alternatively,

$$\Psi := \left\{ \boldsymbol{\psi} : \partial_i\psi_j + \partial_j\psi_i = 0, \quad 1 \leq i, j \leq d \right\}.$$

Here ψ_i for $i = 1, \ldots, d$, denote the components of $\boldsymbol{\psi}$.

Observe now that the space Ψ is defined independently of the Lamé constants λ, μ, and its dimension is 3 if $d = 2$ and 6 if $d = 3$. Define

$$L_\Psi^2(\partial D) := \left\{ \mathbf{f} \in L^2(\partial D) : \int_{\partial D} \mathbf{f} \cdot \boldsymbol{\psi}\, d\sigma = 0 \text{ for all } \boldsymbol{\psi} \in \Psi \right\}, \tag{9.11}$$

a subspace of codimension $d(d + 1)/2$ in $L^2(\partial D)$.

In particular, since Ψ contains constant functions, we get

$$\int_{\partial D} \mathbf{f}\, d\sigma = 0$$

for any $\mathbf{f} \in L_\Psi^2(\partial D)$. The following fact, which immediately follows from (9.2), is useful in later sections.

If $\mathbf{u} \in W^{1,\frac{3}{2}}(D)$ satisfies $\mathcal{L}_{\lambda,\mu}\mathbf{u} = 0$ in D, then $\dfrac{\partial\mathbf{u}}{\partial\nu}\Big|_{\partial D} \in L_\Psi^2(\partial D)\,. \tag{9.12}$

One fundamental result in the theory of linear elasticity using layer potentials is the following invertibility theorem.

Theorem 9.5 ([104]) *The operator $\mathcal{K}_D$ is bounded on $L^2(\partial D)$, and $-(1/2)\,I + \mathcal{K}_D^*$ and $(1/2)\,I + \mathcal{K}_D^*$ are invertible on $L_\Psi^2(\partial D)$ and $L^2(\partial D)$, respectively.*

As a consequence of (9.10) and Theorem 9.5, we are able to prove the following.

Corollary 9.6 ([104]) *For a given $\mathbf{g} \in L_\Psi^2(\partial D)$, the function $\mathbf{u} \in W^{1,2}(D)$ defined by*

$$\mathbf{u}(x) := \mathcal{S}_D\left(-\frac{1}{2}I + \mathcal{K}_D^*\right)^{-1}\mathbf{g} \tag{9.13}$$

is a solution to the problem

$$\begin{cases} \mathcal{L}_{\lambda,\mu}\mathbf{u} = 0 & \text{in } D\,, \\ \left.\dfrac{\partial \mathbf{u}}{\partial \nu}\right|_{\partial D} = \mathbf{g}\,, & (\mathbf{u}|_{\partial D} \in L_\Psi^2(\partial D))\,. \end{cases} \tag{9.14}$$

If $\psi \in \Psi$ and $x \in \mathbb{R}^d \setminus \overline{D}$, then from (9.2) it follows that $\mathcal{D}_D\psi(x) = 0$. Hence by (9.9), ψ satisfies $(-(1/2)\,I + \mathcal{K}_D)\psi = 0$. Since the dimension of the orthogonal complement of the range of the operator $-(1/2)\,I + \mathcal{K}_D^*$ is less than 3 if $d = 2$ and 6 if $d = 3$, which is the dimension of the space Ψ, we obtain the following corollary.

Corollary 9.7 *The null space of $-(1/2)\,I + \mathcal{K}_D$ on $L^2(\partial D)$ is Ψ.*

The following formulation of Korn's inequality will be of interest to us. See Nečas [254] and Ciarlet [96, Theorem 6.3.4].

Lemma 9.8 *Let D be a bounded Lipschitz domain in $\mathbb{R}^d$. Let $\mathbf{u} \in W^{1,2}(D)$ satisfy*

$$\int_D \left(\mathbf{u} \cdot \psi + \nabla\mathbf{u} \cdot \nabla\psi\right) = 0 \quad \text{for all } \psi \in \Psi\,.$$

Then there is a constant C depending only on the Lipschitz character of D such that

$$\int_D \left(|\mathbf{u}|^2 + |\nabla\mathbf{u}|^2\right) dx \leq C \int_D |\nabla\mathbf{u} + \nabla\mathbf{u}^T|^2 \, dx\,. \tag{9.15}$$

9.2 Kelvin Matrix Under Unitary Transformations

Unlike the fundamental solution to the Laplacian given by (2.8), the fundamental solution $\mathbf{\Gamma}$ to $\mathcal{L}_{\lambda,\mu}$ is not invariant under unitary transformations. In this section we find formulae for both $\mathbf{\Gamma}$ and the single layer potential under unitary transformations.

Lemma 9.9 *Let R be a unitary transformation on $\mathbb{R}^d$. Then,*

(i) $\mathcal{L}_{\lambda,\mu}(R^{-1}(\mathbf{u} \circ R)) = R^{-1}(\mathcal{L}_{\lambda,\mu}\mathbf{u}) \circ R$;

(ii) $\left(\dfrac{\partial \mathbf{u}}{\partial \nu}\right) \circ R = R\dfrac{\partial}{\partial \nu}(R^{-1}(\mathbf{u} \circ R))$.

Proof. Since, for a vector $\mathbf{u}$ and a scalar function f,

$$(\nabla \cdot \mathbf{u}) \circ R = \nabla \cdot \left(R^{-1}(\mathbf{u} \circ R)\right) ,$$
$$R^{-1}(\nabla f) \circ R = \nabla(f \circ R) ,$$

we find that

$$
\begin{aligned}
\mathcal{L}_{\lambda,\mu}\left(R^{-1}(\mathbf{u} \circ R)\right) &= \mu\Delta(R^{-1}(\mathbf{u} \circ R)) + (\lambda + \mu)\nabla\nabla \cdot (R^{-1}(\mathbf{u} \circ R)) \\
&= \mu R^{-1}(\Delta(\mathbf{u} \circ R)) + (\lambda + \mu)\nabla((\nabla \cdot \mathbf{u}) \circ R)) \\
&= \mu R^{-1}((\Delta\mathbf{u}) \circ R)) + (\lambda + \mu)R^{-1}(\nabla\nabla \cdot \mathbf{u}) \circ R \\
&= R^{-1}(\mathcal{L}_{\lambda,\mu}\mathbf{u}) \circ R ,
\end{aligned}
$$

which proves part (i).

To prove part (ii), note first that, if N_1 and N_2 are the unit normals to ∂D and $\partial R(D)$, respectively, then $N_2(R(x)) = R(N_1(x))$ for $x \in \partial D$. Therefore, we have

$$
\begin{aligned}
\left(\frac{\partial \mathbf{u}}{\partial \nu}\right) \circ R &= \lambda(\nabla \cdot \mathbf{u} \circ R)N \circ R + \mu((\nabla\mathbf{u}) \circ R + (\nabla\mathbf{u})^T \circ R)N \circ R \\
&= \lambda\nabla \cdot (R^{-1}(\mathbf{u} \circ R))RN + \mu R(R^{-1}(\nabla\mathbf{u}) \circ R + R^{-1}(\nabla\mathbf{u})^T \circ R)RN \\
&= \lambda\nabla \cdot (R^{-1}(\mathbf{u} \circ R))RN + \mu R(\nabla(\mathbf{u} \circ R)R + (\nabla(\mathbf{u} \circ R)^T R)N \\
&= \lambda\nabla \cdot (R^{-1}(\mathbf{u} \circ R))RN + \mu R(\nabla(R^{-1}(\mathbf{u} \circ R)) + (\nabla(R^{-1}(\mathbf{u} \circ R))^T)N \\
&= R\frac{\partial}{\partial \nu}(R^{-1}(\mathbf{u} \circ R)) ,
\end{aligned}
$$

as claimed. $\qquad\qquad\qquad\qquad\qquad\qquad\qquad\qquad\qquad\qquad\qquad\square$

Lemma 9.10 *Suppose that $\mathcal{L}_{\lambda,\mu}\mathbf{u} = 0$ in $\mathbb{R}^d$. If, in addition, $\mathbf{u}$ is bounded for $d = 2$ and behaves like $O(|x|^{-1})$ as $|x| \to +\infty$ for $d = 3$, and $\nabla\mathbf{u} = O(|x|^{1-d})$ as $|x| \to +\infty$, then $\mathbf{u}$ is constant if $d = 2$ and $\mathbf{u} = 0$ if $d = 3$.*

Proof. Let B_r be a ball of radius r centered at 0. Then, by applying (9.7),

$$\mathbf{u}(x) = \mathcal{D}_{B_r}(\mathbf{u}|_{\partial B_r})(x) - \mathcal{S}_{B_r}\left(\frac{\partial \mathbf{u}}{\partial \nu}\bigg|_{\partial B_r}\right)(x) , \quad x \in B_r .$$

Next, we deduce from (9.12) that $\partial\mathbf{u}/\partial\nu \in L^2_{\Psi}(\partial B_r)$, which shows that

$$\int_{\partial B_r} \frac{\partial\mathbf{u}}{\partial\nu}\, d\sigma = 0 \,.$$

Hence $\nabla\mathbf{u}(x) = O(1/r)$ for all $r \to +\infty$ provided that x is in a bounded set and therefore $\mathbf{u}$ is constant, as desired. $\qquad\square$

Lemma 9.11 (Rotation Formula)

$$\mathbf{\Gamma}(R(x)) = R\mathbf{\Gamma}(x)R^{-1}, \quad x \in \mathbb{R}^d. \tag{9.16}$$

Proof.   It follows from Lemma 9.9 (i) that

$$\mathcal{L}_{\lambda,\mu}\big(R^{-1}(\mathbf{\Gamma}\circ R)\big)(x) = R^{-1}(\mathcal{L}_{\lambda,\mu}\mathbf{\Gamma})(R(x)) = \delta_0(R(x))R^{-1} = \delta_0(x)R^{-1} \,.$$

Consequently,
$$\mathcal{L}_{\lambda,\mu}\big(R^{-1}(\mathbf{\Gamma}\circ R) - \mathbf{\Gamma}R^{-1}\big) = 0 \quad \text{in } \mathbb{R}^d \,.$$
Observe that $R^{-1}(\mathbf{\Gamma}\circ R) - \mathbf{\Gamma}R^{-1}$ is bounded if $d = 2$ and behaves like $O(|x|^{-1})$ as $|x| \to +\infty$ if $d = 3$. Moreover,

$$\nabla\big(R^{-1}(\mathbf{\Gamma}\circ R) - \mathbf{\Gamma}R^{-1}\big)(x) - O(|x|^{1-d}) \quad \text{as } |x| \to +\infty \,.$$

Applying Lemma 9.10, we conclude that

$$R^{-1}(\mathbf{\Gamma}\circ R) - \mathbf{\Gamma}R^{-1} = \text{constant} \,,$$

which is obviously zero. $\qquad\square$

As a consequence of (9.16), we obtain the following rotation formula for the single layer potential.

Lemma 9.12 *Let R be a unitary transformation on $\mathbb{R}^d$, and let $\widehat{D}$ be a bounded domain in $\mathbb{R}^d$ and $D = R(\widehat{D})$. Then for any vector potential $\varphi \in L^2(\partial D)$, we have*

$$(\mathcal{S}_D\varphi)(R(x)) = R\mathcal{S}_{\widehat{D}}(R^{-1}(\varphi\circ R))(x) \,, \tag{9.17}$$

$$\frac{\partial(\mathcal{S}_D\varphi)}{\partial\nu}(R(x)) = R\frac{\partial}{\partial\nu}\mathcal{S}_{\widehat{D}}(R^{-1}(\varphi\circ R))(x) \,. \tag{9.18}$$

Proof.   Using (9.16) we compute

$$\begin{aligned}
(\mathcal{S}_D\varphi)(R(x)) &= \int_{\partial D} \mathbf{\Gamma}(R(x) - y)\varphi(y)\, d\sigma(y) \\
&= \int_{\partial\widehat{D}} \mathbf{\Gamma}(R(x) - R(y))\varphi(R(y))\, d\sigma(y) \\
&= R\int_{\partial\widehat{D}} \mathbf{\Gamma}(x - y)R^{-1}\varphi(R(y))\, d\sigma(y) \\
&= R\mathcal{S}_{\widehat{D}}(R^{-1}(\varphi\circ R))(x) \,,
\end{aligned}$$

which proves (9.17).

Applying Lemma 9.9 (ii), we arrive at

$$\frac{\partial}{\partial \nu}(\mathcal{S}_D \varphi)(R(x)) = R\frac{\partial}{\partial \nu}\left(R^{-1}(\mathcal{S}_D\varphi)\circ R\right)(x) .$$

Then (9.18) follows from (9.17) and the above identity. This completes the proof. $\qquad\square$

9.3 Transmission Problem

We suppose that the elastic medium Ω contains a single inclusion D, which is also a bounded Lipschitz domain. Let the constants (λ, μ) denote the background Lamé coefficients, which are the elastic parameters in the absence of any inclusions. Suppose that D has the pair of Lamé constants $(\widetilde{\lambda}, \widetilde{\mu})$ that is different from that of the background elastic body (λ, μ). It is always assumed that

$$\mu > 0, \quad d\lambda + 2\mu > 0, \quad \widetilde{\mu} > 0 \quad \text{and} \quad d\widetilde{\lambda} + 2\widetilde{\mu} > 0 . \tag{9.19}$$

We also assume that

$$(\lambda - \widetilde{\lambda})(\mu - \widetilde{\mu}) \geq 0, \; \left((\lambda - \widetilde{\lambda})^2 + (\mu - \widetilde{\mu})^2 \neq 0\right) . \tag{9.20}$$

We consider the transmission problem

$$\begin{cases} \displaystyle\sum_{j,k,l=1}^{d} \frac{\partial}{\partial x_j}\left(C_{ijkl}\frac{\partial u_k}{\partial x_l}\right) = 0 \quad \text{in } \Omega, \quad i = 1,\ldots,d , \\ \displaystyle\frac{\partial \mathbf{u}}{\partial \nu}\bigg|_{\partial\Omega} = \mathbf{g} , \end{cases} \tag{9.21}$$

where the elasticity tensor $C = (C_{ijkl})$ is given by

$$\begin{aligned} C_{ijkl} := &\left(\lambda\chi(\Omega \setminus D) + \widetilde{\lambda}\chi(D)\right)\delta_{ij}\delta_{kl} \\ &+ \left(\mu\chi(\Omega \setminus D) + \widetilde{\mu}\chi(D)\right)(\delta_{ik}\delta_{jl} + \delta_{il}\delta_{jk}) , \end{aligned} \tag{9.22}$$

and u_k for $k = 1,\ldots,d$, denote the components of the displacement field $\mathbf{u}$.

In order to ensure existence and uniqueness of a solution to (9.21), we assume that $\mathbf{g} \in L^2_{\Psi}(\partial\Omega)$ and seek a solution $\mathbf{u} \in W^{1,2}(\Omega)$ such that $\mathbf{u}|_{\partial\Omega} \in L^2_{\Psi}(\partial\Omega)$. The problem (9.21) is understood in a weak sense, namely, for any $\varphi \in W^{1,2}(\Omega)$, the following equality holds:

$$\sum_{i,j,k,l=1}^{d} \int_{\Omega} C_{ijkl}\frac{\partial u_k}{\partial x_l}\frac{\partial \varphi_i}{\partial x_j}dx = \int_{\partial\Omega} \mathbf{g}\cdot\varphi\,d\sigma ,$$

where φ_i for $i = 1,\ldots,d$, denote the components of φ.

Let $\mathcal{L}_{\widetilde{\lambda},\widetilde{\mu}}$ and $\partial/\partial\widetilde{\nu}$ be the Lamé system and the conormal derivative associated with $(\widetilde{\lambda},\widetilde{\mu})$, respectively. Then, for any $\varphi \in \mathcal{C}_0^\infty(\Omega)$, we compute

$$
\begin{aligned}
0 &= \sum_{i,j,k,l=1}^{d} \int_\Omega C_{ijkl} \frac{\partial u_k}{\partial x_l} \frac{\partial \varphi_i}{\partial x_j} \, dx \\
&= \int_{\Omega\setminus\overline{D}} \lambda(\nabla\cdot\mathbf{u})(\nabla\cdot\boldsymbol{\varphi}) + \frac{\mu}{2}(\nabla\mathbf{u}+\nabla\mathbf{u}^T)\cdot(\nabla\boldsymbol{\varphi}+\nabla\boldsymbol{\varphi}^T)\,dx \\
&\quad + \int_D \widetilde{\lambda}(\nabla\cdot\mathbf{u})(\nabla\cdot\boldsymbol{\varphi}) + \frac{\widetilde{\mu}}{2}(\nabla\mathbf{u}+\nabla\mathbf{u}^T)\cdot(\nabla\boldsymbol{\varphi}+\nabla\boldsymbol{\varphi}^T)\,dx \\
&= -\int_{\Omega\setminus\overline{D}} \mathcal{L}_{\lambda,\mu}\mathbf{u}\cdot\boldsymbol{\varphi}\,dx - \int_{\partial D} \frac{\partial\mathbf{u}}{\partial\nu}\cdot\boldsymbol{\varphi}\,d\sigma - \int_D \mathcal{L}_{\widetilde{\lambda},\widetilde{\mu}}\mathbf{u}\cdot\boldsymbol{\varphi}\,dx + \int_{\partial D}\frac{\partial\mathbf{u}}{\partial\widetilde{\nu}}\cdot\boldsymbol{\varphi}\,d\sigma\,,
\end{aligned}
$$

where the last equality follows from (9.2). Thus (9.21) is equivalent to the following problem:

$$
\begin{cases}
\mathcal{L}_{\lambda,\mu}\mathbf{u} = 0 & \text{in } \Omega\setminus\overline{D}\,, \\[4pt]
\mathcal{L}_{\widetilde{\lambda},\widetilde{\mu}}\mathbf{u} = 0 & \text{in } D\,, \\[4pt]
\mathbf{u}\big|_- = \mathbf{u}\big|_+ & \text{on } \partial D\,, \\[4pt]
\dfrac{\partial\mathbf{u}}{\partial\widetilde{\nu}}\bigg|_- = \dfrac{\partial\mathbf{u}}{\partial\nu}\bigg|_+ & \text{on } \partial D\,, \\[8pt]
\dfrac{\partial\mathbf{u}}{\partial\nu}\bigg|_{\partial\Omega} = \mathbf{g}\,, & \left(\mathbf{u}|_{\partial\Omega} \in L_\Psi^2(\partial\Omega)\right)\,.
\end{cases}
\tag{9.23}
$$

We denote by $\mathcal{S}_D$ and $\widetilde{\mathcal{S}}_D$ the single layer potentials on ∂D corresponding to the Lamé constants (λ,μ) and $(\widetilde{\lambda},\widetilde{\mu})$, respectively.

We use the following solvability theorem due to Escauriaza and Seo [121, Theorem 4].

Theorem 9.13 *Suppose that* $(\lambda-\widetilde{\lambda})(\mu-\widetilde{\mu}) \geq 0$ *and* $0 < \widetilde{\lambda},\widetilde{\mu} < +\infty$. *For any given* $(\mathbf{F},\mathbf{G}) \in W_1^2(\partial D) \times L^2(\partial D)$, *a unique pair* $(\mathbf{f},\mathbf{g}) \in L^2(\partial D) \times L^2(\partial D)$ *exists such that*

$$
\begin{cases}
\widetilde{\mathcal{S}}_D\mathbf{f}\big|_- - \mathcal{S}_D\mathbf{g}\big|_+ = \mathbf{F} & \text{on } \partial D\,, \\[6pt]
\dfrac{\partial}{\partial\widetilde{\nu}}\widetilde{\mathcal{S}}_D\mathbf{f}\bigg|_- - \dfrac{\partial}{\partial\nu}\mathcal{S}_D\mathbf{g}\bigg|_+ = \mathbf{G} & \text{on } \partial D\,,
\end{cases}
\tag{9.24}
$$

and a constant C *exists depending only on* $\lambda,\mu,\widetilde{\lambda},\widetilde{\mu}$, *and the Lipschitz character of* D *such that*

$$
\|\mathbf{f}\|_{L^2(\partial D)} + \|\mathbf{g}\|_{L^2(\partial D)} \leq C\left(\|\mathbf{F}\|_{W_1^2(\partial D)} + \|\mathbf{G}\|_{L^2(\partial D)}\right)\,.
\tag{9.25}
$$

Moreover, if $\mathbf{G} \in L_\Psi^2(\partial D)$, *then* $\mathbf{g} \in L_\Psi^2(\partial D)$.

Proof.   The unique solvability of the integral equation (9.24) was proved in [121]. By (9.12), $\partial \widetilde{\mathcal{S}}_D \mathbf{f}/\partial \widetilde{\nu}|_- \in L^2_\Psi(\partial D)$. Thus, if $\mathbf{G} \in L^2_\Psi(\partial D)$, then $\partial \mathcal{S}_D \mathbf{g}/\partial \nu|_+ \in L^2_\Psi(\partial D)$. Since

$$\mathbf{g} = \frac{\partial}{\partial \nu} \mathcal{S}_D \mathbf{g} \bigg|_+ - \frac{\partial}{\partial \nu} \mathcal{S}_D \mathbf{g} \bigg|_- \, ,$$

then, by (9.10) and $\partial \mathcal{S}_D \mathbf{g}/\partial \nu|_- \in L^2_\Psi(\partial D)$, we conclude that $\mathbf{g} \in L^2_\Psi(\partial D)$. $\square$

Lemma 9.14 *Let $\varphi \in \Psi$. If the pair $(\mathbf{f}, \mathbf{g}) \in L^2(\partial D) \times L^2_\Psi(\partial D)$ is the solution of*

$$\begin{cases} \widetilde{\mathcal{S}}_D \mathbf{f} \big|_- - \mathcal{S}_D \mathbf{g} \big|_+ = \varphi|_{\partial D} \, , \\ \dfrac{\partial}{\partial \widetilde{\nu}} \widetilde{\mathcal{S}}_D \mathbf{f} \bigg|_- - \dfrac{\partial}{\partial \nu} \mathcal{S}_D \mathbf{g} \bigg|_+ = 0 \, , \end{cases} \tag{9.26}$$

then $\mathbf{g} = 0$.

Proof.   Define $\mathbf{u}$ by

$$\mathbf{u}(x) := \begin{cases} \mathcal{S}_D \mathbf{g}(x) \, , & x \in \mathbb{R}^d \setminus \overline{D} \, , \\ \widetilde{\mathcal{S}}_D \mathbf{f}(x) - \varphi(x) \, , & x \in D \, . \end{cases}$$

Since $\mathbf{g} \in L^2_\Psi(\partial D)$, then $\int_{\partial D} \mathbf{g} \, d\sigma = 0$, and hence

$$\mathcal{S}_D \mathbf{g}(x) = O(|x|^{1-d}) \quad \text{as } |x| \to +\infty \, .$$

Therefore $\mathbf{u}$ is the unique solution of

$$\begin{cases} \mathcal{L}_{\lambda,\mu} \mathbf{u} = 0 & \text{in } \mathbb{R}^d \setminus \overline{D} \, , \\ \mathcal{L}_{\widetilde{\lambda},\widetilde{\mu}} \mathbf{u} = 0 & \text{in } D \, , \\ \mathbf{u}|_+ = \mathbf{u}|_- & \text{on } \partial D \, , \\ \dfrac{\partial \mathbf{u}}{\partial \nu} \bigg|_+ = \dfrac{\partial \mathbf{u}}{\partial \widetilde{\nu}} \bigg|_- & \text{on } \partial D \, , \\ \mathbf{u}(x) = O(|x|^{1-d}) & \text{as } |x| \to +\infty \, . \end{cases} \tag{9.27}$$

Using the fact that the trivial solution is the unique solution to (9.27), we see that

$$\mathcal{S}_D \mathbf{g}(x) = 0 \quad \text{for } x \in \mathbb{R}^d \setminus \overline{D} \, .$$

It then follows that $\mathcal{L}_{\lambda,\mu} \mathcal{S}_D \mathbf{g}(x) = 0$ for $x \in D$ and $\mathcal{S}_D \mathbf{g}(x) = 0$ for $x \in \partial D$. Thus, $\mathcal{S}_D \mathbf{g}(x) = 0$ for $x \in D$. Since

$$\mathbf{g} = \frac{\partial(\mathcal{S}_D \mathbf{g})}{\partial \nu} \bigg|_+ - \frac{\partial(\mathcal{S}_D \mathbf{g})}{\partial \nu} \bigg|_- \, ,$$

it is obvious that $\mathbf{g} = 0$. $\square$

We now prove a representation theorem for the solution of the transmission problem (9.23), which will be the main ingredient in deriving the asymptotic expansions in Chapter 11.

Theorem 9.15 *A unique pair $(\varphi, \psi) \in L^2(\partial D) \times L^2_\Psi(\partial D)$ exists such that the solution $\mathbf{u}$ of (9.23) is represented by*

$$\mathbf{u}(x) = \begin{cases} \mathbf{H}(x) + \mathcal{S}_D\psi(x) , & x \in \Omega \setminus \overline{D} , \\ \widetilde{\mathcal{S}}_D\varphi(x) , & x \in D , \end{cases} \tag{9.28}$$

where $\mathbf{H}$ is defined by

$$\mathbf{H}(x) = \mathcal{D}_\Omega(\mathbf{u}|_{\partial\Omega})(x) - \mathcal{S}_\Omega(\mathbf{g})(x) , \quad x \in \mathbb{R}^d \setminus \partial\Omega . \tag{9.29}$$

In fact, the pair (φ, ψ) is the unique solution in $L^2(\partial D) \times L^2_\Psi(\partial D)$ of

$$\begin{cases} \widetilde{\mathcal{S}}_D\varphi\big|_- - \mathcal{S}_D\psi\big|_+ = \mathbf{H}|_{\partial D} & \text{on } \partial D , \\ \dfrac{\partial}{\partial\widetilde{\nu}}\widetilde{\mathcal{S}}_D\varphi\bigg|_- - \dfrac{\partial}{\partial\nu}\mathcal{S}_D\psi\bigg|_+ = \dfrac{\partial\mathbf{H}}{\partial\nu}\bigg|_{\partial D} & \text{on } \partial D . \end{cases} \tag{9.30}$$

A positive constant C exists such that

$$\|\varphi\|_{L^2(\partial D)} + \|\psi\|_{L^2(\partial D)} \leq C\|\mathbf{H}\|_{W_1^2(\partial D)} . \tag{9.31}$$

For any integer n, a positive constant $\hat{C}_n$ exists depending only on c_0 and λ, μ (not on $\widetilde{\lambda}, \widetilde{\mu}$) such that

$$\|\mathbf{H}\|_{\mathcal{C}^n(\overline{D})} \leq C_n\|\mathbf{g}\|_{L^2(\partial\Omega)} . \tag{9.32}$$

Moreover,
$$\mathbf{H}(x) = -\mathcal{S}_D\psi(x) , \quad x \in \mathbb{R}^d \setminus \overline{\Omega} . \tag{9.33}$$

Proof. Let φ and ψ be the unique solutions of (9.30). Then clearly $\mathbf{u}$ defined by (9.28) satisfies the transmission condition [the third and fourth conditions in (9.23)]. By (9.12), $\partial\mathbf{H}/\partial\nu|_{\partial D} \in L^2_\Psi(\partial D)$. Thus, by Theorem 9.13, $\psi \in L^2_\Psi(\partial D)$.

We now prove that $\partial\mathbf{u}/\partial\nu|_{\partial\Omega} = \mathbf{g}$. To this end, we consider the following two-phase transmission problem:

$$\begin{cases} \mathcal{L}_{\lambda,\mu}\mathbf{u} = 0 & \text{in } (\Omega \setminus \overline{D}) \cup (\mathbb{R}^d \setminus \overline{\Omega}) , \\ \mathcal{L}_{\widetilde{\lambda},\widetilde{\mu}}\mathbf{u} = 0 & \text{in } D , \\ \mathbf{u}|_- = \mathbf{u}|_+ \quad \text{and} \quad \dfrac{\partial\mathbf{u}}{\partial\widetilde{\nu}}\bigg|_- = \dfrac{\partial\mathbf{u}}{\partial\nu}\bigg|_+ & \text{on } \partial D , \\ \mathbf{u}|_- - \mathbf{u}|_+ = \mathbf{f} \quad \text{and} \quad \dfrac{\partial\mathbf{u}}{\partial\widetilde{\nu}}\bigg|_- - \dfrac{\partial\mathbf{u}}{\partial\nu}\bigg|_+ = \mathbf{g} & \text{on } \partial\Omega , \\ |x||\mathbf{u}(x)| + |x|^2|\nabla\mathbf{u}(x)| \leq C & \text{as } |x| \to +\infty , \end{cases} \tag{9.34}$$

where $\mathbf{f} = \mathbf{u}|_{\partial\Omega}$. If $\mathbf{v} \in W^{1,2}(\Omega)$ is the solution of (9.23), then $\mathbf{U}_1$, defined by

$$\mathbf{U}_1(x) := \begin{cases} \mathbf{v}(x) , & x \in \Omega , \\ \mathbf{0} , & x \in \mathbb{R}^d \setminus \overline{\Omega} , \end{cases}$$

is a solution of (9.34). On the other hand, it can be easily seen from the jump relations of the layer potentials, (9.9) and (9.10), that $\mathbf{U}_2$ defined by

$$\mathbf{U}_2(x) = \begin{cases} -\mathcal{S}_\Omega(\mathbf{g})(x) + \mathcal{D}_\Omega(\mathbf{u}|_{\partial\Omega})(x) + \mathcal{S}_D\psi(x) , & x \in \mathbb{R}^d \setminus (\overline{D} \cup \partial\Omega) , \\ \widetilde{\mathcal{S}}_D\varphi(x) , & x \in D , \end{cases}$$

is also a solution of (9.34). Thus $\mathbf{U}_1 - \mathbf{U}_2$ is a solution of (9.34) with $\mathbf{f} = 0$ and $\mathbf{g} = 0$. Moreover, $\mathbf{U}_1 - \mathbf{U}_2 \in W^{1,2}(\mathbb{R}^d)$ and therefore, $\mathbf{U}_1 - \mathbf{U}_2 = 0$, which implies, in particular, that $\partial\mathbf{u}/\partial\nu|_{\partial\Omega} = \mathbf{g}$. Indeed, $\mathbf{U}_2(x) = 0$ for $x \in \mathbb{R}^d \setminus \overline{\Omega}$ and hence (9.33) holds.

Now it only remains to prove (9.32). Let

$$\Omega' := \left\{ x \in \Omega : \ \mathrm{dist}(x, \partial\Omega) > c_0 \right\}$$

so that D is compactly contained in Ω'. Then by an identity of Rellich type, that is available for general constant coefficient systems (see [104, Lemma 1.14 (i)]) but is beyond the scope of this book, a constant C exists such that

$$\|\nabla\mathbf{u}\|_{L^2(\partial\Omega)} \leq C\left(\|\mathbf{g}\|_{L^2(\partial\Omega)} + \|\nabla\mathbf{u}\|_{L^2(\Omega\setminus\Omega')} \right) . \tag{9.35}$$

By applying the Korn's inequality (9.15) and the divergence theorem, we find that

$$\begin{aligned} \|\nabla\mathbf{u}\|_{L^2(\Omega\setminus\Omega')} &\leq C\|\nabla\mathbf{u} + \nabla\mathbf{u}^T\|_{L^2(\Omega\setminus\overline{D})} \\ &\leq C \int_\Omega \left(\lambda\chi(\Omega \setminus \overline{D}) + \widetilde{\lambda}\chi(D) \right) |\nabla \cdot \mathbf{u}|^2 \\ &\quad + \frac{1}{2}\left(\mu\chi(\Omega \setminus \overline{D}) + \widetilde{\mu}\chi(D) \right) |\nabla\mathbf{u} + \nabla\mathbf{u}^T|^2 dx \\ &\leq C \int_{\partial\Omega} \mathbf{u} \cdot \frac{\partial\mathbf{u}}{\partial\nu} d\sigma , \end{aligned}$$

where the constants, generically denoted by C, do not depend on $\widetilde{\lambda}, \widetilde{\mu}$. Furthermore, by (9.35) and the Poincaré inequality (2.1), we see that

$$\begin{aligned} \|\mathbf{u}\|_{L^2(\partial\Omega)} &\leq C\|\nabla\mathbf{u}\|_{L^2(\partial\Omega)} \\ &\leq C\left(\|\mathbf{g}\|_{L^2(\partial\Omega)} + \|\mathbf{g}\|_{L^2(\partial\Omega)}\|\mathbf{u}\|_{L^2(\partial\Omega)} \right) , \end{aligned}$$

and hence

$$\|\mathbf{u}\|_{L^2(\partial\Omega)} \leq C\|\mathbf{g}\|_{L^2(\partial\Omega)} . \tag{9.36}$$

Clearly, the desired estimate (9.32) immediately follows from the definition of $\mathbf{H}$ and (9.36). $\square$

We now derive a representation for $\mathbf{u}$ in terms of the background solution. Let $\mathbf{N}(x, y)$ be the Neumann function for $\mathcal{L}_{\lambda,\mu}$ in Ω corresponding to a Dirac mass at y. That is, $\mathbf{N}$ is the solution to

$$
\begin{cases}
\mathcal{L}_{\lambda,\mu}\mathbf{N}(x, y) = -\delta_y(x)I_d & \text{in } \Omega, \\
\left.\dfrac{\partial \mathbf{N}}{\partial \nu}\right|_{\partial\Omega} = -\dfrac{1}{|\partial\Omega|}I_d \,, \\
\mathbf{N}(\cdot, y) \in L^2_{\Psi}(\partial\Omega) & \text{for any } y \in \Omega \,,
\end{cases}
\tag{9.37}
$$

where the differentiations act on the x-variables and I_d is the $d \times d$ identity matrix.

For $\mathbf{g} \in L^2_{\Psi}(\partial\Omega)$, define

$$
\mathbf{U}(x) := \int_{\partial\Omega} \mathbf{N}(x, y)\mathbf{g}(y)\, d\sigma(y) \,, \quad x \in \Omega \,.
\tag{9.38}
$$

Then $\mathbf{U}$ is the solution to (9.14) with D replaced by Ω. On the other hand, by (9.13), the solution to (9.14) is given by

$$
\mathbf{U}(x) := \mathcal{S}_{\Omega}\left(-\frac{1}{2}I + \mathcal{K}^*_{\Omega} \right)^{-1}\mathbf{g}(x) \,.
$$

Thus,

$$
\int_{\partial\Omega} \mathbf{N}(x, y)\mathbf{g}(y)\, d\sigma(y) = \int_{\partial\Omega} \mathbf{\Gamma}(x - y)(-\frac{1}{2}I + \mathcal{K}^*_{\Omega})^{-1}\mathbf{g}(y)\, d\sigma(y) \,,
$$

or equivalently,

$$
\int_{\partial\Omega} \mathbf{N}(x, y)(-\frac{1}{2}I + \mathcal{K}^*_{\Omega})\mathbf{g}(y)\, d\sigma(y) = \int_{\partial\Omega} \mathbf{\Gamma}(x - y)\mathbf{g}(y)\, d\sigma(y) \,, \quad x \in \Omega \,,
$$

for any $\mathbf{g} \in L^2_{\Psi}(\partial\Omega)$. Consequently, it follows that, for any simply connected Lipschitz domain D compactly contained in Ω and for any $\mathbf{g} \in L^2_{\Psi}(\partial D)$, the following identity holds:

$$
\int_{\partial D}(-\frac{1}{2}I + \mathcal{K}_{\Omega})(\mathbf{N}_y)(x)\mathbf{g}(y)\, d\sigma(y) = \int_{\partial D} \mathbf{\Gamma}_y(x)\mathbf{g}(y)\, d\sigma(y) \,,
$$

for all $x \in \partial\Omega$. Therefore, the following lemma has been proved.

Lemma 9.16 *For $y \in \Omega$ and $x \in \partial\Omega$, let $\mathbf{\Gamma}_y(x) := \mathbf{\Gamma}(x - y)$ and $\mathbf{N}_y(x) := \mathbf{N}(x, y)$. Then*

$$
\left(-\frac{1}{2}I + \mathcal{K}_{\Omega} \right)(\mathbf{N}_y)(x) = \mathbf{\Gamma}_y(x) \quad modulo\ \Psi \,.
\tag{9.39}
$$

We fix now some notation. Let

$$
N_D\mathbf{f}(x) := \int_{\partial D} \mathbf{N}(x, y)\mathbf{f}(y)\, d\sigma(y) \,, \quad x \in \overline{\Omega} \,.
$$

Theorem 9.17 *Let* **u** *be the solution to (9.23) and* **U** *the background solution, i.e., the solution to (9.14). Then the following holds:*

$$\mathbf{u}(x) = \mathbf{U}(x) - N_D\psi(x), \quad x \in \partial\Omega, \tag{9.40}$$

where ψ is defined by (9.30).

Proof.   By substituting (9.28) into (9.29), we obtain

$$\mathbf{H}(x) = -\mathcal{S}_\Omega(\mathbf{g})(x) + \mathcal{D}_\Omega\Big(\mathbf{H}|_{\partial\Omega} + (\mathcal{S}_D\psi)|_{\partial\Omega}\Big)(x), \quad x \in \Omega.$$

By using (9.9), we see that

$$(\tfrac{1}{2}I - \mathcal{K}_\Omega)(\mathbf{H}|_{\partial\Omega}) = -(\mathcal{S}_\Omega\mathbf{g})|_{\partial\Omega} + (\tfrac{1}{2}I + \mathcal{K}_\Omega)((\mathcal{S}_D\psi)|_{\partial\Omega}) \quad \text{on } \partial\Omega. \tag{9.41}$$

Since $\mathbf{U}(x) = -\mathcal{S}_\Omega(\mathbf{g})(x) + \mathcal{D}_\Omega(\mathbf{U}|_{\partial\Omega})(x)$ for all $x \in \Omega$, we have

$$(\tfrac{1}{2}I - \mathcal{K}_\Omega)(\mathbf{U}|_{\partial\Omega}) = -(\mathcal{S}_\Omega\mathbf{g})|_{\partial\Omega}. \tag{9.42}$$

By Theorem 9.13 and (9.39), we have

$$(-\tfrac{1}{2}I + \mathcal{K}_\Omega)((N_D\psi)|_{\partial\Omega})(x) = (\mathcal{S}_D\psi)(x), \quad x \in \partial\Omega, \tag{9.43}$$

since $\psi \in L^2_\Psi(\partial D)$. We see from (9.41), (9.42), and (9.43) that

$$(\tfrac{1}{2}I - \mathcal{K}_\Omega)\Big(\mathbf{H}|_{\partial\Omega} - \mathbf{U}|_{\partial\Omega} + (\tfrac{1}{2}I + \mathcal{K}_\Omega)((N_D\psi)|_{\partial\Omega})\Big) = 0 \quad \text{on } \partial\Omega,$$

and hence, by Corollary 9.7, we obtain that

$$\mathbf{H}|_{\partial\Omega} - \mathbf{U}|_{\partial\Omega} + (\tfrac{1}{2}I + \mathcal{K}_\Omega)((N_D\psi)|_{\partial\Omega}) \in \Psi.$$

Note that

$$(\tfrac{1}{2}I + \mathcal{K}_\Omega)((N_D\psi)|_{\partial\Omega}) = (N_D\psi)|_{\partial\Omega} + (\mathcal{S}_D\psi)|_{\partial\Omega},$$

which follows from (9.39). Thus, (9.28) gives

$$\mathbf{u}|_{\partial\Omega} = \mathbf{U}|_{\partial\Omega} - (N_D\psi)|_{\partial\Omega} \quad \text{modulo } \Psi. \tag{9.44}$$

Since all the functions in (9.44) belong to $L^2_\Psi(\partial\Omega)$, we have (9.40). This completes the proof. $\square$

We have a similar representation for solutions of the Dirichlet problem. Let $\mathbf{G}(x, y)$ be the Green's function for the Dirichlet problem, i.e., the solution to

$$\begin{cases} \mathcal{L}_{\lambda,\mu}\mathbf{G}(x,y) = -\delta_y(x)I_d & \text{in } \Omega \,, \\ \mathbf{G}(x,y) = 0 \,, & x \in \partial\Omega \ \text{for any } y \in \partial\Omega \,. \end{cases}$$

Then the function $\mathbf{V}$, for $\mathbf{f} \in W^2_{\frac{1}{2}}(\partial\Omega)$, defined by

$$\mathbf{V}(x) := -\int_{\partial\Omega} \frac{\partial}{\partial\nu_y}\mathbf{G}(x,y)\mathbf{f}(y)\,d\sigma(y) \,,$$

is the solution to the problem

$$\begin{cases} \mathcal{L}_{\lambda,\mu}\mathbf{V} = 0 & \text{in } \Omega \,, \\ \mathbf{V}|_{\partial\Omega} = \mathbf{f} \,. \end{cases}$$

We have the following theorem.

Theorem 9.18 *We have*

$$\left(\frac{1}{2}I + \mathcal{K}^*_\Omega\right)^{-1}\left(\frac{\partial}{\partial\nu}\mathbf{\Gamma}_z\right)(x) = \frac{\partial}{\partial\nu}\mathbf{G}_z(x) \,, \quad x \in \partial\Omega \,, \ z \in \Omega \,.$$

Moreover, let $\mathbf{u}$ be the solution of (9.23) with the Neumann condition on $\partial\Omega$ replaced by the Dirichlet condition $\mathbf{u}|_{\partial\Omega} = \mathbf{f} \in W^2_{\frac{1}{2}}(\partial\Omega)$. Then the following identity holds:

$$\frac{\partial\mathbf{u}}{\partial\nu}(x) = \frac{\partial\mathbf{V}}{\partial\nu}(x) - G_D\psi(x) \,, \quad x \in \partial\Omega \,,$$

where ψ is defined in (9.28) and

$$G_D\psi(x) := \int_{\partial D} \frac{\partial}{\partial\nu}\mathbf{G}(x,y)\psi(y)\,d\sigma(y) \,.$$

Theorem 9.18 can be proved in the same way as Theorem 9.17. In fact, it is simpler because of the solvability of the Dirichlet problem or, equivalently, the invertibility of $(1/2)\,I + \mathcal{K}^*_\Omega$ on $L^2(\partial\Omega)$. So we omit the proof.

9.4 Complex Representation of the Displacement Field

This section is devoted to a representation of the solution of (9.21) by a pair of holomorphic functions in the two-dimensional case. The results of this section will be used to compute the elastic moment tensors in Chapter 10.

The following theorem is from [249]. We include its proof for the sake of the reader.

Theorem 9.19 *Suppose that Ω is a simply connected domain in $\mathbb{R}^2$ (bounded or unbounded) with the Lamé constants λ, μ, and let $\mathbf{u} = (u, v) \in W^{1, \frac{3}{2}}(\Omega)$ be a solution of $\mathcal{L}_{\lambda, \mu} \mathbf{u} = 0$ in Ω. Then there are holomorphic functions φ and ψ in Ω such that*

$$2\mu(u + iv)(z) = \kappa \varphi(z) - z \overline{\varphi'(z)} - \overline{\psi(z)} \,, \quad \kappa = \frac{\lambda + 3\mu}{\lambda + \mu} \,, \quad z = x_1 + ix_2 \,. \quad (9.45)$$

Moreover, the conormal derivative $\partial \mathbf{u} / \partial \nu$ is represented as

$$\left(\left(\frac{\partial \mathbf{u}}{\partial \nu} \right)_1 + i \left(\frac{\partial \mathbf{u}}{\partial \nu} \right)_2 \right) d\sigma = -i\partial \left[\varphi(z) + z \overline{\varphi'(z)} + \overline{\psi(z)} \right] \,, \quad (9.46)$$

where $d\sigma$ is the line element of $\partial\Omega$ and $\partial = (\partial / \partial x_1) \, dx_1 + (\partial / \partial x_2) \, dx_2$. Here $\partial\Omega$ is positively oriented and $\varphi'(z) = d\varphi(z)/dz$.

Proof.   Let $\theta := \nabla \cdot \mathbf{u}$ and

$$X := \lambda\theta + 2\mu\frac{\partial u}{\partial x_1} \,, \quad Y := \lambda\theta + 2\mu\frac{\partial v}{\partial x_2} \,, \quad Z := \mu\left(\frac{\partial v}{\partial x_1} + \frac{\partial u}{\partial x_2} \right) \, {}^1 \,.$$

An elementary calculation shows that the equation $\mathcal{L}_{\lambda, \mu} \mathbf{u} = 0$ is equivalent to

$$\frac{\partial X}{\partial x_1} + \frac{\partial Z}{\partial x_2} = 0 \quad \text{and} \quad \frac{\partial Z}{\partial x_1} + \frac{\partial Y}{\partial x_2} = 0 \,. \quad (9.47)$$

Thus there are two functions A and B such that

$$\nabla B = (-Z, X) \quad \text{and} \quad \nabla A = (Y, -Z) \,.$$

In particular, $\partial A/\partial x_2 = \partial B/\partial x_1$, and hence, there is a function[2] U such that $\nabla U = (A, B)$. Thus,

$$X = \frac{\partial^2 U}{\partial x_2^2} \,, \quad Y = \frac{\partial^2 U}{\partial x_1^2} \,, \quad Z = -\frac{\partial^2 U}{\partial x_1 \partial x_2} \,. \quad (9.48)$$

By taking the x_1-derivative of the first component of $\mathcal{L}_{\lambda, \mu} \mathbf{u}$ and the x_2-derivative of the second, we can see that

$$\frac{\partial}{\partial x_1}(\Delta u) + \frac{\partial}{\partial x_2}(\Delta v) = 0 \,.$$

It then follows that

$$\Delta(X + Y) = 2(\lambda + \mu)\left[\frac{\partial}{\partial x_1}(\Delta u) + \frac{\partial}{\partial x_2}(\Delta v) \right] = 0 \,.$$

---

[1] These notations are slightly different from those of [249].

[2] This function U is called the stress function or the Airy function.

Thus U is biharmonic, namely, $\Delta\Delta U = 0$. In short, we proved that there is a biharmonic function U such that

$$\lambda\theta + 2\mu\frac{\partial u}{\partial x_1} = \frac{\partial^2 U}{\partial x_2^2} \ , \ \lambda\theta + 2\mu\frac{\partial v}{\partial x_2} = \frac{\partial^2 U}{\partial x_1^2} \ , \ \mu\left(\frac{\partial v}{\partial x_1} + \frac{\partial u}{\partial x_2}\right) = -\frac{\partial^2 U}{\partial x_1\partial x_2} \ . \tag{9.49}$$

We claim that two holomorphic functions in Ω, φ and f exist, such that

$$2U(z) = \bar{z}\varphi(z) + z\overline{\varphi(z)} + f(z) + \overline{f(z)} \ , \quad z \in \Omega \ . \tag{9.50}$$

In fact, let $P := \Delta U$. Then P is harmonic in Ω. Let Q be a harmonic conjugate of P so that $P + iQ$ is holomorphic in Ω. Such a function exists since Ω is simply connected. See Lemma 2.1 (ii). Let $\varphi = p + iq$ be a holomorphic function in Ω so that $4\varphi'(z) = P(z) + iQ(z)$. Then,

$$\frac{\partial p}{\partial x_1} = \frac{1}{4}P \ , \quad \frac{\partial p}{\partial x_2} = -\frac{1}{4}Q \ , \tag{9.51}$$

which yields

$$\Delta(U - \Re(\bar{z}\varphi)) = P - \Re\varphi'(z) = 0 \ .$$

Therefore, a function f holomorphic in Ω exists such that

$$U - \Re(\bar{z}\varphi) = \Re f(z) \ ,$$

as was to be shown.

Next, adding the first two equations in (9.49), we obtain $2(\lambda+\mu)\theta = \Delta U = P$. It then follows from the first equation in (9.49) and (9.51) that

$$2\mu\frac{\partial u}{\partial x_1} = -\frac{\partial^2 U}{\partial x_1^2} + \frac{2(\lambda + 2\mu)}{\lambda + \mu}\frac{\partial p}{\partial x_1} \ .$$

Likewise, we obtain

$$2\mu\frac{\partial v}{\partial x_2} = -\frac{\partial^2 U}{\partial x_2^2} + \frac{2(\lambda + 2\mu)}{\lambda + \mu}\frac{\partial q}{\partial x_2} \ ,$$

and therefore

$$2\mu u = -\frac{\partial U}{\partial x_1} + \frac{2(\lambda + 2\mu)}{\lambda + \mu}p + f_1(x_2) \ ,$$

$$2\mu v = -\frac{\partial U}{\partial x_2} + \frac{2(\lambda + 2\mu)}{\lambda + \mu}q + f_2(x_1) \ .$$

Substitute these equations into the third equation in (9.49), and apply the Cauchy–Riemann equation $\partial p/\partial x_2 = -\partial q/\partial x_1$ to show that

$$f_1'(x_2) + f_2'(x_1) = 0 \ ,$$

which implies that

$$f_1(x_2) = ax_2 + b , \quad f_2(x_1) = -ax_1 + c ,$$

for some constants a, b, c. Thus we obtain

$$2\mu(u + iv)(x_1, x_2) = -\frac{\partial U}{\partial x_1} - i\frac{\partial U}{\partial x_2} + \frac{2(\lambda + 2\mu)}{\lambda + \mu}(p + iq) + a(x_2 - ix_1) + b + ic .$$

It then follows from (9.50) that

$$2\mu(u + iv)(x_1, x_2) = \frac{\lambda + 3\mu}{\lambda + \mu}\varphi(z) - z\overline{\varphi(z)} + \overline{\psi'(z)} - aiz + b + ic ,$$

where $\psi(z) = f'(z)$. By adding constants to φ and ψ to define new φ and ψ, we get (9.45).

Turning to the proof of (9.46), we first observe that

$$\frac{\partial \mathbf{u}}{\partial \nu} = \left(XN_1 + ZN_2, ZN_1 + YN_2 \right) ,$$

where $N = (N_1, N_2)$. Since $(-N_2, N_1)$ is a positively oriented tangential vector field on $\partial\Omega$, we have

$$-N_2 ds = dx_1, \quad N_1 ds = dx_2 . \tag{9.52}$$

It then follows from (9.48) that

$$\begin{aligned}
&\left(\left(\frac{\partial \mathbf{u}}{\partial \nu}\right)_1 + i\left(\frac{\partial \mathbf{u}}{\partial \nu}\right)_2 \right) d\sigma \\
&= \left(\frac{\partial^2 U}{\partial x_2^2} dx_2 + \frac{\partial^2 U}{\partial x_1 \partial x_2} dx_1 \right) - i\left(\frac{\partial^2 U}{\partial x_1 \partial x_2} dx_2 + \frac{\partial^2 U}{\partial x_1^2} dx_1 \right) \\
&= \partial\left(\frac{\partial U}{\partial x_2} - i\frac{\partial U}{\partial x_1} \right) .
\end{aligned}$$

Now, (9.46) follows from (9.50). This completes the proof. $\square$

We now prove that a similar theorem holds for the solution of (9.23).

Theorem 9.20 *Suppose $d = 2$. Let $\mathbf{u} = (u, v)$ be the solution of (9.23), and let $\mathbf{u}_e := \mathbf{u}|_{\mathbb{C} \setminus D}$ and $\mathbf{u}_i := \mathbf{u}|_D$. Then there are functions φ_e and ψ_e holomorphic in $\Omega \setminus \overline{D}$ and φ_i and ψ_i holomorphic in D such that*

$$2\mu(u_e + iv_e)(z) = \kappa\varphi_e(z) - z\overline{\varphi'_e(z)} - \overline{\psi_e(z)} , \quad z \in \mathbb{C} \setminus \overline{D} , \tag{9.53}$$

$$2\tilde{\mu}(u_i + iv_i)(z) = \tilde{\kappa}\varphi_i(z) - z\overline{\varphi'_i(z)} - \overline{\psi_i(z)} , \quad z \in D , \tag{9.54}$$

where

$$\kappa = \frac{\lambda + 3\mu}{\lambda + \mu} , \qquad \widetilde{\kappa} = \frac{\widetilde{\lambda} + 3\widetilde{\mu}}{\widetilde{\lambda} + \widetilde{\mu}} . \tag{9.55}$$

Moreover, the following holds on ∂D:

$$\frac{1}{2\mu}\left(\kappa\varphi_e(z) - z\overline{\varphi_e'(z)} - \overline{\psi_e(z)} \right) = \frac{1}{2\widetilde{\mu}}\left(\widetilde{\kappa}\varphi_i(z) - z\overline{\varphi_i'(z)} - \overline{\psi_i(z)} \right) , \tag{9.56}$$

$$\varphi_e(z) + z\overline{\varphi_e'(z)} + \overline{\psi_e(z)} = \varphi_i(z) + z\overline{\varphi_i'(z)} + \overline{\psi_i(z)} + c , \tag{9.57}$$

where c is a constant.

Proof. By Theorem 9.15, a unique pair $(\varphi, \psi) \in L^2(\partial D) \times L^2_{\Psi}(\partial D)$ exists such that

$$\mathbf{u}_e(x) = \mathbf{H}(x) + \mathcal{S}_D\psi(x) , \quad x \in \Omega \setminus \overline{D} ,$$
$$\mathbf{u}_i(x) = \widetilde{\mathcal{S}}_D\varphi(x) , \quad x \in D .$$

Since $\mathcal{L}_{\lambda,\mu}\mathbf{H} = 0$ in Ω and $\mathcal{L}_{\widetilde{\lambda},\widetilde{\mu}}\widetilde{\mathcal{S}}_D\varphi = 0$ in D, by Theorem 9.19, $\mathbf{H}$ and $\widetilde{\mathcal{S}}_D\varphi$ have the desired representation by holomorphic functions. So, in order to prove (9.53), it suffices to show that there are functions f and g holomorphic in $\Omega \setminus \overline{D}$ such that

$$2\mu\left[(\mathcal{S}_D\psi)_1 + i(\mathcal{S}_D\psi)_2\right](z) = \kappa f(z) - z\overline{f'(z)} - \overline{g(z)} , \quad z \in \Omega \setminus \overline{D} . \tag{9.58}$$

Observe that for $i = 1, 2$,

$$(\mathcal{S}_D\psi)_i(x) = \frac{A}{2\pi} \int_{\partial D} \ln|x - y|\psi_i(y)\, d\sigma(y)$$
$$- \frac{B}{2\pi} \sum_{j=1}^{2} \int_{\partial D} \frac{(x_i - y_i)(x_j - y_j)}{|x - y|^2}\psi_j(y)\, d\sigma(y) .$$

Hence

$$\left[(\mathcal{S}_D\psi)_1 + i(\mathcal{S}_D\psi)_2\right](x) = \frac{A}{2\pi} \int_{\partial D} \ln|x - y|\left[\psi_1(y) + i\psi_2(y)\right] d\sigma(y)$$
$$- \frac{B}{2\pi} \int_{\partial D} \frac{(x_1 - y_1) + i(x_2 - y_2)}{|x - y|^2}\left[(x_1 - y_1)\psi_1(y) + (x_2 - y_2)\psi_2(y)\right] d\sigma(y) .$$

Let $z = x_1 + ix_2$, $\zeta = y_1 + iy_2$, and $\psi = \psi_1 + i\psi_2$. Then

$$\left[(\mathcal{S}_D\psi)_1 + i(\mathcal{S}_D\psi)_2\right](z) = \frac{A}{2\pi}\int_{\partial D}\ln|z-\zeta|\psi(\zeta)\,d\sigma(\zeta)$$

$$-\frac{B}{2\pi}\int_{\partial D}\frac{z-\zeta}{|z-\zeta|^2}\left[(z-\zeta)\overline{\psi(\zeta)} + \overline{(z-\zeta)}\psi(\zeta)\right]d\sigma(\zeta)$$

$$= \frac{A}{4\pi}\int_{\partial D}\ln(z-\zeta)\psi(\zeta)\,d\sigma(\zeta) - \frac{B}{4\pi}z\int_{\partial D}\frac{\overline{\psi(\zeta)}}{z-\zeta}\,d\sigma(\zeta)$$

$$+ \frac{A}{4\pi}\int_{\partial D}\overline{\ln(z-\zeta)}\psi(\zeta)\,d\sigma(\zeta) + \frac{B}{4\pi}\int_{\partial D}\frac{\overline{\zeta\psi(\zeta)}}{z-\zeta}\,d\sigma(\zeta) - \frac{B}{4\pi}\int_{\partial D}\psi(\zeta)\,d\sigma(\zeta)\,.$$

Observe that
$$\frac{A}{B} = \frac{\lambda+3\mu}{\lambda+\mu}\,.$$

Then (9.58) follows with f defined by

$$f(z) := \frac{B}{8\mu\pi}\int_{\partial D}\ln(z-\zeta)\psi(\zeta)\,d\sigma(\zeta)\,, \tag{9.59}$$

and g defined in an obvious way. It should be noted that f defined by (9.59) is holomorphic outside D. This is because $\psi \in L^2_\Psi(\partial D)$, which implies that $\int_{\partial D}\psi\,d\sigma = 0$.

The equation (9.56) is identical to the third equation in (9.23). By the fourth equation in (9.23) and (9.46), we get

$$\partial\left[\varphi_e(z) + z\overline{\varphi'_e(z)} + \overline{\psi_e(z)}\right] = \partial\left[\varphi_i(z) + z\overline{\varphi'_i(z)} + \overline{\psi_i(z)}\right]\,,$$

from which (9.57) follows immediately. This finishes the proof. $\square$

9.5 Periodic Green's Function

We now construct a periodic Green's function (with period one in each direction) for the Lamé system in the two-dimensional case.

Lemma 9.21 *Define* $\mathbf{G} = (G_{pq})_{p,q=1,2}$ *by*

$$G_{pq}(x) = \frac{1}{4\pi^2\mu}\sum_{n=(n_1,n_2)\neq 0}\left[-\frac{1}{|n|^2}\delta_{pq} + \frac{\lambda+\mu}{\lambda+2\mu}\frac{n_p n_q}{|n|^4}\right]e^{i2\pi n\cdot x}\,. \tag{9.60}$$

Then $\mathbf{G}$ *is periodic and satisfies*

$$\mathcal{L}_{\lambda,\mu}\mathbf{G}(x) = \sum_{n\in\mathbb{Z}^2}\delta_0(x+n)I - I,\quad x\in\mathbb{R}^2\,, \tag{9.61}$$

where I *is the identity matrix. Moreover, a smooth function* $\mathbf{R}$ *exists such that*

$$\mathbf{G}(x) = \mathbf{\Gamma}(x) + \mathbf{R}(x), \quad x \in Y \ .$$

The function $\mathbf{R}$ has the following Taylor expansion at the origin:

$$\mathbf{R}(x_1, x_2) = \mathbf{R}(0) + \frac{1}{2} \begin{pmatrix} ax_1^2 + bx_2^2 & 2cx_1x_2 \\ 2cx_1x_2 & bx_1^2 + ax_2^2 \end{pmatrix} + O(|x|^4) \ , \tag{9.62}$$

where b is given by

$$b = -\frac{1}{2\mu} + \frac{\lambda + \mu}{4\mu(\lambda + 2\mu)} \left(\frac{2\pi}{3} + 16\pi^2 \sum_{n=1}^{+\infty} \frac{n^2 e^{-2\pi n}}{(1 - e^{-2\pi n})^2} - 8\pi \sum_{n=1}^{+\infty} \frac{n e^{-2\pi n}}{1 - e^{-2\pi n}} \right) , \tag{9.63}$$

and a and c are defined by

$$a + b = -\frac{\lambda + 3\mu}{2\mu(2\mu + \lambda)}, \quad a + c = -\frac{1}{2(2\mu + \lambda)} \ . \tag{9.64}$$

Proof.   We seek a periodic solution $\mathbf{G}$ of

$$\mathcal{L}_{\lambda,\mu}\mathbf{G}(x) = \sum_{n \in \mathbb{Z}^2} \delta_0(x + n)I - I, \quad x \in \mathbb{R}^2 \ . \tag{9.65}$$

Taking the divergence of (9.65), we have

$$(\lambda + 2\mu)\Delta \nabla \cdot \mathbf{G} = \sum_{n \in \mathbb{Z}^2} \nabla \delta_0(x + n) \ .$$

Thus, by Lemma 2.39,

$$\nabla \cdot \mathbf{G} = \frac{1}{\lambda + 2\mu} \nabla G \quad \text{modulo constants} \ .$$

Inserting this equation into (9.65) gives

$$\mu \Delta G_{pq} = -\frac{\lambda + \mu}{\lambda + 2\mu} \partial_p \partial_q G + \delta_{pq} \Big(\sum_{n \in \mathbb{Z}^2} \delta_0(x + n) - 1 \Big), \quad p, q = 1, 2 \ .$$

Let $\{G_{pq}^n\}_{n \in \mathbb{Z}^2, n \neq 0}$ be the Fourier coefficients of G_{pq}. It follows from the Poisson summation formula (2.92) that

$$G_{pq}^n = \frac{1}{4\pi^2 \mu} \left[-\frac{\delta_{pq}}{|n|^2} + \frac{\lambda + \mu}{\lambda + 2\mu} \frac{n_p n_q}{|n|^4} \right], \quad n = (n_1, n_2) \in \mathbb{Z}^2, n \neq 0, p, q = 1, 2 \ .$$

Thus, (9.60) follows. We also have

$$\sum_{n \in \mathbb{Z}^2, n \neq 0} G_{pq}^n e^{i2\pi n \cdot x} = \frac{1}{4\pi^2 \mu} \left[-\delta_{pq} \sum_{n \in \mathbb{Z}^2, n \neq 0} \frac{e^{i2\pi n \cdot x}}{|n|^2} \right.$$

$$\left. + \frac{\lambda + \mu}{\lambda + 2\mu} \sum_{n \in \mathbb{Z}^2, n \neq 0} \frac{n_p n_q e^{i2\pi n \cdot x}}{|n|^4} \right]$$

$$= \delta_{pq} \frac{1}{\mu} \left(\frac{1}{2\pi} \ln|x| + R_0(x) \right) + \frac{\lambda + \mu}{4\pi^2 \mu(\lambda + 2\mu)} \gamma_{pq}(x) \ ,$$

where

$$\gamma_{pq}(x) = \sum_{n \in \mathbb{Z}^2, n \neq 0} \frac{n_p n_q e^{i2\pi n \cdot x}}{|n|^4} \ .$$

Note that $\gamma_{22}(x_1, x_2) = \gamma_{11}(x_2, x_1)$ and $\gamma_{12}(x_1, x_2) = \gamma_{21}(x_2, x_1)$ for all $x = (x_1, x_2)$. We also note that

$$\gamma_{11}(x) + \gamma_{22}(x) = \sum_{n \in \mathbb{Z}^2, n \neq 0} \frac{e^{i2\pi n \cdot x}}{|n|^2} = -4\pi^2 \left(\frac{1}{2\pi} \ln |x| + R_0(x) \right) , \qquad (9.66)$$

as shown in (2.94).

In order to prove (9.62), it then suffices to compute $\gamma_{11}(x)$ and $\gamma_{12}(x)$. We have

$$\gamma_{11}(x) = \sum_{n_1 \neq 0} \frac{e^{i2\pi n_1 x_1}}{n_1^2} + \sum_{n_2 \neq 0} e^{i2\pi n_2 x_2} \sum_{n_1 \in \mathbb{Z}} \frac{e^{i2\pi n_1 x_1}}{n_1^2 + n_2^2}$$
$$- \sum_{n_2 \neq 0} e^{i2\pi n_2 x_2} n_2^2 \sum_{n_1 \in \mathbb{Z}} \frac{e^{i2\pi n_1 x_1}}{(n_1^2 + n_2^2)^2} \ .$$

Let us invoke the summation identities (2.96) and (2.97). To compute the series $\sum_{n_1 \in \mathbb{Z}} e^{i2\pi n_1 x_1}/(n_1^2 + n_2^2)^2$, we use (2.114). Let $P(z) := (z^2 + n_2^2)^2$. Then the zeros of $P(z)$ are $\pm i n_2$, and from (2.114), it immediately follows that

$$\sum_{n_1 \in \mathbb{Z}} \frac{e^{i2\pi n_1 x_1}}{(n_1^2 + n_2^2)^2} = -\frac{\pi^2}{n_2^2} x_1 \left(\frac{e^{-2\pi x_1 n_2}}{e^{-2\pi n_2} - 1} + \frac{e^{2\pi x_1 n_2}}{e^{2\pi n_2} - 1} \right)$$
$$+ \frac{\pi^2}{n_2^2} \left(\frac{e^{-2\pi n_2} e^{-2\pi x_1 n_2}}{(e^{-2\pi n_2} - 1)^2} + \frac{e^{2\pi n_2} e^{2\pi x_1 n_2}}{(e^{2\pi n_2} - 1)^2} \right) - \frac{\pi}{2n_2^3} \left(\frac{e^{-2\pi x_1 n_2}}{e^{-2\pi n_2} - 1} - \frac{e^{2\pi x_1 n_2}}{e^{2\pi n_2} - 1} \right) .$$

We then calculate

$$\gamma_{11}(x) = \frac{\pi^2}{3} - 2\pi^2 x_1 + 2\pi^2 x_1^2 + 2\pi \sum_{n_2=1}^{+\infty} \frac{\cos(2\pi n_2 x_2)}{n_2} \frac{\cosh \pi (2x_1 - 1) n_2}{\sinh \pi n_2}$$
$$+ \pi^2 x_1 \sum_{n_2 \neq 0} e^{i2\pi n_2 x_2} \left(\frac{e^{-2\pi x_1 n_2}}{e^{-2\pi n_2} - 1} + \frac{e^{2\pi x_1 n_2}}{e^{2\pi n_2} - 1} \right)$$
$$+ \frac{\pi}{2} \sum_{n_2 \neq 0} \frac{e^{i2\pi n_2 x_2}}{n_2} \left(\frac{e^{-2\pi x_1 n_2}}{e^{-2\pi n_2} - 1} - \frac{e^{2\pi x_1 n_2}}{e^{2\pi n_2} - 1} \right) + r_0(x) ,$$

to arrive at

$$\gamma_{11}(x) = \frac{\pi^2}{3} - 2\pi^2 x_1 + 2\pi^2 x_1^2 + 2\pi \left(\pi x_1 - \ln 2 - \frac{1}{2} \ln(\sinh^2 \pi x_1 + \sin^2 \pi x_2) \right)$$
$$- 2\pi^2 x_1 \sum_{n_2=1}^{+\infty} \cos(2\pi n_2 x_2) e^{-2\pi x_1 n_2} - \pi \sum_{n_2=1}^{+\infty} \frac{\cos(2\pi n_2 x_2)}{n_2} e^{-2\pi x_1 n_2}$$
$$+ r_0(x) + r_1(x) + r_2(x) + r_3(x) , \qquad (9.67)$$

where

$$r_0(x) = -\pi^2 \sum_{n_2 \neq 0} e^{i2\pi n_2 x_2} \left(\frac{e^{-2\pi n_2} e^{-2\pi x_1 n_2}}{(e^{-2\pi n_2} - 1)^2} + \frac{e^{2\pi n_2} e^{2\pi x_1 n_2}}{(e^{2\pi n_2} - 1)^2} \right)$$

$$= -2\pi^2 \sum_{n_2=1}^{+\infty} \cos(2\pi n_2 x_2) \left(\frac{e^{-2\pi n_2} e^{-2\pi x_1 n_2}}{(e^{-2\pi n_2} - 1)^2} + \frac{e^{2\pi n_2} e^{2\pi x_1 n_2}}{(e^{2\pi n_2} - 1)^2} \right) ,$$

$$r_1(x) = 2\pi \sum_{n_2=1}^{+\infty} \frac{\cos 2\pi n_2 x_2}{n_2} \frac{e^{2\pi n_2 x_1} + e^{-2\pi n_2 x_1}}{e^{2\pi n_2} - 1} ,$$

$$r_2(x) = 2\pi^2 x_1 \sum_{n_2=1}^{+\infty} \cos(2\pi n_2 x_2) \left(e^{-2\pi x_1 n_2} + \frac{e^{-2\pi x_1 n_2}}{e^{-2\pi n_2} - 1} + \frac{e^{2\pi x_1 n_2}}{e^{2\pi n_2} - 1} \right) ,$$

and

$$r_3(x) = \pi \sum_{n_2=1}^{+\infty} \frac{\cos(2\pi n_2 x_2)}{n_2} \left(e^{-2\pi x_1 n_2} + \frac{e^{-2\pi x_1 n_2}}{e^{-2\pi n_2} - 1} - \frac{e^{2\pi x_1 n_2}}{e^{2\pi n_2} - 1} \right) .$$

Because of the term $e^{-2\pi n_2}$, one can easily see that r_0, r_1, r_2, and r_3 are C^∞-functions. On the other hand, we have

$$2 \sum_{n_2=1}^{+\infty} \cos(2\pi n_2 x_2) e^{-2\pi x_1 n_2} = \frac{x_1}{\pi(x_1^2 + x_2^2)} + r_4(x) , \tag{9.68}$$

for $x_1 > 0$, where r_4 is a C^∞-function.

In short, using formulae (2.97) and (9.68), we obtain from (9.67) that $G_{11} = \Gamma_{11} + R_{11}$, where R_{11} is a smooth function. From (9.61), (9.66), and the Taylor expansions of the remainders r_0, r_1, r_2, r_3, and r_4, an elementary calculation shows that the Taylor expansion of R_{11} at 0 is given by

$$R_{11}(x) = R_{11}(0) + \frac{1}{2}(ax_1^2 + bx_2^2) + O(|x|^4) ,$$

where b is defined by (9.63) and

$$a + b = -\frac{\lambda + 3\mu}{2\mu(2\mu + \lambda)} ,$$

as stated in (9.64).

The formula for $\gamma_{12}(x)$ can be obtained in the exactly same way. This completes the proof. $\qquad\square$

We now define the periodic single and double layer potentials of the density function $\varphi \in L_0^2(\partial D)$ associated with the Lamé parameters (λ, μ) by

$$\mathcal{G}_D\varphi(x) := \int_{\partial D} \mathbf{G}(x-y)\varphi(y)d\sigma(y), \quad x \in Y \ .$$

By (9.62), we have

$$\mathcal{G}_D\varphi(x) = \mathcal{S}_D\varphi(x) + \int_{\partial D} \mathbf{R}(x-y)\varphi(y)d\sigma(y), \quad x \in Y \ ,$$

where $\mathcal{R}_D\varphi := \int_{\partial D} \mathbf{R}(x-y)\varphi(y)d\sigma(y)$ is a smoothing operator. Therefore, it follows from (9.10) that

$$\left.\frac{\partial(\mathcal{G}_D\varphi)}{\partial\nu}\right|_+ - \left.\frac{\partial(\mathcal{G}_D\varphi)}{\partial\nu}\right|_- = \varphi \quad \text{on } \partial D \ . \tag{9.69}$$

Consider $\mathbf{w}_k^l = (w_{kp}^l)_{p=1,2}$ to be the solution to

$$\begin{cases} \nabla \cdot (C\mathcal{E}(\mathbf{w}_k^l)) = 0 \quad \text{in } Y \ , \\ \mathbf{w}_k^l - x_k\mathbf{e}_l \quad \text{is periodic with period 1} \ , \\ \displaystyle\int_Y (\mathbf{w}_k^l - x_k\mathbf{e}_l)\, dx = 0 \ , \end{cases} \tag{9.70}$$

where

$$\mathcal{E}(\mathbf{u}) := \frac{1}{2}(\nabla\mathbf{u} + \nabla\mathbf{u}^T) \quad \text{for } \mathbf{u} \in W^{1,2}(Y) \ .$$

Observe that $C\mathcal{E}(\mathbf{w}_k^l) = \sum_{p,n=1}^2 C_{ijpn}\partial w_{kp}^l/\partial x_n$ for $i,j = 1,2$.

Analogously to Theorems 2.41 and 2.45, the following result holds, giving a decomposition formula of the solution of the periodic transmission problem (9.70).

Theorem 9.22 *For $k,l = 1,2$, the solution $\mathbf{w}_k^l$ of (9.70) is represented by*

$$\mathbf{w}_k^l(x) = C + \begin{cases} x_k\mathbf{e}_l + \mathcal{G}_D\psi_k^l(x), & x \in Y \setminus \overline{D} \ , \\ \widetilde{\mathcal{S}}_D\varphi_k^l(x), & x \in D \ , \end{cases} \tag{9.71}$$

where the pair $(\varphi_k^l, \psi_k^l) \in L^2(\partial D) \times L^2(\partial D)$ is the unique solution to

$$\begin{cases} \widetilde{\mathcal{S}}_D\varphi_k^l|_- - \mathcal{G}_D\psi_k^l|_+ = x_k\mathbf{e}_l|_{\partial D} \ , \\ \left.\dfrac{\partial}{\partial\widetilde{\nu}}\widetilde{\mathcal{S}}_D\varphi_k^l\right|_- - \left.\dfrac{\partial}{\partial\nu}\mathcal{G}_D\psi_k^l\right|_+ = \left.\dfrac{\partial(x_k\mathbf{e}_l)}{\partial\nu}\right|_{\partial D} \ . \end{cases} \tag{9.72}$$

The constant C is chosen so that the condition $\int_Y(\mathbf{w}_k^l - x_k\mathbf{e}_l)\, dx = 0$ is fulfilled. Moreover, $\psi_k^l \in L_\Psi^2(\partial D)$ and

$$\|\varphi_k^l\|_{L^2(\partial D)} + \|\psi_k^l\|_{L^2(\partial D)} \leq C\|x_k\mathbf{e}_l\|_{W_1^2(\partial D)} \ . \tag{9.73}$$

Here $L_\Psi^2(\partial D)$ is defined by (9.11).

Proof.   It suffices to prove the unique solvability of the integral equation (9.72). By Theorem 9.13, a unique pair $(\mathbf{f}, \mathbf{g}) \in L^2(\partial D) \times L^2(\partial D)$ exists satisfying

$$\begin{cases} \widetilde{\mathcal{S}}_D\mathbf{f}\big|_- - \mathcal{S}_D\mathbf{g}\big|_+ = x_k\mathbf{e}_l\big|_{\partial D} \,, \\[2mm] \dfrac{\partial}{\partial\widetilde{\nu}}\widetilde{\mathcal{S}}_D\mathbf{f}\bigg|_- - \dfrac{\partial}{\partial\nu}\mathcal{S}_D\mathbf{g}\bigg|_+ = \dfrac{\partial(x_k\mathbf{e}_l)}{\partial\nu}\bigg|_{\partial D} \,. \end{cases}$$

Since $\mathcal{G}_D = \mathcal{S}_D + \mathcal{R}_D$ and $\mathcal{R}_D$ is compact on $L^2(\partial D)$, uniqueness and existence of $(\boldsymbol{\varphi}_k^l, \boldsymbol{\psi}_k^l)$ follow from the Fredholm alternative.

Since $\partial(x_k\mathbf{e}_l)/\partial\nu \in L^2_{\Psi}(\partial D)$, (9.69) gives that $\boldsymbol{\psi}_k^l \in L^2_{\Psi}(\partial D)$. In fact, by (9.72) we have $\partial\mathcal{G}_D\boldsymbol{\psi}_k^l/\partial\nu|_+ \in L^2_{\Psi}(\partial D)$ and hence, by (9.69), $\boldsymbol{\psi}_k^l \in L^2_{\Psi}(\partial D)$. $\square$

9.6 Further Results and Open Problems

Results similar to those presented in this chapter can be obtained for the Stokes system of linearized hydrostatics. See [124]. Some results on the periodic Green's function given in this chapter can be applied to the mathematical theory of phononic crystals [270].

One interesting problem is to obtain a global uniqueness result similar to Theorem 3.4 for the determination of disk-shaped elastic inclusions with one boundary measurement. Apparently, there will be some difficulties with simplifying the expressions of the integral operators $\mathcal{K}_D$ and $\mathcal{K}_D^*$ when D is a disk in the plane or a ball in three-dimensional space, but this problem looks like a solvable one.

Li and Nirenberg proved that the stress for linear elasticity stays bounded if the Lamé parameters are bounded [217]. It would be very interesting to characterize the blow-up rate of the stress when the inclusions are either hard ones or holes, i.e., when the Young's modulus is either $+\infty$ or zero.

10

Elastic Moment Tensor

Introduction

In this chapter, we extend the concept of generalized polarization tensors
(GPTs) to linear elasticity defining generalized elastic moment tensors (EMTs).
We investigate some important properties of the first-order EMT such as symmetry and positive-definiteness. We also obtain estimations of its eigenvalues
and compute EMTs associated with ellipses, elliptic holes, and hard inclusions
of elliptic shape.

10.1 Asymptotic Expansion in Free Space

As in the electrostatic case, [see (4.3)], the elastic moment tensors describe the
perturbation of the displacement field due to the presence of elastic inclusions.
To see this let us consider a transmission problem in free space.

Let B be a bounded Lipschitz domain in $\mathbb{R}^d$, $d = 2, 3$. Consider the following transmission problem:

$$\begin{cases} \displaystyle\sum_{j,k,l=1}^{d} \frac{\partial}{\partial x_j}\left(C_{ijkl}\frac{\partial u_k}{\partial x_l}\right) = 0 & \text{in } \mathbb{R}^d, \quad i = 1,\ldots,d, \\[2mm] \mathbf{u}(x) - \mathbf{H}(x) = O(|x|^{1-d}) & \text{as } |x| \to +\infty, \end{cases} \tag{10.1}$$

where

$$C_{ijkl} = \left(\lambda\,\chi(\mathbb{R}^d \setminus B) + \widetilde{\lambda}\,\chi(B)\right)\delta_{ij}\delta_{kl} + \left(\mu\,\chi(\mathbb{R}^d \setminus B) + \widetilde{\mu}\,\chi(B)\right)(\delta_{ik}\delta_{jl} + \delta_{il}\delta_{jk}),$$

and $\mathbf{H}$ is a vector-valued function satisfying $\mathcal{L}_{\lambda,\mu}\mathbf{H} = 0$ in $\mathbb{R}^d$. In a way similar
to the proof of Theorem 9.15, we can show that the solution $\mathbf{u}$ to (10.1) is
represented as

$$\mathbf{u}(x) = \begin{cases} \mathbf{H}(x) + \mathcal{S}_B\boldsymbol{\psi}(x) \,, & x \in \mathbb{R}^d \setminus \overline{B} \,, \\ \widetilde{\mathcal{S}}_B\boldsymbol{\varphi}(x) \,, & x \in B \,, \end{cases} \tag{10.2}$$

for a unique pair $(\boldsymbol{\varphi}, \boldsymbol{\psi}) \in L^2(\partial B) \times L^2_{\widetilde{\Psi}}(\partial B)$, which satisfies

$$\begin{cases} \widetilde{\mathcal{S}}_B\boldsymbol{\varphi}\big|_- - \mathcal{S}_B\boldsymbol{\psi}\big|_+ = \mathbf{H}|_{\partial B} & \text{on } \partial B \,, \\ \dfrac{\partial}{\partial\widetilde{\nu}}\widetilde{\mathcal{S}}_B\boldsymbol{\varphi}\bigg|_- - \dfrac{\partial}{\partial\nu}\mathcal{S}_B\boldsymbol{\psi}\bigg|_+ = \dfrac{\partial\mathbf{H}}{\partial\nu}\bigg|_{\partial B} & \text{on } \partial B \,. \end{cases} \tag{10.3}$$

Suppose that the origin $0 \in B$ and expand $\mathbf{H}$ in terms of Taylor series to write

$$\begin{aligned} \mathbf{H}(x) &= \Big(\sum_{\alpha \in \mathbb{N}^d} \frac{1}{\alpha!}\partial^\alpha H_1(0)x^\alpha, \ldots, \sum_{\alpha \in \mathbb{N}^d} \frac{1}{\alpha!}\partial^\alpha H_d(0)x^\alpha \Big) \\ &= \sum_{j=1}^{d} \sum_{\alpha \in \mathbb{N}^d} \frac{1}{\alpha!}\partial^\alpha H_j(0)\, x^\alpha \mathbf{e}_j \,, \end{aligned}$$

where $\{\mathbf{e}_j\}_{j=1}^d$ is the standard basis for $\mathbb{R}^d$. This series converges uniformly and absolutely on any compact set. For multi-index $\alpha \in \mathbb{N}^d$ and $j = 1, \ldots, d$, let the pair $(\mathbf{f}_\alpha^j, \mathbf{g}_\alpha^j)$ in $L^2(\partial B) \times L^2(\partial B)$ be the solution of

$$\begin{cases} \widetilde{\mathcal{S}}_B\mathbf{f}_\alpha^j\big|_- - \mathcal{S}_B\mathbf{g}_\alpha^j\big|_+ = x^\alpha\mathbf{e}_j|_{\partial B} \,, \\ \dfrac{\partial}{\partial\widetilde{\nu}}\widetilde{\mathcal{S}}_B\mathbf{f}_\alpha^j\bigg|_- - \dfrac{\partial}{\partial\nu}\mathcal{S}_B\mathbf{g}_\alpha^j\bigg|_+ = \dfrac{\partial(x^\alpha\mathbf{e}_j)}{\partial\nu}|_{\partial B} \,. \end{cases} \tag{10.4}$$

Then, by linearity, we get

$$\boldsymbol{\psi} = \sum_{j=1}^{d} \sum_{\alpha \in \mathbb{N}^d} \frac{1}{\alpha!}\partial^\alpha H_j(0)\, \mathbf{g}_\alpha^j \,. \tag{10.5}$$

By a Taylor expansion, we have

$$\boldsymbol{\Gamma}(x - y) = \sum_{\beta \in \mathbb{N}^d} \frac{1}{\beta!}\partial^\beta\boldsymbol{\Gamma}(x)y^\beta, \quad y \text{ in a compact set}, \quad |x| \to +\infty \,. \tag{10.6}$$

Combining (10.2), (10.5), and (10.6) yields the expansion

$$\mathbf{u}(x) = \mathbf{H}(x) + \sum_{j=1}^{d} \sum_{\alpha \in \mathbb{N}^d} \sum_{\beta \in \mathbb{N}^d} \frac{1}{\alpha!\beta!}\partial^\alpha H_j(0)\partial^\beta\boldsymbol{\Gamma}(x) \int_{\partial B} y^\beta\mathbf{g}_\alpha^j(y)\, d\sigma(y) \,, \tag{10.7}$$

which is valid for all x with $|x| > R$, where R is such that $B \subset B_R(0)$.

We now introduce the notion of EMTs as was defined in [36].

Definition 10.1 (Elastic moment tensors) *For multi-index $\alpha \in \mathbb{N}^d$ and $j = 1, \ldots, d$, let the pair $(\mathbf{f}_\alpha^j, \mathbf{g}_\alpha^j)$ in $L^2(\partial B) \times L^2(\partial B)$ be the solution of (10.4). For $\beta \in \mathbb{N}^d$, the EMT $M_{\alpha\beta}^j$, $j = 1, \ldots, d$, associated with the domain B and Lamé parameters (λ, μ) for the background and $(\widetilde{\lambda}, \widetilde{\mu})$ for B is defined by*

$$M_{\alpha\beta}^j = (m_{\alpha\beta1}^j, \ldots, m_{\alpha\beta d}^j) = \int_{\partial B} y^\beta \mathbf{g}_\alpha^j(y) \, d\sigma(y) \ .$$

We note the analogy of the EMTs with the polarization tensor studied in Chapter 4. For holes and hard inclusions in a homogeneous elastic body, Maz'ya and Nazarov introduced the notion of Pólya–Szegö tensor in connection with the asymptotic expansion for energy due to existence of a small hole or a hard inclusion [228]. See also [245] and [216]. This tensor is exactly the one defined by (10.4) when $|\alpha| = |\beta| = 1$ and B is a hard inclusion ($\widetilde{\mu} = +\infty$) or a hole ($\widetilde{\lambda} = \widetilde{\mu} = 0$).

Theorem 10.2 *Let $\mathbf{u}$ be the solution of (10.1). Then for all x with $|x| > R$ where $B \subset B_R(0)$, the displacement field $\mathbf{u}$ has the expansion*

$$\mathbf{u}(x) = \mathbf{H}(x) + \sum_{j=1}^d \sum_{|\alpha| \geq 1} \sum_{|\beta| \geq 1} \frac{1}{\alpha! \beta!} \partial^\alpha H_j(0) \partial^\beta \mathbf{\Gamma}(x) M_{\alpha\beta}^j \ . \tag{10.8}$$

Proof. We first show that, if $\alpha = 0$, then $\mathbf{g}_0^j = 0$ for $j = 1, \ldots, d$. To this end, recall that $(\mathbf{f}_0^j, \mathbf{g}_0^j)$ is the unique solution to

$$\begin{cases} \widetilde{\mathcal{S}}_B \mathbf{f}_0^j\big|_- - \mathcal{S}_B \mathbf{g}_0^j\big|_+ = \mathbf{e}_j\big|_{\partial B} \ , \\[2mm] \dfrac{\partial}{\partial \widetilde{\nu}} \widetilde{\mathcal{S}}_B \mathbf{f}_0^j\bigg|_- - \dfrac{\partial}{\partial \nu} \mathcal{S}_B \mathbf{g}_0^j\bigg|_+ = 0 \ . \end{cases} \tag{10.9}$$

Thus, by Lemma 9.14, $\mathbf{g}_0^j = 0$. Note that $\sum_{j=1}^d \sum_{|\alpha|=l} \frac{1}{\alpha!} \partial^\alpha H_j(0) \mathbf{g}_\alpha^j$ is the solution of the integral equation (10.4) when the right-hand side is given by the function

$$\mathbf{u} := \sum_{j=1}^d \sum_{|\alpha|=l} \frac{1}{\alpha!} \partial^\alpha H_j(0) x^\alpha \mathbf{e}_j \ .$$

Moreover, this function is a solution of $\mathcal{L}_{\lambda,\mu} \mathbf{u} = 0$ in B and, therefore, $\partial \mathbf{u}/\partial \nu|_{\partial B} \in L_{\Psi}^2(\partial B)$. Hence, by Theorem 9.13, we obtain that

$$\sum_{j=1}^d \sum_{|\alpha|=l} \frac{1}{\alpha!} \partial^\alpha H_j(z) \mathbf{g}_\alpha^j \in L_{\Psi}^2(\partial B) \ .$$

In particular, we have

$$\sum_{j=1}^d \sum_{|\alpha|=l} \frac{1}{\alpha!} \partial^\alpha H_j(z) \int_{\partial B} \mathbf{g}_\alpha^j(y) \, d\sigma(y) = 0 \quad \forall \, l \ .$$

Now (10.8) follows from (10.7). This completes the proof. $\square$

The asymptotic expansion formula (10.8) shows that the perturbations of the displacement field in $\mathbb{R}^d$ due to the presence of an inclusion B are completely described by the EMTs $M^j_{\alpha\beta}$.

When $|\alpha| = |\beta| = 1$, we make a slight change of notation: When $\alpha = \mathbf{e}_i$ and $\beta = \mathbf{e}_p$ $(i, p = 1, \ldots, d)$, put

$$m^{ij}_{pq} := m^j_{\alpha\beta q} , \quad q, j = 1, \ldots, d .$$

So, if we set $\mathbf{f}^j_i := \mathbf{f}^j_\alpha$ and $\mathbf{g}^j_i := \mathbf{g}^j_\alpha$, then

$$\begin{cases} \widetilde{\mathcal{S}}_B \mathbf{f}^j_i \big|_- - \mathcal{S}_B \mathbf{g}^j_i \big|_+ = x_i \mathbf{e}_j |_{\partial B} , \\ \dfrac{\partial}{\partial \widetilde{\nu}} \widetilde{\mathcal{S}}_B \mathbf{f}^j_i \bigg|_- - \dfrac{\partial}{\partial \nu} \mathcal{S}_B \mathbf{g}^j_i \bigg|_+ = \dfrac{\partial(x_i \mathbf{e}_j)}{\partial \nu} \big|_{\partial B} , \end{cases} \tag{10.10}$$

and

$$m^{ij}_{pq} = \int_{\partial B} x_p \mathbf{e}_q \cdot \mathbf{g}^j_i \, d\sigma . \tag{10.11}$$

Lemma 10.3 *Suppose that* $0 < \widetilde{\lambda}, \widetilde{\mu} < +\infty$. *For* $p, q, i, j = 1, \ldots, d$,

$$m^{ij}_{pq} = \int_{\partial B} \left[-\frac{\partial(x_p \mathbf{e}_q)}{\partial \nu} + \frac{\partial(x_p \mathbf{e}_q)}{\partial \widetilde{\nu}} \right] \cdot \mathbf{u} \, d\sigma , \tag{10.12}$$

where $\mathbf{u}$ *is the unique solution of the transmission problem*

$$\begin{cases} \mathcal{L}_{\lambda,\mu} \mathbf{u} = 0 & \text{in } \mathbb{R}^d \setminus \overline{B} , \\ \mathcal{L}_{\widetilde{\lambda},\widetilde{\mu}} \mathbf{u} = 0 & \text{in } B , \\ \mathbf{u}|_+ - \mathbf{u}|_- = 0 & \text{on } \partial B , \\ \dfrac{\partial \mathbf{u}}{\partial \nu} \bigg|_+ - \dfrac{\partial \mathbf{u}}{\partial \widetilde{\nu}} \bigg|_- = 0 & \text{on } \partial B , \\ \mathbf{u}(x) - x_i \mathbf{e}_j = O(|x|^{1-d}) & \text{as } |x| \to +\infty . \end{cases} \tag{10.13}$$

Proof.   Note first that $\mathbf{u}$ defined by

$$\mathbf{u}(x) := \begin{cases} \mathcal{S}_B \mathbf{g}^j_i(x) + x_i \mathbf{e}_j, & x \in \mathbb{R}^d \setminus \overline{B} , \\ \widetilde{\mathcal{S}}_B \mathbf{f}^j_i(x) , & x \in B , \end{cases}$$

is the solution of (10.13). Using (9.10) and (10.10), we compute

$$
\begin{aligned}
m_{pq}^{ij} &= \int_{\partial B} x_p \mathbf{e}_q \cdot \mathbf{g}_i^j \, d\sigma \\
&= \int_{\partial B} x_p \mathbf{e}_q \cdot \left[\frac{\partial}{\partial \nu} \mathcal{S}_B \mathbf{g}_i^j \Big|_+ - \frac{\partial}{\partial \nu} \mathcal{S}_B \mathbf{g}_i^j \Big|_- \right] d\sigma \\
&= - \int_{\partial B} x_p \mathbf{e}_q \cdot \frac{\partial (x_i \mathbf{e}_j)}{\partial \nu} \, d\sigma - \int_{\partial B} x_p \mathbf{e}_q \cdot \left[\frac{\partial}{\partial \nu} \mathcal{S}_B \mathbf{g}_i^j \Big|_- - \frac{\partial}{\partial \widetilde{\nu}} \widetilde{\mathcal{S}}_B \mathbf{f}_i^j \Big|_- \right] d\sigma \\
&= - \int_{\partial B} \frac{\partial (x_p \mathbf{e}_q)}{\partial \nu} \cdot x_i \mathbf{e}_j \, d\sigma - \int_{\partial B} \left[\frac{\partial (x_p \mathbf{e}_q)}{\partial \nu} \cdot \mathcal{S}_B \mathbf{g}_i^j - \frac{\partial (x_p \mathbf{e}_q)}{\partial \widetilde{\nu}} \cdot \widetilde{\mathcal{S}}_B \mathbf{f}_i^j \right] d\sigma \\
&= \int_{\partial B} \left[- \frac{\partial (x_p \mathbf{e}_q)}{\partial \nu} + \frac{\partial (x_p \mathbf{e}_q)}{\partial \widetilde{\nu}} \right] \cdot \widetilde{\mathcal{S}}_B \mathbf{f}_i^j \, d\sigma \, ,
\end{aligned}
$$

and hence (10.12) is established. $\qquad\square$

10.2 Properties of EMTs

In this section, we investigate some important properties of the first-order EMT $M = (m_{pq}^{ij})$ such as symmetry and positive-definiteness. These properties of EMTs were first proved in [36]. It is worth mentioning that these properties make M an (anisotropic in general) elasticity tensor. We first define a bilinear form on a domain B corresponding to the Lamé parameters λ, μ by

$$
\langle \mathbf{u}, \mathbf{v} \rangle_B^{\lambda, \mu} := \int_B \left[\lambda (\nabla \cdot \mathbf{u})(\nabla \cdot \mathbf{v}) + \frac{\mu}{2} (\nabla \mathbf{u} + \nabla \mathbf{u}^T) \cdot (\nabla \mathbf{v} + \nabla \mathbf{v}^T) \right] dx \, .
$$

The corresponding quadratic form is defined by

$$
Q_B^{\lambda, \mu}(\mathbf{u}) := \langle \mathbf{u}, \mathbf{u} \rangle_B^{\lambda, \mu}.
$$

If $\mathcal{L}_{\lambda, \mu} \mathbf{u} = 0$, then

$$
\int_{\partial B} \frac{\partial \mathbf{u}}{\partial \nu} \cdot \mathbf{v} \, d\sigma = \langle \mathbf{u}, \mathbf{v} \rangle_B^{\lambda, \mu} \, .
$$

Proposition 10.4 *Suppose that $\mu \neq \widetilde{\mu}$. Given a non-zero symmetric matrix $a = (a_{ij})$, define $\boldsymbol{\varphi}_a$, $\mathbf{f}_a$, and $\mathbf{g}_a$ by*

$$
\boldsymbol{\varphi}_a := (a_{ij}) x = \sum_{i,j=1}^d a_{ij} x_j \mathbf{e}_i \, , \quad \mathbf{f}_a := \sum_{i,j=1}^d a_{ij} \mathbf{f}_i^j \, , \quad \mathbf{g}_a := \sum_{i,j=1}^d a_{ij} \mathbf{g}_i^j \, .
\tag{10.14}
$$

Define $\bar{a}$ by

$$
\bar{a} := \frac{\widetilde{\mu} + \mu}{\widetilde{\mu} - \mu} \left[a - \frac{\operatorname{Tr}(a)}{d} I_d \right] + \frac{d(\widetilde{\lambda} + \lambda) + 2(\widetilde{\mu} + \mu)}{d(\widetilde{\lambda} - \lambda) + 2(\widetilde{\mu} - \mu)} \frac{\operatorname{Tr}(a)}{d} I_d \, ,
\tag{10.15}
$$

where I_d is the $d \times d$ identity matrix. Then

$$
\langle \bar{a}, Ma \rangle = \langle \widetilde{\mathcal{S}}_B \mathbf{f}_a, \widetilde{\mathcal{S}}_B \mathbf{f}_a \rangle_B^{\widetilde{\lambda}, \widetilde{\mu}} + \langle \mathcal{S}_B \mathbf{g}_a, \mathcal{S}_B \mathbf{g}_a \rangle_{\mathbb{R}^d \backslash B}^{\lambda, \mu} + \langle \boldsymbol{\varphi}_a, \boldsymbol{\varphi}_a \rangle_B^{\lambda, \mu} \, .
\tag{10.16}
$$

Recall that $\langle a, b \rangle = a \cdot b = \sum_{ij} a_{ij} b_{ij}$ for $d \times d$ matrices $a = (a_{ij})$ and $b = (b_{ij})$.

Proof. Set, for convenience, $\varphi = \varphi_a$, $\mathbf{f} = \mathbf{f}_a$, and $\mathbf{g} = \mathbf{g}_a$. Then these functions clearly satisfy

$$\begin{cases} \widetilde{\mathcal{S}}_B \mathbf{f} - \mathcal{S}_B \mathbf{g} = \varphi|_{\partial B} \, , \\ \dfrac{\partial}{\partial \widetilde{\nu}} \widetilde{\mathcal{S}}_B \mathbf{f} \Big|_- - \dfrac{\partial}{\partial \nu} \mathcal{S}_B \mathbf{g} \Big|_+ = \dfrac{\partial \varphi}{\partial \nu} \Big|_{\partial B} \, . \end{cases} \tag{10.17}$$

For $j = 1, 2$, define

$$\varphi_1 := \left[(a_{ij}) - \frac{\mathrm{Tr}(a_{ij})}{d} I_d \right] x \quad \text{and} \quad \varphi_2 := \frac{\mathrm{Tr}(a_{ij})}{d} x \, . \tag{10.18}$$

Then $\varphi = \varphi_1 + \varphi_2$. Define $\mathbf{f}_j$ and $\mathbf{g}_j$, $j = 1, 2$, by

$$\begin{cases} \widetilde{\mathcal{S}}_B \mathbf{f}_j - \mathcal{S}_B \mathbf{g}_j = \varphi_j|_{\partial B} \, , \\ \dfrac{\partial}{\partial \widetilde{\nu}} \widetilde{\mathcal{S}}_B \mathbf{f}_j \Big|_- - \dfrac{\partial}{\partial \nu} \mathcal{S}_B \mathbf{g}_j \Big|_+ = \dfrac{\partial \varphi_j}{\partial \nu} \Big|_{\partial B} \, . \end{cases} \tag{10.19}$$

It is clear that $\mathbf{f} = \mathbf{f}_1 + \mathbf{f}_2$ and $\mathbf{g} = \mathbf{g}_1 + \mathbf{g}_2$. We now claim that

$$\langle \bar{a}, M a \rangle = \frac{\widetilde{\mu} + \mu}{\widetilde{\mu} - \mu} \int_{\partial B} \varphi_1 \cdot \mathbf{g} \, d\sigma + \frac{d(\widetilde{\lambda} + \lambda) + 2(\widetilde{\mu} + \mu)}{d(\widetilde{\lambda} - \lambda) + 2(\widetilde{\mu} - \mu)} \int_{\partial B} \varphi_2 \cdot \mathbf{g} \, d\sigma \, . \tag{10.20}$$

In fact, we have

$$\langle \bar{a}, M a \rangle = \sum_{i,j,p,q=1}^{d} \bar{a}_{pq} m_{pq}^{ij} a_{ij}$$

$$= \int_{pB} \Big(\sum_{pq} \bar{a}_{pq} x_p \mathbf{e}_q \Big) \cdot \Big(\sum_{ij} a_{ij} \mathbf{g}_i^j \Big) d\sigma \, .$$

But

$$\sum_{pq} \bar{a}_{pq} x_p \mathbf{e}_q = \frac{\widetilde{\mu} + \mu}{\widetilde{\mu} - \mu} \varphi_1 + \frac{d(\widetilde{\lambda} + \lambda) + 2(\widetilde{\mu} + \mu)}{d(\widetilde{\lambda} - \lambda) + 2(\widetilde{\mu} - \mu)} \varphi_2 \, ,$$

and therefore (10.20) holds.

Next, using the jump relation (9.10) and (10.17), we compute that

$$\int_{\partial B} \varphi_j \cdot \mathbf{g} \, d\sigma = \int_{\partial B} \varphi_j \cdot \left[\frac{\partial}{\partial \nu} \mathcal{S}_B \mathbf{g} \Big|_+ - \frac{\partial}{\partial \nu} \mathcal{S}_B \mathbf{g} \Big|_- \right] d\sigma \tag{10.21}$$

$$= - \int_{\partial B} \varphi_j \cdot \frac{\partial \varphi}{\partial \nu} \, d\sigma - \int_{\partial B} \varphi_j \cdot \left[\frac{\partial}{\partial \nu} \mathcal{S}_B \mathbf{g} \Big|_- - \frac{\partial}{\partial \widetilde{\nu}} \widetilde{\mathcal{S}}_B \mathbf{f} \Big|_- \right] d\sigma$$

$$= - \int_{\partial B} \varphi_j \cdot \frac{\partial \varphi}{\partial \nu} \, d\sigma - \int_{\partial B} \left[\frac{\partial \varphi_j}{\partial \nu} \cdot \mathcal{S}_B \mathbf{g} - \frac{\partial \varphi_j}{\partial \widetilde{\nu}} \cdot \widetilde{\mathcal{S}}_B \mathbf{f} \right] d\sigma$$

$$= \int_{\partial B} \left[-\frac{\partial \varphi_j}{\partial \nu} + \frac{\partial \varphi_j}{\partial \widetilde{\nu}} \right] \cdot \widetilde{\mathcal{S}}_B \mathbf{f} \, d\sigma \, .$$

Observe that $\nabla \cdot \boldsymbol{\varphi}_1 = 0$. Put $\alpha := \widetilde{\mu}/\mu$. Then, from the definition of the conormal derivative $\partial/\partial\nu$, we can immediately see that

$$\frac{\partial \boldsymbol{\varphi}_1}{\partial \nu} - \frac{\partial \boldsymbol{\varphi}_1}{\partial \widetilde{\nu}} = (1 - \alpha)\frac{\partial \boldsymbol{\varphi}_1}{\partial \nu} = \frac{1 - \alpha}{\alpha}\frac{\partial \boldsymbol{\varphi}_1}{\partial \widetilde{\nu}} . \tag{10.22}$$

A combination of (10.17), (10.19), and (10.21), together with the second relation of (10.22), yields

$$-\frac{\alpha}{1-\alpha}\int_{\partial B}\boldsymbol{\varphi}_1 \cdot \mathbf{g}\, d\sigma = \int_{\partial B}\frac{\partial \boldsymbol{\varphi}_1}{\partial \widetilde{\nu}} \cdot \widetilde{\mathcal{S}}_B\mathbf{f}\, d\sigma = \int_{\partial B}\boldsymbol{\varphi}_1 \cdot \frac{\partial}{\partial \widetilde{\nu}}\widetilde{\mathcal{S}}_B\mathbf{f}\Big|_{-}\, d\sigma$$

$$= \int_{\partial B}\widetilde{\mathcal{S}}_B\mathbf{f}_1 \cdot \frac{\partial}{\partial \widetilde{\nu}}\widetilde{\mathcal{S}}_B\mathbf{f}\Big|_{-}\, d\sigma - \int_{\partial B}\mathcal{S}_B\mathbf{g}_1 \cdot \frac{\partial}{\partial \nu}\mathcal{S}_B\mathbf{g}\Big|_{+}\, d\sigma - \int_{\partial B}\mathcal{S}_B\mathbf{g}_1 \cdot \frac{\partial \boldsymbol{\varphi}}{\partial \nu}\, d\sigma$$

$$= \langle \widetilde{\mathcal{S}}_B\mathbf{f}_1, \widetilde{\mathcal{S}}_B\mathbf{f}\rangle_B^{\widetilde{\lambda},\widetilde{\mu}} + \langle \mathcal{S}_B\mathbf{g}_1, \mathcal{S}_B\mathbf{g}\rangle_{\mathbb{R}^d\setminus B}^{\lambda,\mu} - \langle \mathcal{S}_B\mathbf{g}_1, \boldsymbol{\varphi}\rangle_B^{\lambda,\mu} .$$

On the other hand, it follows from (10.17), (10.21), and the first relation of (10.22) that

$$-\frac{1}{1-\alpha}\int_{\partial B}\boldsymbol{\varphi}_1 \cdot \mathbf{g}\, d\sigma = \int_{\partial B}\frac{\partial \boldsymbol{\varphi}_1}{\partial \nu} \cdot \widetilde{\mathcal{S}}_B\mathbf{f}\, d\sigma$$

$$= \int_{\partial B}\frac{\partial \boldsymbol{\varphi}_1}{\partial \nu} \cdot \mathcal{S}_B\mathbf{g}\, d\sigma + \int_{\partial B}\frac{\partial \boldsymbol{\varphi}_1}{\partial \nu} \cdot \boldsymbol{\varphi}\, d\sigma$$

$$= \langle \boldsymbol{\varphi}_1, \mathcal{S}_B\mathbf{g}\rangle_B^{\lambda,\mu} + \langle \boldsymbol{\varphi}_1, \boldsymbol{\varphi}\rangle_B^{\lambda,\mu} .$$

By adding the above two identities, we obtain that

$$-\frac{1+\alpha}{1-\alpha}\int_{\partial B}\boldsymbol{\varphi}_1 \cdot \mathbf{g}\, d\sigma$$

$$= \langle \widetilde{\mathcal{S}}_B\mathbf{f}_1, \widetilde{\mathcal{S}}_B\mathbf{f}\rangle_B^{\widetilde{\lambda},\widetilde{\mu}} + \langle \mathcal{S}_B\mathbf{g}_1, \mathcal{S}_B\mathbf{g}\rangle_{\mathbb{R}^d\setminus B}^{\lambda,\mu} + \langle \boldsymbol{\varphi}_1, \boldsymbol{\varphi}\rangle_B^{\lambda,\mu} \tag{10.23}$$

$$- \langle \mathcal{S}_B\mathbf{g}_1, \boldsymbol{\varphi}\rangle_B^{\lambda,\mu} + \langle \boldsymbol{\varphi}_1, \mathcal{S}_B\mathbf{g}\rangle_B^{\lambda,\mu} .$$

Observe that

$$\frac{1+\alpha}{1-\alpha} = \frac{\mu + \widetilde{\mu}}{\mu - \widetilde{\mu}} .$$

Put

$$\beta := \frac{d\lambda + 2\mu}{d(\lambda - \widetilde{\lambda}) + 2(\mu - \widetilde{\mu})} \quad \text{and} \quad \widetilde{\beta} := \frac{d\widetilde{\lambda} + 2\widetilde{\mu}}{d(\lambda - \widetilde{\lambda}) + 2(\mu - \widetilde{\mu})} .$$

It can be easily seen that

$$\frac{\partial \boldsymbol{\varphi}_2}{\partial \nu} - \frac{\partial \boldsymbol{\varphi}_2}{\partial \widetilde{\nu}} = \frac{1}{\beta}\frac{\partial \boldsymbol{\varphi}_2}{\partial \nu} = \frac{1}{\widetilde{\beta}}\frac{\partial \boldsymbol{\varphi}_2}{\partial \widetilde{\nu}} . \tag{10.24}$$

Following the same lines as in the derivation of (10.23), we obtain

$$- (\beta + \widetilde{\beta}) \int_{\partial B} \boldsymbol{\varphi}_2 \cdot \mathbf{g}\, d\sigma$$

$$= \langle \widetilde{\mathcal{S}}_B \mathbf{f}_2, \widetilde{\mathcal{S}}_B \mathbf{f} \rangle_B^{\widetilde{\lambda},\widetilde{\mu}} + \langle \mathcal{S}_B \mathbf{g}_2, \mathcal{S}_B \mathbf{g} \rangle_{\mathbb{R}^d \backslash B}^{\lambda,\mu} + \langle \boldsymbol{\varphi}_2, \boldsymbol{\varphi} \rangle_B^{\lambda,\mu} \qquad (10.25)$$

$$- \langle \mathcal{S}_B \mathbf{g}_2, \boldsymbol{\varphi} \rangle_B^{\lambda,\mu} + \langle \boldsymbol{\varphi}_2, \mathcal{S}_B \mathbf{g} \rangle_B^{\lambda,\mu}\, ,$$

which together with (10.23) gives

$$- \frac{1 + \alpha}{1 - \alpha} \int_{\partial B} \boldsymbol{\varphi}_1 \cdot \mathbf{g}\, d\sigma - (\beta + \widetilde{\beta}) \int_{\partial B} \boldsymbol{\varphi}_2 \cdot \mathbf{g}\, d\sigma$$

$$= \langle \widetilde{\mathcal{S}}_B \mathbf{f}, \widetilde{\mathcal{S}}_B \mathbf{f} \rangle_B^{\widetilde{\lambda},\widetilde{\mu}} + \langle \mathcal{S}_B \mathbf{g}, \mathcal{S}_B \mathbf{g} \rangle_{\mathbb{R}^d \backslash B}^{\lambda,\mu} + \langle \boldsymbol{\varphi}, \boldsymbol{\varphi} \rangle_B^{\lambda,\mu} - \langle \mathcal{S}_B \mathbf{g}, \boldsymbol{\varphi} \rangle_B^{\lambda,\mu} + \langle \boldsymbol{\varphi}, \mathcal{S}_B \mathbf{g} \rangle_B^{\lambda,\mu}$$

$$= \langle \widetilde{\mathcal{S}}_B \mathbf{f}, \widetilde{\mathcal{S}}_B \mathbf{f} \rangle_B^{\widetilde{\lambda},\widetilde{\mu}} + \langle \mathcal{S}_B \mathbf{g}, \mathcal{S}_B \mathbf{g} \rangle_{\mathbb{R}^d \backslash B}^{\lambda,\mu} + \langle \boldsymbol{\varphi}, \boldsymbol{\varphi} \rangle_B^{\lambda,\mu}\, .$$

Then the final formula (10.16) follows from (10.20), which completes the proof. $\qquad\qquad\square$

Theorem 10.5 (Symmetry) *For $p, q, i, j = 1, \ldots, d$, the following holds:*

$$m_{pq}^{ij} = m_{qp}^{ij}\, , \quad m_{pq}^{ij} = m_{pq}^{ji}\, , \quad \text{and} \quad m_{pq}^{ij} = m_{ij}^{pq}\, . \qquad (10.26)$$

Proof. By Theorem 9.13 and the definition (10.4) of $\mathbf{g}_i^j$, we obtain that $\mathbf{g}_i^j \in L_{\Psi}^2(\partial B)$. Since $x_p \mathbf{e}_q - x_q \mathbf{e}_p \in \Psi$, we have

$$\int_{\partial B} (x_p \mathbf{e}_q - x_q \mathbf{e}_p) \cdot \mathbf{g}_i^j \, d\sigma = 0\, .$$

The first identity of (10.26) immediately follows from the above identity.

Since $x_i \mathbf{e}_j - x_j \mathbf{e}_i \in \Psi$, we have $\partial(x_i \mathbf{e}_j - x_j \mathbf{e}_i)/\partial \nu = 0$ on ∂B. Let $\mathbf{g} := \mathbf{g}_i^j - \mathbf{g}_j^i$ and $\mathbf{f} := \mathbf{f}_i^j - \mathbf{f}_j^i$. Then the pair $(\mathbf{f}, \mathbf{g})$ satisfies

$$\begin{cases} \widetilde{\mathcal{S}}_B \mathbf{f}|_- - \mathcal{S}_B \mathbf{g}|_+ = (x_i \mathbf{e}_j - x_j \mathbf{e}_i)|_{\partial B}\, , \\[2mm] \left. \dfrac{\partial}{\partial \widetilde{\nu}} \widetilde{\mathcal{S}}_B \mathbf{f} \right|_- - \left. \dfrac{\partial}{\partial \nu} \mathcal{S}_B \mathbf{g} \right|_+ = 0\, . \end{cases}$$

Lemma 9.14 shows that $\mathbf{g} = 0$ or $\mathbf{g}_i^j = \mathbf{g}_j^i$. This proves the second identity of (10.26).

It stems from the first and second identities of (10.26) that

$$\langle a, Mb \rangle = \frac{1}{4} \langle a + a^T, M(b + b^T) \rangle$$

for any matrices a, b. Therefore, in order to prove the third identity in (10.26), it suffices to show that

$$\langle a, Mb \rangle = \langle b, Ma \rangle \quad \text{for all symmetric matrices } a, b\, .$$

Let a, b be two symmetric matrices. Define $\varphi_a, \mathbf{f}_a, \mathbf{g}_a, \varphi_{aj}, \mathbf{f}_{aj}, \mathbf{g}_{aj}$, $j = 1, 2$, as in (10.14), (10.18), and (10.19). Define $\varphi_b, \mathbf{f}_b, \mathbf{g}_b, \varphi_{bj}, \mathbf{f}_{bj}, \mathbf{g}_{bj}$, $j = 1, 2$, likewise. Then,

$$\langle a, Mb \rangle = \int_{\partial B} \varphi_a \cdot \mathbf{g}_b \, d\sigma = \int_{\partial B} \varphi_{a1} \cdot \mathbf{g}_b \, d\sigma + \int_{\partial B} \varphi_{a2} \cdot \mathbf{g}_b \, d\sigma \ .$$

By (10.21), we have

$$\int_{\partial B} \varphi_{aj} \cdot \mathbf{g}_b \, d\sigma = \int_{\partial B} \left[\frac{\partial \varphi_{aj}}{\partial \nu} - \frac{\partial \varphi_{aj}}{\partial \widetilde{\nu}} \right] \cdot \widetilde{\mathcal{S}}_B \mathbf{f}_b \, d\sigma \quad \text{for } j = 1, 2 \ . \tag{10.27}$$

Let α, β, and $\widetilde{\beta}$ be as before. The system of equations (10.19), the first relation in (10.22), and (10.27) give that

$$-\frac{1}{1 - \alpha} \int_{\partial B} \varphi_{a1} \cdot \mathbf{g}_b \, d\sigma$$
$$= \int_{\partial B} \frac{\partial \varphi_{a1}}{\partial \nu} \cdot \widetilde{\mathcal{S}}_B \mathbf{f}_b \, d\sigma \tag{10.28}$$
$$= \int_{\partial B} \frac{\partial (\varphi_{a1} + \mathcal{S}_B \mathbf{g}_{a1})}{\partial \nu} \Big|_- \cdot (\mathcal{S}_B \mathbf{g}_a \mid \varphi_a) \, d\sigma$$
$$- \int_{\partial B} \frac{\partial (\mathcal{S}_B \mathbf{g}_{a1})}{\partial \nu} \Big|_- \cdot (\mathcal{S}_B \mathbf{g}_a + \varphi_a) \, d\sigma \ .$$

On the other hand, we see from (10.19), the second relation in (10.22), and (10.27) that

$$-\frac{\alpha}{1 - \alpha} \int_{\partial B} \varphi_{a1} \cdot \mathbf{g}_b \, d\sigma$$
$$= \int_{\partial B} \frac{\partial \varphi_{a1}}{\partial \widetilde{\nu}} \cdot \widetilde{\mathcal{S}}_B \mathbf{f}_b \, d\sigma = \int_{\partial B} \varphi_{a1} \cdot \frac{\partial (\widetilde{\mathcal{S}}_B \mathbf{f}_b)}{\partial \widetilde{\nu}} \Big|_- \, d\sigma \tag{10.29}$$
$$= \int_{\partial B} \widetilde{\mathcal{S}}_B \mathbf{f}_{a1} \cdot \frac{\partial (\widetilde{\mathcal{S}}_B \mathbf{f}_b)}{\partial \widetilde{\nu}} \Big|_- \, d\sigma$$
$$- \int_{\partial B} \mathcal{S}_B \mathbf{g}_{a1} \cdot \frac{\partial (\mathcal{S}_B \mathbf{g}_b)}{\partial \nu} \Big|_+ \, d\sigma - \int_{\partial B} \mathcal{S}_B \mathbf{g}_{a1} \cdot \frac{\partial \varphi_b}{\partial \nu} \, d\sigma \ .$$

Next, subtracting (10.29) from (10.28), we obtain

$$\int_{\partial B} \varphi_{a1} \cdot \mathbf{g}_b \, d\sigma$$
$$= \int_{\partial B} \frac{\partial (\varphi_{a1} + \mathcal{S}_B \mathbf{g}_{a1})}{\partial \nu} \Big|_- \cdot (\mathcal{S}_B \mathbf{g}_a + \varphi_a) \, d\sigma \tag{10.30}$$
$$- \int_{\partial B} \widetilde{\mathcal{S}}_B \mathbf{f}_{a1} \cdot \frac{\partial (\widetilde{\mathcal{S}}_B \mathbf{f}_b)}{\partial \widetilde{\nu}} \Big|_- \, d\sigma$$

$$- \int_{\partial B} \mathcal{S}_B \mathbf{g}_{a1} \cdot \left[\frac{\partial(\mathcal{S}_B \mathbf{g}_b)}{\partial \nu} \Big|_- - \frac{\partial(\mathcal{S}_B \mathbf{g}_b)}{\partial \nu} \Big|_+ \right] d\sigma \; .$$

$$= \langle \varphi_{a1} + \mathcal{S}_B \mathbf{g}_{a1}, \varphi_b + \mathcal{S}_B \mathbf{g}_b \rangle_B^{\lambda, \mu} - \langle \widetilde{\mathcal{S}}_B \mathbf{f}_{a1}, \widetilde{\mathcal{S}}_B \mathbf{f}_b \rangle_B^{\widetilde{\lambda}, \widetilde{\mu}} - \int_{\partial B} \mathcal{S}_B \mathbf{g}_{a1} \cdot \mathbf{g}_b \, d\sigma \; .$$

Note that $\beta - \widetilde{\beta} = 1$. Using (10.24), we write

$$\int_{\partial B} \varphi_{a2} \cdot \mathbf{g}_b \, d\sigma = \langle \varphi_{a2} + \mathcal{S}_B \mathbf{g}_{a2}, \varphi_b + \mathcal{S}_B \mathbf{g}_b \rangle_B^{\lambda, \mu} \tag{10.31}$$

$$- \langle \widetilde{\mathcal{S}}_B \mathbf{f}_{a2}, \widetilde{\mathcal{S}}_B \mathbf{f}_b \rangle_B^{\widetilde{\lambda}, \widetilde{\mu}} - \int_{\partial B} \mathcal{S}_B \mathbf{g}_{a2} \cdot \mathbf{g}_b \, d\sigma \; .$$

Then, by adding (10.30) and (10.31), we find that

$$\int_{\partial B} \varphi_a \cdot \mathbf{g}_b \, d\sigma = \langle \varphi_a + \mathcal{S}_B \mathbf{g}_a, \varphi_b + \mathcal{S}_B \mathbf{g}_b \rangle_B^{\lambda, \mu} \tag{10.32}$$

$$- \langle \widetilde{\mathcal{S}}_B \mathbf{f}_a, \widetilde{\mathcal{S}}_B \mathbf{f}_b \rangle_B^{\widetilde{\lambda}, \widetilde{\mu}} - \int_{\partial B} \mathcal{S}_B \mathbf{g}_a \cdot \mathbf{g}_b \, d\sigma \; .$$

Since

$$\int_{\partial B} \mathcal{S}_B \mathbf{g}_a \cdot \mathbf{g}_b \, d\sigma = \int_{\partial B} \mathbf{g}_a \cdot \mathcal{S}_B \mathbf{g}_b \, d\sigma \; ,$$

identity (10.32) obviously implies that

$$\langle a, Mb \rangle = \int_{\partial B} \varphi_a \cdot \mathbf{g}_b \, d\sigma = \int_{\partial B} \varphi_b \cdot \mathbf{g}_a \, d\sigma = \langle b, Ma \rangle \; ,$$

which completes the proof. $\qquad\qquad\qquad\qquad\qquad\qquad\qquad\qquad\quad \square$

Theorem 10.6 (Positive-definiteness) *Suppose that (9.20) holds. If $\widetilde{\mu} > \mu$ ($\widetilde{\mu} < \mu$, resp.), then M is positive- (negative-, resp.) definite on the space of symmetric matrices. Let κ be an eigenvalue of M. Then there are constants C_1 and C_2 depending only on $\lambda, \mu, \widetilde{\lambda}, \widetilde{\mu}$ and the Lipschitz character of B such that*

$$C_1 |B| \leq |\kappa| \leq C_2 |B| \; .$$

Proof. Let $\varphi = ax$, as before. Since

$$\langle \varphi, \varphi \rangle_B^{\lambda, \mu} = \left(\lambda \mathrm{Tr}(a_{ij})^2 + 2\mu \sum_{ij} a_{ij}^2 \right) |B| \; ,$$

(10.16) yields

$$\langle \bar{a}, Ma \rangle \geq 2\mu |B| \, \|a\|^2 \; ,$$

where $\|a\|^2 = \sum_{ij} a_{ij}^2$. On the other hand, we can obtain an upper bound for m_{pq}^{ij} from its definition. In fact, let $z \in B$. Since $\int_{\partial B} \mathbf{g}_i^j \, d\sigma = 0$, we have

$$m_{pq}^{ij} = \int_{\partial B} x_p \mathbf{e}_q \cdot \mathbf{g}_i^j(x)\, d\sigma = \int_{\partial B} (x_p - z_p)\mathbf{e}_q \cdot \mathbf{g}_i^j(x)\, d\sigma \ .$$

It then follows from (9.30) that

$$\begin{aligned}
|m_{pq}^{ij}|^2 &\le \int_{\partial B} (x_p - z_p)^2\, d\sigma \int_{\partial B} |\mathbf{g}_i^j|^2\, d\sigma \\
&\le C \mathrm{diam}(B)^2 |\partial B| \left(\|x_j \mathbf{e}_i\|_{L^2(\partial B)}^2 + \|\nabla(x_j \mathbf{e}_i)\|_{L^2(\partial B)}^2 \right) \\
&\le C \mathrm{diam}(B)^2 |\partial B|^2 \ .
\end{aligned}$$

Thus, if B satisfies the geometric condition: $\mathrm{diam}(B)|\partial B| \le C_0 |B|$, we can verify that

$$|m_{pq}^{ij}| \le C|B|$$

where the constant C depends on $\lambda, \mu, \widetilde{\lambda}, \widetilde{\mu}$ and C_0. Observe that C_0 depends on the Lipschitz character of B. Hence

$$\langle \bar{a}, Ma \rangle \le C|B| \|a\|^2 \ .$$

Therefore, there is a constant C depending on $\lambda, \mu, \widetilde{\lambda}, \widetilde{\mu}$ and the Lipschitz character of B such that

$$\mu|B|\, \|a\|^2 \le \langle \bar{a}, Ma \rangle \le C|B|\, \|a\|^2 \ . \tag{10.33}$$

Let κ be an eigenvalue of the tensor M, and let the matrix a be its corresponding eigenvector. Then $\langle \bar{a}, Ma \rangle = \kappa \langle \bar{a}, a \rangle$ and

$$\langle \bar{a}, a \rangle = \frac{\widetilde{\mu} + \mu}{\widetilde{\mu} - \mu} \left| a - \frac{\mathrm{Tr}(a)}{d} I_d \right|^2 + \frac{d(\widetilde{\lambda} + \lambda) + 2(\widetilde{\mu} + \mu)}{d(\widetilde{\lambda} - \lambda) + 2(\widetilde{\mu} - \mu)} \left| \frac{\mathrm{Tr}(a)}{d} I_d \right|^2 \ . \tag{10.34}$$

Suppose that $\widetilde{\mu} > \mu$. Then by (9.20), $d(\widetilde{\lambda} - \lambda) + 2(\widetilde{\mu} - \mu) > 0$. Let

$$K_1 := \min \left(\frac{\widetilde{\mu} + \mu}{\widetilde{\mu} - \mu}, \frac{d(\widetilde{\lambda} + \lambda) + 2(\widetilde{\mu} + \mu)}{d(\widetilde{\lambda} - \lambda) + 2(\widetilde{\mu} - \mu)} \right) \ ,$$

$$K_2 := \max \left(\frac{\widetilde{\mu} + \mu}{\widetilde{\mu} - \mu}, \frac{d(\widetilde{\lambda} + \lambda) + 2(\widetilde{\mu} + \mu)}{d(\widetilde{\lambda} - \lambda) + 2(\widetilde{\mu} - \mu)} \right) \ .$$

Then

$$K_1 |B|\, \|a\|^2 \le \langle \bar{a}, a \rangle \le K_2 |B|\, \|a\|^2 \ ,$$

and therefore, estimates (10.33) imply that $\kappa > 0$ and

$$\frac{C_1}{K_2} |B| \le \kappa \le \frac{C_2}{K_1} |B| \ .$$

When $\widetilde{\mu} < \mu$, we obtain, by a word for word translation of the previous proof, that $\kappa < 0$ and similar upper and lower bounds for $|\kappa|$ hold. The proof is complete. $\square$

Theorem 10.6 shows that the eigenvalues of M carry information on the size of the corresponding domain. We now prove that some components of M also carry the same information.

If $(a_{ij}) = \frac{1}{2}(E_{ij} + E_{ji})$, $i \neq j$, then $\varphi = (x_j \mathbf{e}_i + x_i \mathbf{e}_j)/2$. Hence, by (10.16), we obtain

$$m_{ij}^{ij} = \frac{\widetilde{\mu} - \mu}{\widetilde{\mu} + \mu}\left[Q_B^{\widetilde{\lambda},\widetilde{\mu}}(\widetilde{\mathcal{S}}_B \mathbf{f}_i^j) + Q_{\mathbb{R}^d \backslash B}^{\lambda,\mu}(\mathcal{S}_B \mathbf{g}_i^j) + \mu|B|\right] .$$

It then follows that

$$\left|m_{ij}^{ij}\right| \geq \mu \left|\frac{\mu - \widetilde{\mu}}{\mu + \widetilde{\mu}}\right| |B| .$$

Thus, we have the following corollary.

Corollary 10.7 *Suppose $i \neq j$. Then a constant C exists depending only on $\lambda, \mu, \widetilde{\lambda}, \widetilde{\mu}$, and the Lipschitz character of B such that*

$$\mu \left|\frac{\mu - \widetilde{\mu}}{\mu + \widetilde{\mu}}\right| |B| \leq \left|m_{ij}^{ij}\right| \leq C|B| . \tag{10.35}$$

10.3 EMTs Under Linear Transformations

In this section we derive formulae for EMTs under linear transformations.

Lemma 10.8 *Let B be a bounded domain in $\mathbb{R}^d$, and let $[m_{pq}^{ij}(B)]$ denote the EMT associated with B. Then*

$$m_{pq}^{ij}(\epsilon B) = \epsilon^d m_{pq}^{ij}(B) , \quad i,j,p,q = 1,\ldots,d .$$

Proof. Let $(\mathbf{f}_i^j, \mathbf{g}_i^j)$ and $(\boldsymbol{\varphi}_i^j, \boldsymbol{\psi}_i^j)$ be the solution of (10.10) on ∂B and $\partial(\epsilon B)$, respectively. We claim that

$$\boldsymbol{\psi}_i^j(\epsilon x) = \mathbf{g}_i^j(x), \quad x \in \partial B . \tag{10.36}$$

If $d = 3$, then (10.36) simply follows from a homogeneity argument. In fact, in three dimensions, the Kelvin matrix $\boldsymbol{\Gamma}(x)$ is homogeneous of degree -1. Thus for any $\mathbf{f}$,

$$\mathcal{S}_{\epsilon B}\mathbf{f}(\epsilon x) = \epsilon \mathcal{S}_B \mathbf{f}_\epsilon(x), \quad x \in \partial B ,$$

$$\frac{\partial(\mathcal{S}_{\epsilon B}\mathbf{f})}{\partial \nu}(\epsilon x) = \frac{\partial(\mathcal{S}_B \mathbf{f}_\epsilon)}{\partial \nu}(x) , \quad x \in \partial B ,$$

where $\mathbf{f}_\epsilon(x) = \mathbf{f}(\epsilon x)$. Then (10.36) follows from the uniqueness of a solution to (10.10).

In two dimensions, note first the easy to prove fact:

$$\boldsymbol{\Gamma}(\epsilon x) = \frac{A}{2\pi} \ln \epsilon \, I_d + \boldsymbol{\Gamma}(x) \ .$$

Since the pair $((\boldsymbol{\varphi}_i^j)_\epsilon, (\boldsymbol{\psi}_i^j)_\epsilon)$ satisfies

$$\begin{cases} \widetilde{\mathcal{S}}_B(\boldsymbol{\varphi}_i^j)_\epsilon \Big|_- + \dfrac{A}{2\pi}\dfrac{\ln \epsilon}{\epsilon} \displaystyle\int_{\partial B} (\boldsymbol{\varphi}_i^j)_\epsilon \, d\sigma - \mathcal{S}_B(\boldsymbol{\psi}_i^j)_\epsilon \Big|_+ = x_i \mathbf{e}_j |_{\partial B} \ , \\[3mm] \dfrac{\partial}{\partial \widetilde{\nu}} \widetilde{\mathcal{S}}_B(\boldsymbol{\varphi}_i^j)_\epsilon \Big|_- - \dfrac{\partial}{\partial \nu} \mathcal{S}_B(\boldsymbol{\psi}_i^j)_\epsilon \Big|_+ = \dfrac{\partial(x_i \mathbf{e}_j)}{\partial \nu} |_{\partial B} \ , \end{cases}$$

we have

$$\begin{cases} \widetilde{\mathcal{S}}_B \left[(\boldsymbol{\varphi}_i^j)_\epsilon - \mathbf{f}_i^j \right] \Big|_- - \mathcal{S}_B \left[(\boldsymbol{\psi}_i^j)_\epsilon - \mathbf{g}_i^j \right] \Big|_+ = \text{constant} \\[3mm] \dfrac{\partial}{\partial \widetilde{\nu}} \widetilde{\mathcal{S}}_B \left[(\boldsymbol{\varphi}_i^j)_\epsilon - \mathbf{f}_i^j \right] \Big|_- - \dfrac{\partial}{\partial \nu} \mathcal{S}_B \left[(\boldsymbol{\psi}_i^j)_\epsilon - \mathbf{g}_i^j \right] \Big|_+ = 0 \end{cases} \quad \text{on } \partial B \ .$$

We then obtain (10.36) from Lemma 9.14. Armed with this identity, we now write

$$\begin{aligned} m_{pq}^{ij}(\epsilon B) &= \int_{\partial(\epsilon B)} x_p \mathbf{e}_q \cdot \mathbf{g}_i^j(\epsilon B) \, d\sigma \\ &= \epsilon^d \int_{\partial B} x_p \mathbf{e}_q \cdot \mathbf{g}_i^j(B) \, d\sigma = \epsilon^d m_{pq}^{ij}(B) \ , \end{aligned}$$

to arrive at the desired conclusion. $\qquad\square$

Lemma 10.9 *Let $R = (r_{ij})$ be a unitary transformation in $\mathbb{R}^d$, and let $\widehat{B}$ be a bounded Lipschitz domain in $\mathbb{R}^d$ and $B = R(\widehat{B})$. Let m_{pq}^{ij} and $\widehat{m}_{pq}^{ij}$, $i, j, p, q = 1, \ldots, d$, denote the EMTs associated with B and $\widehat{B}$, respectively. Then,*

$$m_{pq}^{ij} = \sum_{u,v=1}^{d} \sum_{k,l=1}^{d} r_{pu} r_{qv} r_{ik} r_{jl} \widehat{m}_{uv}^{kl} \ . \tag{10.37}$$

Proof. For $i, j = 1, \ldots, d$, let $(\mathbf{f}_i^j, \mathbf{g}_i^j)$ and $(\widehat{\mathbf{f}}_i^j, \widehat{\mathbf{g}}_i^j)$ be the solutions of (10.10) on ∂B and $\partial \widehat{B}$, respectively. By Lemmas 9.9 (ii) and 9.12,

$$\widetilde{\mathcal{S}}_{\widehat{B}}(R^{-1}(\mathbf{f}_i^j \circ R)) \Big|_- - \mathcal{S}_{\widehat{B}}(R^{-1}(\mathbf{g}_i^j \circ R)) \Big|_+ = R^{-1}((x_i \mathbf{e}_j) \circ R)|_{\partial \widehat{B}} \ ,$$

$$\frac{\partial}{\partial \widetilde{\nu}} \widetilde{\mathcal{S}}_{\widehat{B}}(R^{-1}(\mathbf{f}_i^j \circ R)) \Big|_- - \frac{\partial}{\partial \nu} \mathcal{S}_{\widehat{B}}(R^{-1}(\mathbf{g}_i^j \circ R)) \Big|_+ = \frac{\partial}{\partial \nu}(R^{-1}((x_i \mathbf{e}_j) \circ R))|_{\partial \widehat{B}} \ .$$

It is easy to see that

$$R^{-1}\big((x_i\mathbf{e}_j)\circ R\big) = R(x)_i R^{-1}(\mathbf{e}_j) = \sum_{k,l=1}^{d} r_{ik}r_{jl}(x_k\mathbf{e}_l)\,, \quad i,j = 1,\ldots,d\,.$$

It then follows from the uniqueness of a solution to the integral equation (10.4) that

$$R^{-1}(\mathbf{g}_i^j \circ R) = \sum_{k,l=1}^{d} r_{ik}r_{jl}\widehat{\mathbf{g}}_k^l\,, \quad i,j = 1,\ldots,d\,.$$

By (10.11) and a change of variables, we have

$$\begin{aligned}
m_{pq}^{ij} &= \int_{\partial B} x_p\mathbf{e}_q \cdot \mathbf{g}_i^j\, d\sigma \\
&= \int_{\partial \widehat{B}} R^{-1}\big((x_p\mathbf{e}_q)\circ R\big) \cdot R^{-1}(\mathbf{g}_i^j \circ R)\, d\sigma \\
&= \int_{\partial \widehat{B}} \sum_{u,v=1}^{d} r_{pu}r_{qv}(x_u\mathbf{e}_v) \cdot \sum_{k,l=1}^{d} r_{ik}r_{jl}\widehat{\mathbf{g}}_k^l\, d\sigma \\
&= \sum_{u,v=1}^{d}\sum_{k,l=1}^{d} r_{pu}r_{qv}r_{ik}r_{jl}\widehat{m}_{uv}^{kl}\,.
\end{aligned}$$

The proof is complete. $\qquad\qquad\square$

The formula (10.37) can be written in more condensed form. Let M and $\widehat{M}$ be the EMTs associated with B and $\widehat{B}$, respectively. Since $\widehat{M}$ is a linear transformation on the space of $d \times d$ symmetric matrices, it has $d(d+1)/2$ eigen-matrices, say $A_1,\ldots,A_{d(d+1)/2}$, and can be represented as

$$\widehat{M} = A_1 \otimes A_1 + \cdots + A_d \otimes A_{d(d+1)/2}\,.$$

The relation (10.37) can be written as

$$M = RA_1 R^T \otimes RA_1 R^T + \cdots + RA_{d(d+1)/2}R^T \otimes RA_{d(d+1)/2}R^T\,. \qquad (10.38)$$

In two dimensions, the unitary transformation R is given by the rotation:

$$R = R_\theta = \begin{pmatrix} r_{11} & r_{12} \\ r_{21} & r_{22} \end{pmatrix} = \begin{pmatrix} \cos\theta & -\sin\theta \\ \sin\theta & \cos\theta \end{pmatrix}\,.$$

The following corollary follows from (10.37), after elementary but tedious computations.

Corollary 10.10 *Let $B = R_\theta(\widehat{B})$ and (m_{pq}^{ij}) and $(\widehat{m}_{pq}^{ij})$ denote the EMTs for B and $\widehat{B}$, respectively. Then,*

$$
\begin{cases}
m_{11}^{11} = \cos^4\theta\,\widehat{m}_{11}^{11} + \dfrac{1}{2}\sin^2(2\theta)\widehat{m}_{22}^{11} + \sin^2(2\theta)\widehat{m}_{12}^{12} + \sin^4\theta\,\widehat{m}_{22}^{22}\,, \\[2ex]
m_{12}^{11} = \sin\theta\cos^3\theta\,\widehat{m}_{11}^{11} - \dfrac{1}{4}\sin(4\theta)\widehat{m}_{22}^{11} - \dfrac{1}{2}\sin(4\theta)\widehat{m}_{12}^{12} - \sin^3\theta\cos\theta\,\widehat{m}_{22}^{22}\,, \\[2ex]
m_{22}^{11} = \dfrac{1}{2}\sin^2(2\theta)\widehat{m}_{11}^{11} + (1 - \dfrac{1}{2}\sin^2(2\theta))\widehat{m}_{22}^{11} - \sin^2(2\theta)\widehat{m}_{12}^{12} + \dfrac{1}{2}\sin^2(2\theta)\widehat{m}_{22}^{22}\,, \\[2ex]
m_{12}^{12} = \dfrac{1}{2}\sin^2(2\theta)\widehat{m}_{11}^{11} - \dfrac{1}{2}\sin^2(2\theta)\widehat{m}_{22}^{11} + \cos^2(2\theta)\widehat{m}_{12}^{12} + \dfrac{1}{4}\sin^2(2\theta)\widehat{m}_{22}^{22}\,, \\[2ex]
m_{22}^{12} = \sin^3\theta\cos\theta\,\widehat{m}_{11}^{11} + \dfrac{1}{4}\sin(4\theta)\widehat{m}_{22}^{11} + \dfrac{1}{2}\sin(4\theta)\widehat{m}_{12}^{12} - \sin\theta\cos^3\theta\,\widehat{m}_{22}^{22}\,, \\[2ex]
m_{22}^{22} = \sin^4\theta\,\widehat{m}_{11}^{11} + \dfrac{1}{2}\sin^2(2\theta)\widehat{m}_{22}^{11} + \sin^2(2\theta)\widehat{m}_{12}^{12} + \cos^4\theta\,\widehat{m}_{22}^{22}\,.
\end{cases}
\tag{10.39}
$$

Corollary 10.10 has an interesting consequence. If B is a disk, then $m_{pq}^{ij} = \widehat{m}_{pq}^{ij}$, $i,j,p,q = 1,2$, for any θ. Thus, we can observe from the first identity in (10.39) that

$$
m_{11}^{11} = m_{22}^{22} = m_{22}^{11} + 2m_{12}^{12}\,.
\tag{10.40}
$$

It then follows from the second and the fifth identity in (10.39) that

$$
m_{12}^{11} = m_{22}^{12} = 0\,.
$$

Thus we have the following lemma.

Lemma 10.11 *If B is a disk, then the EMT (m_{pq}^{ij}) is isotropic and given by*

$$
m_{pq}^{ij} = m_{22}^{11}\delta_{ij}\delta_{pq} + m_{12}^{12}(\delta_{ip}\delta_{jq} + \delta_{iq}\delta_{jp})\,, \quad i,j,p,q = 1,2\,.
\tag{10.41}
$$

We also obtain the following lemma from Corollary 10.10.

Lemma 10.12 *Suppose that either $m_{12}^{11}+m_{22}^{12}$ or $m_{11}^{11}-m_{22}^{22}$ is not zero. Then*

$$
\frac{m_{12}^{11} + m_{22}^{12}}{m_{11}^{11} - m_{22}^{22}} = \frac{1}{2}\tan 2\theta\,.
\tag{10.42}
$$

Proof. We can easily see from (10.39) that

$$
m_{11}^{11} - m_{22}^{22} = \cos 2\theta(\widehat{m}_{11}^{11} - \widehat{m}_{22}^{22})\,, \quad m_{12}^{11} + m_{22}^{12} = \frac{1}{2}\sin 2\theta(\widehat{m}_{11}^{11} - \widehat{m}_{22}^{22})\,.
$$

Thus, (10.42) holds, as claimed. $\square$

10.4 EMTs for Ellipses

In this section we compute the EMTs associated with an ellipse. We suppose that the ellipse takes the form

$$B : \frac{x_1^2}{a^2} + \frac{x_2^2}{b^2} = 1 \,, \quad a,b > 0 \,. \tag{10.43}$$

The EMTs for general ellipses can be found using (10.39).

Suppose that B is an ellipse of the form (10.43). Let (λ, μ) and $(\widetilde{\lambda}, \widetilde{\mu})$ be the Lamé constants for $\mathbb{R}^2 \setminus \overline{B}$ and B, respectively. We will be looking for the solution of (10.13).

Let $\mathbf{u} = (u, v)$ be a solution to (10.13), and let $\mathbf{u}_e := \mathbf{u}|_{\mathbb{R}^2 \setminus B}$ and $\mathbf{u}_i := \mathbf{u}|_B$. By Theorem 9.20, there are functions φ_e and ψ_e holomorphic in $\mathbb{C} \setminus \overline{B}$ and φ_i and ψ_i holomorphic in B such that

$$2\mu(u_e + iv_e)(z) = \kappa\varphi_e(z) - z\overline{\varphi_e'(z)} - \overline{\psi_e(z)} \,, \quad z \in \mathbb{C} \setminus \overline{B} \,, \tag{10.44}$$

$$2\widetilde{\mu}(u_i + iv_i)(z) = \widetilde{\kappa}\varphi_i(z) - z\overline{\varphi_i'(z)} - \overline{\psi_i(z)} \,, \quad z \in B \,, \tag{10.45}$$

where κ and $\widetilde{\kappa}$ are given by (9.55) and

$$\begin{cases} \dfrac{1}{2\mu}\left(\kappa\varphi_e(z) - z\overline{\varphi_e'(z)} - \overline{\psi_e(z)}\right) = \dfrac{1}{2\widetilde{\mu}}\left(\widetilde{\kappa}\varphi_i(z) - z\overline{\varphi_i'(z)} - \overline{\psi_i(z)}\right) \,, \\ \varphi_e(z) + z\overline{\varphi_e'(z)} + \overline{\psi_e(z)} = \varphi_i(z) + z\overline{\varphi_i'(z)} + \overline{\psi_i(z)} + c \quad \text{on } \partial B \,, \end{cases} \tag{10.46}$$

where c is a constant. In order to find such $\varphi_e, \psi_e, \varphi_i, \psi_i$, we use elliptic coordinates, as done in [249]. Let

$$r := \frac{1}{2}(a + b) \,, \quad m := \frac{a - b}{a + b} \,, \tag{10.47}$$

and define

$$z = x_1 + ix_2 = \omega(\zeta) := r\left(\zeta + \frac{m}{\zeta}\right) \,.$$

Then ω maps the exterior of the unit disk onto $\mathbb{C} \setminus \overline{B}$.

Lemma 10.13 *Suppose that $m > 0$. For a given pair of complex numbers α and β, there are unique complex numbers A, B, C, E, F such that the functions $\varphi_e, \psi_e, \varphi_i,$ and ψ_i defined by*

$$\varphi_e \circ \omega(\zeta) = r\left[\alpha\zeta + \frac{A}{\zeta}\right] \,, \quad |\zeta| > 1 \,,$$

$$\psi_e \circ \omega(\zeta) = r\left[\beta\zeta + \frac{B}{\zeta} + \frac{C\zeta}{\zeta^2 - m}\right] \,, \quad |\zeta| > 1 \,, \tag{10.48}$$

$$\varphi_i(z) = Ez \,, \quad z \in B \,,$$

$$\psi_i(z) = Fz \,, \quad z \in B \,,$$

satisfy the conditions (9.56) and (9.57). Here, the constant c in (9.57) can be taken to be zero. In fact, $A, B, C, E,$ and F are the unique solutions of the algebraic equations

$$\begin{cases}
\dfrac{\kappa}{\mu}\alpha - \dfrac{1}{\mu}\Big(\dfrac{\overline{A}}{m} + \overline{B}\Big) = \dfrac{\widetilde{\kappa}E - \overline{E}}{\widetilde{\mu}} - \dfrac{m}{\widetilde{\mu}}\overline{F} \,, \\[2mm]
\alpha + \Big(\dfrac{\overline{A}}{m} + \overline{B}\Big) = E + \overline{E} + m\overline{F} \,, \\[2mm]
\dfrac{\kappa}{\mu}A - \dfrac{1}{\mu}\big(m\overline{\alpha} + \overline{\beta}\big) = m\dfrac{\widetilde{\kappa}E - \overline{E}}{\widetilde{\mu}} - \dfrac{1}{\widetilde{\mu}}\overline{F} \,, \\[2mm]
A + \big(m\overline{\alpha} + \overline{\beta}\big) = m(E + \overline{E}) + \overline{F} \,, \\[2mm]
(m^2 + 1)\alpha - \big(m + \dfrac{1}{m}\big)A + C = 0 \,.
\end{cases} \tag{10.49}$$

Proof. Since
$$\frac{\overline{\omega(\zeta)}}{\omega'(\zeta)} = \frac{\zeta^2 + m}{\zeta(1 - m\zeta^2)} \,, \qquad |\zeta| = 1 \,,$$

we can check by elementary but tedious computations that the transmission conditions (10.46) are equivalent to the algebraic equations (10.49). It is easy to check that (10.49) has a unique solution $A, B, C, E,$ and F, provided that $m > 0$. The proof is complete. $\qquad\square$

For a given pair of complex numbers α and β, let $\mathbf{u} = (u, v)$ be the solution defined by φ and ψ given by (10.48). Define

$$\begin{cases}
m_{pq}(\alpha, \beta) := \displaystyle\int_{\partial B} \frac{\partial(x_p \mathbf{e}_q)}{\partial \nu} \cdot (u_e, v_e)\, d\sigma \,, \\[3mm]
\widetilde{m}_{pq}(\alpha, \beta) := \displaystyle\int_{\partial B} \frac{\partial(x_p \mathbf{e}_q)}{\partial \widetilde{\nu}} \cdot (u_e, v_e)\, d\sigma \,.
\end{cases} \tag{10.50}$$

In order to compute the first-order EMT m_{pq}^{ij} associated with B, we need to find the solution of (10.13), which behaves at infinity like $x_i \mathbf{e}_j$. Let $\alpha = \alpha_1 + i\alpha_2$, *etc.*, and observe that the exterior solution $u_e + iv_e$ behaves at infinity like

$$\begin{aligned}
u_e(z) + iv_e(z) = \frac{1}{2\mu}\Big[&(\kappa\alpha_1 - \alpha_1 - \beta_1)x + (-\kappa\alpha_2 - \alpha_2 + \beta_2)y\Big] \\
+ \frac{i}{2\mu}\Big[&(\kappa\alpha_2 + \alpha_2 + \beta_2)x + (\kappa\alpha_1 - \alpha_1 + \beta_1)y\Big] \\
&+ O(|z|^{-1}) \,.
\end{aligned} \tag{10.51}$$

Therefore, to compute m_{pq}^{11}, for example, we need to take $\alpha = \mu/(\kappa - 1)$ and $\beta = -\mu$. In view of (10.12) and (10.51), we see that

$$\begin{cases}
m_{pq}^{11} = -m_{pq}\Big(\dfrac{\mu}{\kappa - 1}, -\mu\Big) + \widetilde{m}_{pq}\Big(\dfrac{\mu}{\kappa - 1}, -\mu\Big) \,, \\[3mm]
m_{pq}^{22} = -m_{pq}\Big(\dfrac{\mu}{\kappa - 1}, \mu\Big) + \widetilde{m}_{pq}\Big(\dfrac{\mu}{\kappa - 1}, \mu\Big) \,, \\[3mm]
m_{pq}^{12} = -m_{pq}\Big(\dfrac{i\mu}{\kappa + 1}, i\mu\Big) + \widetilde{m}_{pq}\Big(\dfrac{i\mu}{\kappa + 1}, i\mu\Big) \,.
\end{cases} \tag{10.52}$$

We now compute $m_{pq}(\alpha, \beta)$. For $p, q = 1, 2$, let $a = a_{pq}$ and $b = b_{pq}$ be complex numbers such that $f(z) = az$ and $g(z) = bz$ satisfy

$$2\mu((x_p\mathbf{e}_q)_1 + i(x_p\mathbf{e}_q)_2) = \kappa f(z) - z\overline{f'(z)} - \overline{g(z)}, \quad z \in \mathbb{C}. \tag{10.53}$$

In fact, the pair (a, b) is given by

$$(a, b) = \begin{cases} (\dfrac{\mu}{\kappa - 1}, -\mu) & \text{if } (p, q) = (1, 1), \\[2mm] (\dfrac{\mu}{\kappa - 1}, \mu) & \text{if } (p, q) = (2, 2), \\[2mm] (\dfrac{i\mu}{\kappa + 1}, i\mu) & \text{if } (p, q) = (1, 2). \end{cases} \tag{10.54}$$

Then, by (9.46), we get

$$\left(\left(\frac{\partial(x_p\mathbf{e}_q)}{\partial\nu} \right)_1 + i \left(\frac{\partial(x_p\mathbf{e}_q)}{\partial\nu} \right)_2 \right) d\sigma \tag{10.55}$$

$$= -i\partial\left[f(z) + z\overline{f'(z)} + \overline{g(z)} \right] = -i\partial\left[2\Re az + \bar{b}\bar{z} \right]. \tag{10.56}$$

Therefore

$$\begin{aligned} m_{pq}(\alpha, \beta) &= \Re \int_{\partial B} \left(\left(\frac{\partial(x_p\mathbf{e}_q)}{\partial\nu} \right)_1 + i \left(\frac{\partial(x_p\mathbf{e}_q)}{\partial\nu} \right)_2 \right) (u_e - iv_e)\, d\sigma \\ &= \Re \frac{-i}{2\mu} \int_{\partial B} \left[\kappa\overline{\varphi_e(z)} - \bar{z}\varphi_e'(z) - \psi_e(z) \right] \partial\left[2\Re az + \bar{b}\bar{z} \right] \\ &= \Re \frac{-i}{2\tilde{\mu}} \int_{\partial B} \left[\tilde{\kappa}\overline{\varphi_i(z)} - \bar{z}\varphi_i'(z) - \psi_i(z) \right] \left[2\Re adz + \bar{b}d\bar{z} \right], \end{aligned}$$

where the last equality comes from (10.46). It then follows from (10.48) that

$$\begin{aligned} m_{pq}(\alpha, \beta) &= \Re \frac{-i}{2\tilde{\mu}} \int_{\partial B} \left[(\tilde{\kappa}\overline{E} - E)\bar{z} - Fz \right] \left[2\Re adz + \bar{b}d\bar{z} \right] \\ &= \Re \frac{\pi}{\tilde{\mu}} \left[2\Re a(\tilde{\kappa}\overline{E} - E) + \bar{b}F \right]. \end{aligned} \tag{10.57}$$

Following the same arguments, we obtain that

$$\widetilde{m}_{pq}(\alpha, \beta) = \Re \frac{\pi}{\mu} \left[2\Re\tilde{a}(\kappa\overline{E} - E) + \bar{\tilde{b}}F \right], \tag{10.58}$$

where $(\tilde{a}, \tilde{b})$ is defined by (10.54) with μ, κ replaced by $\tilde{\mu}, \tilde{\kappa}$.

Denote the solutions of (10.49), which depend on given α and β, by $A = A_1 + iA_2 = A(\alpha, \beta)$, *etc.* Then we see from (10.52), (10.54), (10.57), and (10.58) that

$$\frac{\widetilde{\mu}}{|B|}\left[-m_{pq}(\alpha,\beta)+\widetilde{m}_{pq}(\alpha,\beta)\right]$$

$$=\begin{cases}(\widetilde{\kappa}-1)(\widetilde{\lambda}-\lambda+\widetilde{\mu}-\mu)E_1-(\widetilde{\mu}-\mu)F_1 & \text{if } p=q=1\,,\\[4pt](\widetilde{\mu}-\mu)F_2 & \text{if } p\neq q\,,\\[4pt](\widetilde{\kappa}-1)(\widetilde{\lambda}-\lambda+\widetilde{\mu}-\mu)E_1+(\widetilde{\mu}-\mu)F_1 & \text{if } p=q=2\,.\end{cases}\qquad(10.59)$$

For given α,β, we solve the system of linear equations (10.49) to find $E(\alpha,\beta)$ and $F(\alpha,\beta)$. Then, using (10.52) and (10.59), we can find m_{pq}^{ij}, $i,j,p,q=1,2$.

In short, we have the following theorem.

Theorem 10.14 *Suppose that $0<\widetilde{\lambda},\widetilde{\mu}<+\infty$. Let B be the ellipse of the form (10.43). Then,*

$$m_{11}^{12}=m_{22}^{12}=0\,,\qquad(10.60)$$

and $m_{11}^{11},m_{22}^{22},m_{22}^{11},m_{12}^{12}$ can be computed by making use of (10.49), (10.52), and (10.59). The remaining terms are determined by the symmetry properties (10.26). The EMTs for rotated ellipses can be found using (10.39).

Proof. It suffices to show (10.60). Since the coefficients of (10.49) are real, $E_1(\alpha,\beta)=F_1(\alpha,\beta)=0$ if α and β are purely imaginary, and $E_2(\alpha,\beta)=F_2(\alpha,\beta)=0$ if α and β are real. Thus (10.60) follows from (10.52) and (10.59). This completes the proof. $\qquad\square$

Since the meaning of (10.49) is not clear when $m=0$, i.e., when B is a disk, we now compute the first-order EMT for a disk. If B is a disk of radius one, we can easily check that (10.13) admits a unique solution $\mathbf{u}=(u,v)$ given by φ and ψ that are defined by

$$\varphi_e(z)=\alpha z+\frac{A}{z}\,,\quad |z|>1\,,$$

$$\psi_e(z)=\beta z+\frac{B}{z}+\frac{C}{z^3}\,,\quad |z|>1,$$

$$\varphi_i(z)=Ez\,,\quad |z|<1\,,$$

$$\psi_i(z)=Fz\,,\quad |z|<1\,,\qquad(10.61)$$

where the coefficients A,B,C,E,F satisfy

$$\begin{cases}A=C=\dfrac{\widetilde{\mu}-\mu}{\kappa\widetilde{\mu}+\mu}\bar{\beta}\,,\\[10pt]B=\dfrac{\mu(\widetilde{\kappa}+1)}{\mu-\widetilde{\mu}}E-\bar{\alpha}-\dfrac{\kappa\widetilde{\mu}+\mu}{\mu-\widetilde{\mu}}\alpha\,,\\[10pt]E=\dfrac{\widetilde{\mu}(\kappa+1)}{(\widetilde{\kappa}-1)\mu+2\widetilde{\mu}}\Re\alpha+i\dfrac{\widetilde{\mu}(\kappa+1)}{\mu(\widetilde{\kappa}+1)}\Im\alpha\,,\\[10pt]F=\dfrac{\widetilde{\mu}(\kappa+1)}{\kappa\widetilde{\mu}+\mu}\beta\,.\end{cases}\qquad(10.62)$$

We then obtain the following theorem from (10.52) and (10.59).

Theorem 10.15 *Let B be a disk. Then*

$$
\begin{cases}
m_{22}^{11} = |B|\mu \left[\dfrac{(\widetilde{\kappa} - 1)(\kappa + 1)(\widetilde{\lambda} - \lambda + \widetilde{\mu} - \mu)}{(\widetilde{\kappa}\mu + 2\widetilde{\mu} - \mu)(\kappa - 1)} - \dfrac{(\widetilde{\mu} - \mu)(\kappa + 1)}{\kappa\widetilde{\mu} + \mu} \right] , \\[2ex]
m_{12}^{12} = |B|\mu \dfrac{(\kappa + 1)(\widetilde{\mu} - \mu)}{\kappa\widetilde{\mu} + \mu} ,
\end{cases}
$$

where κ and $\widetilde{\kappa}$ are given by (9.55). The remaining terms are determined by (10.41) and the symmetry properties (10.26).

10.5 EMTs for Elliptic Holes and Hard Ellipses

In this section we compute EMTs for elliptic holes and hard inclusions of elliptic shape. By a hole we mean that $\widetilde{\lambda} = \widetilde{\mu} = 0$, whereas by a hard inclusion we mean that $\widetilde{\mu} = +\infty$. In other words, Young's modulus tends to $+\infty$, whereas Poisson's ratio tends to 0. Young's modulus, E, and Poisson's ratio, ν, are defined to be

$$
E = \frac{\mu(2\mu + d\lambda)}{\lambda + \mu}, \quad \nu = \frac{\lambda}{2(\lambda + \mu)} .
$$

We note that the EMTs associated with elliptic holes with $\widetilde{\lambda} = \widetilde{\mu} = 0$ were computed in [216] and [242].

Let us first deal with hard inclusions. If $\widetilde{\mu} = +\infty$, we obtain from (10.49) that

$$
\begin{cases}
\kappa\alpha - \left(\dfrac{\overline{A}}{m} + \overline{B} \right) = 0 , \\[2ex]
\alpha + \left(\dfrac{\overline{A}}{m} + \overline{B} \right) = E + \overline{E} + m\overline{F} , \\[2ex]
\kappa A - \left(m\overline{\alpha} + \overline{\beta} \right) = 0 , \\[2ex]
A + \left(m\overline{\alpha} + \overline{\beta} \right) = m(E + \overline{E}) + \overline{F} ,
\end{cases}
$$

where m is given by (10.47), and hence,

$$
\begin{cases}
E + \overline{E} + m\overline{F} = (\kappa + 1)\alpha , \\[2ex]
m(E + \overline{E}) + \overline{F} = \dfrac{\kappa + 1}{\kappa}(m\overline{\alpha} + \overline{\beta}) .
\end{cases}
$$

Thus,

$$
\begin{cases}
E + \overline{E} = \dfrac{\kappa + 1}{1 - m^2} \left[\alpha - \dfrac{m^2}{\kappa}\overline{\alpha} - \dfrac{m}{\kappa}\overline{\beta} \right] , \\[2ex]
\overline{F} = \dfrac{\kappa + 1}{1 - m^2} \left[-m\alpha + \dfrac{m}{\kappa}\overline{\alpha} + \dfrac{1}{\kappa}\overline{\beta} \right] .
\end{cases}
$$

Observe that the first equation has a solution only when α and β are real.

As $\widetilde{\mu} \to +\infty$, $\widetilde{\kappa} \to 3$, and hence, we obtain from (10.59) that

$$\frac{1}{|B|}\left[m_{pq}(\alpha,\beta) - \widetilde{m}_{pq}(\alpha,\beta)\right] = \begin{cases} -2E_1 + F_1 & \text{if } p = q = 1 , \\ -F_2 & \text{if } p \neq q , \\ -2E_1 - F_1 & \text{if } p = q = 2 . \end{cases} \tag{10.63}$$

If $\alpha = \mu/(\kappa - 1)$ and $\beta = -\mu$, then

$$\begin{cases} E + \overline{E} = \dfrac{\mu(\kappa+1)}{1-m^2}\left[\dfrac{1}{\kappa-1} - \dfrac{m^2}{\kappa(\kappa-1)} + \dfrac{m}{\kappa}\right] , \\ \overline{F} = \dfrac{\mu(\kappa+1)}{1-m^2}\left[-\dfrac{m}{\kappa-1} + \dfrac{m}{\kappa(\kappa-1)} - \dfrac{1}{\kappa}\right] . \end{cases}$$

Thus we arrive at

$$m_{11}^{11} = -m_{pq}\left(\frac{\mu}{\kappa-1}, -\mu\right) + \widetilde{m}_{pq}\left(\frac{\mu}{\kappa-1}, -\mu\right) = |B|\frac{\mu(\kappa+1)(m-2\kappa+1)}{(m-1)\kappa(\kappa-1)} .$$

Similarly, we can compute m_{pq}^{ij} using (10.52) and (10.63). The result of these computations is summarized in the following theorem.

Theorem 10.16 *Let B be the ellipse of the form (10.43), and suppose that $\widetilde{\mu} = +\infty$. Then, in addition to (10.60),*

$$\begin{cases} m_{11}^{11} = |B|\dfrac{\mu(\kappa+1)(m-2\kappa+1)}{(m-1)\kappa(\kappa-1)} , \\ m_{22}^{22} = |B|\dfrac{\mu(\kappa+1)(m+2\kappa-1)}{(m+1)\kappa(\kappa-1)} , \\ m_{22}^{11} = |B|\dfrac{\mu(\kappa+1)}{\kappa(\kappa-1)} , \\ m_{12}^{12} = |B|\dfrac{\mu(\kappa+1)}{\kappa+m^2} , \end{cases} \tag{10.64}$$

where m and κ are given by (10.47) and (9.55), respectively. The remaining terms are determined by the symmetry properties (10.26). The EMTs for rotated ellipses can be found using (10.39).

Let us now compute the EMTs for holes. To this end, we need to change the presentation of formula (10.59). By equating the first and third equations in (10.49), we obtain from (10.57) and (10.58) that

$$m_{pq}(\alpha,\beta) - \widetilde{m}_{pq}(\alpha,\beta)$$

$$= \frac{\pi}{(1-m^2)\mu}\Re\left[2\Re(a-\widetilde{a})\left(\kappa(\alpha-mA) + \left(m^2\bar{\alpha} - \frac{\bar{A}}{m} + m\bar{\beta} - \bar{B}\right)\right)\right.$$

$$\left. + (\bar{b} - \bar{\widetilde{b}})\left(\kappa(m\alpha - A) + (m\bar{\alpha} - \bar{A} + \bar{\beta} - m\bar{B})\right)\right] . \tag{10.65}$$

If $\widetilde{\lambda} = \widetilde{\mu} = 0$, then $E = F = 0$ in (10.49). Thus,

$$
\begin{cases}
\alpha + \left(\dfrac{\overline{A}}{m} + \overline{B}\right) = 0\,, \\[2mm]
A + \left(m\overline{\alpha} + \overline{\beta}\right) = 0\,, \\[2mm]
(m^2 + 1)\alpha - \left(m + \dfrac{1}{m}\right)A + C = 0\,.
\end{cases}
\tag{10.66}
$$

Since $\widetilde{a} = \widetilde{b} = 0$, it follows from (10.65) and (10.66) that

$$
m_{pq}(\alpha, \beta) = \frac{\pi(\kappa + 1)}{(1 - m^2)\mu} \Re\left[\bar{a}(2\Re a + \bar{b}m) + (m\alpha + \beta)(2\Re am + \bar{b})\right].
$$

We now obtain the following theorem from (10.52) and (10.54), after elementary but tedious computations.

Theorem 10.17 *Let B be the ellipse of the form (10.43), and suppose that $\widetilde{\lambda} = \widetilde{\mu} = 0$. Then, in addition to (10.60),*

$$
\begin{cases}
m_{11}^{11} = -|B|\dfrac{\mu(\kappa + 1)}{(1 - m^2)(\kappa - 1)^2}\left[2(1 + m^2) - 4m(\kappa - 1) + (\kappa - 1)^2\right], \\[3mm]
m_{22}^{22} = -|B|\dfrac{\mu(\kappa + 1)}{(1 - m^2)(\kappa - 1)^2}\left[2(1 + m^2) + 4m(\kappa - 1) + (\kappa - 1)^2\right], \\[3mm]
m_{22}^{11} = |B|\dfrac{\mu(\kappa + 1)}{(1 - m^2)(\kappa - 1)^2}\left[-2(1 + m^2) + (\kappa - 1)^2\right], \\[3mm]
m_{12}^{12} = -|B|\dfrac{\mu(\kappa + 1)}{1 - m^2}\,.
\end{cases}
\tag{10.67}
$$

The remaining terms are determined by the symmetry properties (10.26). The EMTs for rotated ellipses can be found using (10.39).

As an immediate consequence of Theorem 10.16 and Theorem 10.17, we obtain the following result.

Corollary 10.18 *Let B be a disk. If $\widetilde{\lambda} = \widetilde{\mu} = 0$, then*

$$
\begin{cases}
m_{22}^{11} = |B|\dfrac{\mu(\kappa + 1)}{(\kappa - 1)^2}\left[-2 + (\kappa - 1)^2\right], \\[3mm]
m_{12}^{12} = -|B|\mu(\kappa + 1)\,.
\end{cases}
$$

If $\widetilde{\mu} = +\infty$, then

$$
\begin{cases}
m_{22}^{11} = |B|\dfrac{\mu(\kappa + 1)}{\kappa(\kappa - 1)}\,, \\[3mm]
m_{12}^{12} = |B|\dfrac{\mu(\kappa + 1)}{\kappa}\,.
\end{cases}
$$

10.6 Further Results and Open Problems

Quite recently the elastic moment tensors for ellipses and ellipsoids were explicitly computed in [30] using a different method based on the layer potentials.

Capdeboscq and Kang [79] derived Hashin–Shtrikman bounds for the first-order elastic moment tensor that are analogous to (4.43) and (4.44). See also Lipton [222]. Capdeboscq and Kang also applied these bounds to estimate the size of diametrically small unknown elastic inclusions. An interesting and still open question concerns the optimality of these bounds.

In [17], the notion of viscosity moment tensor has been introduced. The viscosity moment tensor V associated with an incompressible inclusion B inside an incompressible object is given by

$$V := \lim_{\lambda,\widetilde{\lambda}\to\infty} PMP \, ,$$

where M is the elastic moment tensor associated with the inclusion and P is the orthogonal projection from the space of symmetric matrices onto the space of symmetric matrices of trace zero. It turns out that there are several conjectured relations between V and the polarization tensor associated with the same domain B and the conductivity contrast $k = \widetilde{\mu}/\mu$. We refer the interested reader to [114].

11

Full Asymptotic Expansions of the Displacement Field

Introduction

We suppose that the elastic medium occupies a bounded domain Ω in $\mathbb{R}^d$, with a connected Lipschitz boundary $\partial\Omega$. Let the constants (λ, μ) denote the background Lamé coefficients, which are the elastic parameters in the absence of any inclusions. Suppose that the elastic inclusion D in Ω is given by $D = \epsilon B + z$, where B is a bounded Lipschitz domain in $\mathbb{R}^d$. We assume that $c_0 > 0$ exists such that $\inf_{x \in D} \text{dist}(x, \partial\Omega) > c_0$.

Suppose that D has the pair of Lamé constants $(\widetilde{\lambda}, \widetilde{\mu})$ satisfying (9.19) and (9.20). The purpose of this chapter is to find a complete asymptotic expansion for the displacement field in terms of the reference Lamé constants, the location, and the shape of the inclusion D. This expansion describes the perturbation of the solution caused by the presence of D. Our derivations are rigorous and based on layer potential techniques. The asymptotic expansion in this chapter is valid for elastic inclusions with Lipschitz boundaries. Based on this asymptotic expansion we will derive in Chapter 12 formulae to obtain accurate reconstructions of the location and the order of magnitude of the elastic inclusion. The formulae are explicit and can be easily implemented numerically.

11.1 Full Asymptotic Expansions

We first observe that, if D is of the form $D = \epsilon B + z$, then the constant C in (9.30) depends on ϵ. However, for such a domain, we can obtain the following lemma by scaling both the integral equation (9.24) and the estimate (9.30).

Lemma 11.1 *For any given* $(\mathbf{F}, \mathbf{G}) \in W_1^2(\partial D) \times L^2(\partial D)$, *let* $(\mathbf{f}, \mathbf{g}) \in L^2(\partial D) \times L^2(\partial D)$ *be the solution of (9.24). Then a constant C exists depending only on* λ, μ, $\widetilde{\lambda}$, $\widetilde{\mu}$, *and the Lipschitz character of B, but not on ϵ, such that*

$$\|\mathbf{g}\|_{L^2(\partial D)} \leq C\left(\epsilon^{-1}\|\mathbf{F}\|_{L^2(\partial D)} + \|\frac{\partial \mathbf{F}}{\partial T}\|_{L^2(\partial D)} + \|\mathbf{G}\|_{L^2(\partial D)}\right) . \qquad (11.1)$$

Here $\partial/\partial T$ denotes the tangential derivative.

Proof. Assuming without loss of generality that $z = 0$, we scale $x = \epsilon y$, $y \in B$. Let $\mathbf{f}_\epsilon(y) = \mathbf{f}(\epsilon y)$, $y \in \partial B$, etc. Let (φ, ψ) be the solution to the integral equation

$$\begin{cases} \widetilde{\mathcal{S}}_B\varphi|_- - \mathcal{S}_B\psi|_+ = \epsilon^{-1}\mathbf{F}_\epsilon & \text{on } \partial B , \\ \dfrac{\partial}{\partial\widetilde{\nu}}\widetilde{\mathcal{S}}_B\varphi\bigg|_- - \dfrac{\partial}{\partial\nu}\mathcal{S}_B\psi\bigg|_+ = \mathbf{G}_\epsilon & \text{on } \partial B . \end{cases}$$

Following the lines as in the proof of (10.36), we can show that $\mathbf{g}_\epsilon = \psi$. It then follows from (9.30) that

$$\|\mathbf{g}_\epsilon\|_{L^2(\partial B)} = \|\psi_\epsilon\|_{L^2(\partial B)} \leq C\left(\|\epsilon^{-1}\mathbf{F}_\epsilon\|_{W_1^2(\partial B)} + \|\mathbf{G}_\epsilon\|_{L^2(\partial B)} \right) ,$$

where C does not depend on ϵ. By scaling back using $x = \epsilon y$, we obtain (11.1). This completes the proof. $\square$

Let $\mathbf{u}$ be the solution of (9.23). In this chapter, we derive an asymptotic formula for $\mathbf{u}$ as ϵ goes to 0 in terms of the background solution $\mathbf{U}$, that is, the solution of (9.14).

Recall that $\mathbf{u}$ is represented as

$$\mathbf{u}(x) = \mathbf{U}(x) - N_D\psi(x) , \quad x \in \partial\Omega , \tag{11.2}$$

where ψ is defined by (9.30). See (9.40). Let $\mathbf{H}$ be the function defined in (9.29). For a given integer n, define $\mathbf{H}^{(n)}$ by

$$\mathbf{H}^{(n)}(x) := \sum_{|\alpha|=0}^n \frac{1}{\alpha!}\partial^\alpha\mathbf{H}(z)(x-z)^\alpha$$

$$= \left(\sum_{|\alpha|=0}^n \frac{1}{\alpha!}\partial^\alpha H_1(z)(x-z)^\alpha ,\dots , \sum_{|\alpha|=0}^n \frac{1}{\alpha!}\partial^\alpha H_d(z)(x-z)^\alpha \right)$$

$$= \sum_{j=1}^d \sum_{|\alpha|=0}^n \frac{1}{\alpha!}\partial^\alpha H_j(z)(x-z)^\alpha\mathbf{e}_j .$$

Define φ_n and ψ_n in $L^2(\partial D)$ by

$$\begin{cases} \widetilde{\mathcal{S}}_D\varphi_n|_- - \mathcal{S}_D\psi_n|_+ = \mathbf{H}^{(n)}|_{\partial D} , \\ \dfrac{\partial}{\partial\widetilde{\nu}}\widetilde{\mathcal{S}}_D\varphi_n\bigg|_- - \dfrac{\partial}{\partial\nu}\mathcal{S}_D\psi_n\bigg|_+ = \dfrac{\partial\mathbf{H}^{(n)}}{\partial\nu}|_{\partial D} , \end{cases}$$

and set

$$\varphi := \varphi_n + \varphi_R \quad \text{and} \quad \psi := \psi_n + \psi_R .$$

Since $(\boldsymbol{\varphi}_R, \boldsymbol{\psi}_R)$ is the solution of the integral equation (9.24) with $\mathbf{F} = \mathbf{H} - \mathbf{H}^{(n)}$ and $\mathbf{G} = \partial(\mathbf{H} - \mathbf{H}^{(n)})/\partial\nu$, it follows from (11.1) that

$$\|\boldsymbol{\psi}_R\|_{L^2(\partial D)} \le C\big(\epsilon^{-1}\|\mathbf{H} - \mathbf{H}^{(n)}\|_{L^2(\partial D)} + \|\nabla(\mathbf{H} - \mathbf{H}^{(n)})\|_{L^2(\partial D)}\big) . \tag{11.3}$$

By (9.32),

$$\epsilon^{-1}\|\mathbf{H} - \mathbf{H}^{(n)}\|_{L^2(\partial D)} + \|\nabla(\mathbf{H} - \mathbf{H}^{(n)})\|_{L^2(\partial D)}$$

$$\le |\partial D|^{1/2}\Big[\epsilon^{-1}\|\mathbf{H} - \mathbf{H}^{(n)}\|_{L^\infty(\partial D)} + \|\nabla(\mathbf{H} - \mathbf{H}^{(n)})\|_{L^\infty(\partial D)}\Big]$$

$$\le \|\mathbf{H}\|_{\mathcal{C}^{n+1}(\overline{D})}\epsilon^n|\partial D|^{1/2}$$

$$\le C\|\mathbf{g}\|_{L^2(\partial\Omega)}\epsilon^n|\partial D|^{1/2} ,$$

and therefore,

$$\|\boldsymbol{\psi}_R\|_{L^2(\partial D)} \le C\|\mathbf{g}\|_{L^2(\partial\Omega)}\epsilon^n|\partial D|^{1/2} , \tag{11.4}$$

where C is independent of ϵ.

By (11.2), we obtain that

$$\mathbf{u}(x) = \mathbf{U}(x) - N_D\boldsymbol{\psi}_n(x) - N_D\boldsymbol{\psi}_R(x) , \quad x \in \partial\Omega . \tag{11.5}$$

The first two terms in (11.5) are the main terms in our asymptotic expansion, and the last term is the error term. We claim that the error term is $O(\epsilon^{n+d})$. In fact, since $\boldsymbol{\psi}, \boldsymbol{\psi}_n \in L^2_\Psi(\partial D)$, in particular, $\int_{\partial D} \boldsymbol{\psi}\,d\sigma = \int_{\partial D} \boldsymbol{\psi}_n\,d\sigma = 0$, and we have $\int_{\partial D} \boldsymbol{\psi}_R\,d\sigma = 0$. It then follows from (11.4) that, for $x \in \partial\Omega$,

$$|N_D\boldsymbol{\psi}_R(x)| = \left|\int_{\partial D} \big(\mathbf{N}(x - y) - \mathbf{N}(x - z)\big)\boldsymbol{\psi}_R(y)\,d\sigma(y)\right|$$

$$\le C\epsilon|\partial D|^{1/2}\|\boldsymbol{\psi}_R\|_{L^2(\partial D)}$$

$$\le C\|\mathbf{g}\|_{L^2(\partial\Omega)}\epsilon^{n+d} .$$

In order to expand the second term in (11.5), we first define some auxiliary functions. Let $D_0 := D - z$, the translate of D by $-z$. For multi-index $\alpha \in \mathbb{N}^d$ and $j = 1,\ldots,d$, define $\boldsymbol{\varphi}_\alpha^j$ and $\boldsymbol{\psi}_\alpha^j$ by

$$\begin{cases} \widetilde{\mathcal{S}}_{D_0}\boldsymbol{\varphi}_\alpha^j\big|_- - \mathcal{S}_{D_0}\boldsymbol{\psi}_\alpha^j\big|_+ = x^\alpha\mathbf{e}_j|_{\partial D_0} , \\[2mm] \dfrac{\partial}{\partial\nu}\widetilde{\mathcal{S}}_{D_0}\boldsymbol{\varphi}_\alpha^j\bigg|_- - \dfrac{\partial}{\partial\nu}\mathcal{S}_{D_0}\boldsymbol{\psi}_\alpha^j\bigg|_+ = \dfrac{\partial(x^\alpha\mathbf{e}_j)}{\partial\nu}\big|_{\partial D_0} . \end{cases} \tag{11.6}$$

Then the linearity and the uniqueness of the solution to (11.6) yield

$$\boldsymbol{\psi}_n(x) = \sum_{j=1}^{d}\sum_{|\alpha|=0}^{n} \frac{1}{\alpha!}\partial^\alpha H_j(z)\boldsymbol{\psi}_\alpha^j(x - z) , \quad x \in \partial D .$$

Recall that $D_0 = \epsilon B$ and $(\mathbf{f}_\alpha^j, \mathbf{g}_\alpha^j)$ is the solution of (10.4). Then, following the same lines as in the proof of (10.36), we can see that

$$\boldsymbol{\psi}_\alpha^j(x) = \epsilon^{|\alpha|-1}\mathbf{g}_\alpha^j(\epsilon^{-1}x) \,,$$

and hence

$$\boldsymbol{\psi}_n(x) = \sum_{j=1}^{d}\sum_{|\alpha|=0}^{n}\frac{1}{\alpha!}\partial^\alpha H_j(z)\epsilon^{|\alpha|-1}\mathbf{g}_\alpha^j(\epsilon^{-1}(x-z))\,, \quad x \in \partial D\,.$$

We thus get

$$N_D\boldsymbol{\psi}_n(x) = \sum_{j=1}^{d}\sum_{|\alpha|=0}^{n}\frac{1}{\alpha!}\partial^\alpha H_j(z)\epsilon^{|\alpha|+d-2}\int_{\partial B}\mathbf{N}(x,z+\epsilon y)\mathbf{g}_\alpha^j(y)\,d\sigma(y)\,.$$

$$(11.7)$$

We now consider the asymptotic expansion of $\mathbf{N}(x, z + \epsilon y)$ as $\epsilon \to 0$. We remind the reader that $x \in \partial\Omega$ and $z + \epsilon y \in \partial D$. By (9.39), we have the following relation:

$$\left(-\frac{1}{2}I + \mathcal{K}_\Omega\right)\left[\mathbf{N}(\cdot, \epsilon y + z)\right](x) = \boldsymbol{\Gamma}(x - z - \epsilon y)\,, \quad x \in \partial\Omega, \quad \text{modulo } \Psi\,.$$

Since

$$\boldsymbol{\Gamma}(x - \epsilon y) = \sum_{|\beta|=0}^{+\infty}\frac{1}{\beta!}\epsilon^{|\beta|}\partial^\beta(\boldsymbol{\Gamma}(x))y^\beta\,,$$

we get, modulo Ψ,

$$\left(-\frac{1}{2}I + \mathcal{K}_\Omega\right)\left[\mathbf{N}(\cdot, \epsilon y + z)\right](x) = \sum_{|\beta|=0}^{+\infty}\frac{1}{\beta!}\epsilon^{|\beta|}\partial^\beta(\boldsymbol{\Gamma}(x - z))y^\beta$$

$$= \left(-\frac{1}{2}I + \mathcal{K}_\Omega\right)\left[\sum_{|\beta|=0}^{+\infty}\frac{1}{\beta!}\epsilon^{|\beta|}\partial_z^\beta\mathbf{N}(\cdot, z)y^j\right](x)\,.$$

Since $\mathbf{N}(\cdot, w) \in L_\Psi^2(\partial\Omega)$ for all $w \in \Omega$, we have the following asymptotic expansion of the Neumann function.

Lemma 11.2 *For $x \in \partial\Omega$, $z \in \Omega$, $y \in \partial B$, and $\epsilon \to 0$,*

$$\mathbf{N}(x, \epsilon y + z) = \sum_{|\beta|=0}^{+\infty}\frac{1}{\beta!}\epsilon^{|\beta|}\partial_z^\beta\mathbf{N}(x, z)y^\beta\,.$$

It then follows from (11.7) that

$$N_D\boldsymbol{\psi}_n(x)$$

$$= \sum_{j=1}^{d}\sum_{|\alpha|=0}^{n}\frac{1}{\alpha!}\partial^\alpha H_j(z)\epsilon^{|\alpha|+d-2}\sum_{|\beta|=0}^{+\infty}\frac{1}{\beta!}\epsilon^{|\beta|}\partial_z^\beta\mathbf{N}(x,z)\int_{\partial B}y^\beta\mathbf{g}_\alpha^j(y)\,d\sigma(y)\,.$$

Note that $\sum_{j=1}^{d}\sum_{|\alpha|=l}\frac{1}{\alpha!}\partial^\alpha H_j(z)\mathbf{g}_\alpha^j$ is the solution of (9.30) when the right-hand side is given by the function

$$\mathbf{u} = \sum_{j=1}^{d}\sum_{|\alpha|=l}\frac{1}{\alpha!}\partial^\alpha H_j(z)x^\alpha \mathbf{e}_j \ .$$

Moreover, this function is a solution of $\mathcal{L}_{\lambda,\mu}\mathbf{u} = 0$ in B and, therefore, $\partial\mathbf{u}/\partial\nu|_{\partial B} \in L_\Psi^2(\partial B)$. Hence, by Theorem 9.13, we obtain that

$$\sum_{j=1}^{d}\sum_{|\alpha|=l}\frac{1}{\alpha!}\partial^\alpha H_j(z)\mathbf{g}_\alpha^j \in L_\Psi^2(\partial B) \ .$$

In particular, we have

$$\sum_{j=1}^{d}\sum_{|\alpha|=l}\frac{1}{\alpha!}\partial^\alpha H_j(z)\int_{\partial B}\mathbf{g}_\alpha^j(y)\,d\sigma(y) = 0 \quad \forall\, l \ .$$

On the other hand, $\mathbf{g}_0^j = 0$ by Lemma 9.14. We finally obtain by combining these facts with the above identity that

$$N_D\psi_n(x) = \sum_{j=1}^{d}\sum_{|\alpha|=1}^{n}\sum_{|\beta|=1}^{+\infty}\frac{\epsilon^{|\alpha|+|\beta|+d-2}}{\alpha!\beta!}\partial^\alpha H_j(z)\partial_z^\beta\mathbf{N}(x,z)\int_{\partial B}y^\beta\mathbf{g}_\alpha^j(y)\,d\sigma(y) \ . \tag{11.8}$$

We then see from the definition of the elastic moment tensors, (11.5), and (11.8) that

$$\mathbf{u}(x) = \mathbf{U}(x) - \sum_{j=1}^{d}\sum_{|\alpha|=1}^{n}\sum_{|\beta|=1}^{n-|\alpha|+1}\frac{\epsilon^{|\alpha|+|\beta|+d-2}}{\alpha!\beta!}\partial^\alpha H_j(z)\partial_z^\beta\mathbf{N}(x,z)M_{\alpha\beta}^j$$
$$+O(\epsilon^{n+d}) \ , \quad x \in \partial\Omega \ . \tag{11.9}$$

Observe that formula (11.9) still uses the function $\mathbf{H}$, which depends on ϵ. Therefore the remaining task is to transform this formula into a formula that is expressed using only the background solution $\mathbf{U}$.

By (9.7), $\mathbf{U} = -\mathcal{S}_\Omega(\mathbf{g}) + \mathcal{D}_\Omega(\mathbf{U}|_{\partial\Omega})$ in Ω. Thus substitution of (11.9) into (9.29) yields that, for any $x \in \Omega$,

$$\mathbf{H}(x) = -\mathcal{S}_\Omega(\mathbf{g})(x) + \mathcal{D}_\Omega(\mathbf{u}|_{\partial\Omega})(x)$$
$$= \mathbf{U}(x) - \sum_{j=1}^{d}\sum_{|\alpha|=1}^{n}\sum_{|\beta|=1}^{n-|\alpha|+1}\frac{\epsilon^{|\alpha|+|\beta|+d-2}}{\alpha!\beta!}\partial^\alpha H_j(z)\mathcal{D}_\Omega(\partial_z^\beta\mathbf{N}(.,z))(x)M_{\alpha\beta}^j$$
$$+ O(\epsilon^{n+d}) \ . \tag{11.10}$$

In (11.10) the remainder $O(\epsilon^{n+d})$ is uniform in the $\mathcal{C}^k$-norm on any compact subset of Ω for any k, and therefore,

$$\partial^\gamma \mathbf{H}(z) + \sum_{j=1}^d \sum_{|\alpha|=1}^n \sum_{|\beta|=1}^{n-|\alpha|+1} \epsilon^{|\alpha|+|\beta|+d-2} \partial^\alpha H_j(z) P^j_{\alpha\beta\gamma} = \partial^\gamma \mathbf{U}(z) + O(\epsilon^{n+d}) ,$$

$$(11.11)$$

for all $\gamma \in \mathbb{N}^d$ with $|\gamma| \le n$, where

$$P^j_{\alpha\beta\gamma} = \frac{1}{\alpha!\beta!} \partial^\gamma \mathcal{D}_\Omega(\partial_z^\beta \mathbf{N}(.,z))(x)|_{x=z} M^j_{\alpha\beta} .$$

We now introduce a linear transformation that transforms $\partial^\alpha \mathbf{H}(z)$ into $\partial^\alpha \mathbf{U}(z)$. Let

$$N := d \sum_{k=1}^n \frac{(k+1)(k+2)}{2} ,$$

and define the linear transformation $\mathcal{P}_\epsilon$ on $\mathbb{R}^N$ by

$$\mathcal{P}_\epsilon : (\mathbf{v}_\gamma)_{\gamma \in \mathbb{N}^d, |\gamma| \le n} \mapsto \left(\mathbf{v}_\gamma + \sum_{j=1}^d \sum_{|\alpha|=1}^n \sum_{|\beta|=1}^{n-|\alpha|+1} \epsilon^{|\alpha|+|\beta|+d-2} v_\alpha^j P^j_{\alpha\beta\gamma} \right)_{\gamma \in \mathbb{N}^d, |\gamma| \le n} .$$

Observe that

$$\mathcal{P}_\epsilon = I - \epsilon^d \mathcal{P}_1 - \ldots - \epsilon^{n+d-1} \mathcal{P}_n ,$$

where the definitions of $\mathcal{P}_j$ are obvious. Clearly, for small enough ϵ, $\mathcal{P}_\epsilon$ is invertible. We now define $\mathcal{Q}_i$, $i = 1, \ldots, n-1$, by

$$\mathcal{P}_\epsilon^{-1} = I + \epsilon^d \mathcal{Q}_1 + \ldots + \epsilon^{n+d-1} \mathcal{Q}_n + O(\epsilon^{n+d}) .$$

It then follows from (11.11) that

$$((\partial^\gamma \mathbf{H})(z))_{|\gamma| \le n} = \left(I + \sum_{i=1}^{n-d} \epsilon^{i+2} \mathcal{Q}_i \right) \left(((\partial^\gamma \mathbf{U})(z))_{|\gamma| \le n} \right) + O(\epsilon^n) ,$$

which yields the main result of this chapter.

Theorem 11.3 *Let $\mathbf{u}$ be the solution of (9.21) and $\mathbf{U}$ be the background solution. The following pointwise asymptotic expansion on $\partial\Omega$ holds:*

$$\mathbf{u}(x) = \mathbf{U}(x)$$
$$- \sum_{j=1}^d \sum_{|\alpha|=1}^n \sum_{|\beta|=1}^{n-|\alpha|+1} \frac{\epsilon^{|\alpha|+|\beta|+d-2}}{\alpha!\beta!} \left(\left(I + \sum_{i=1}^{n-d} \epsilon^{i+2} \mathcal{Q}_i \right)((\partial^\gamma \mathbf{U})(z)) \right)_\alpha^j \partial_z^\beta \mathbf{N}(x,z) M^j_{\alpha\beta}$$
$$+ O(\epsilon^{n+d}) , \quad x \in \partial\Omega .$$

$$(11.12)$$

The operator $\mathcal{Q}_j$ describes the interaction between the inclusion and $\partial\Omega$. It is interesting to compare (11.12) with formula (10.8) in free space. In (10.8) no $\mathcal{Q}_j$ is involved. This is because free space does not have any boundary.

If $n = d$, (11.12) takes a simpler form: For $x \in \partial\Omega$,

$$\mathbf{u}(x) = \mathbf{U}(x) - \sum_{j=1}^{d} \sum_{|\alpha|=1}^{d} \sum_{|\beta|=1}^{d+1-|\alpha|} \frac{\epsilon^{|\alpha|+|\beta|+d-2}}{\alpha!\beta!} (\partial^\alpha U_j)(z)\partial_z^\beta \mathbf{N}(x,z) M_{\alpha\beta}^j + O(\epsilon^{2d}) \ .$$

$$(11.13)$$

Observe that no $\mathcal{Q}_j$ appears in (11.13). This is because D is well separated from $\partial\Omega$.

The coefficient of the leading-order term, namely, the ϵ^d-term of the expansion, is

$$\sum_{j,p,q=1}^{d} (\partial_p U_j)(z)\partial_{z_q} N_{ij}(x,z) m_{pq}^{ij}, \quad i = 1,\ldots,d \ .$$

By Theorem 10.6, this term is bounded below and above by constant multiples of

$$\|\nabla U(z)\| \left[\sum_{q,j=1}^{d} |\partial_{z_q} N_{ij}(x,z)|^2 \right]^{1/2} ,$$

for $i = 1,\ldots,d$, and these constants are independent of ϵ.

When there are multiple well-separated inclusions

$$D_s = \epsilon B_s + z_s, \quad s = 1,\cdots,m \ ,$$

where $|z_s - z_{s'}| > 2c_0$ for some $c_0 > 0$, $s \neq s'$, then by iterating formula (11.13), we obtain the following theorem.

Theorem 11.4 *The following asymptotic expansion holds uniformly for $x \in \partial\Omega$:*

$$\mathbf{u}(x) = \mathbf{U}(x)$$
$$- \sum_{s=1}^{m} \sum_{j=1}^{d} \sum_{|\alpha|=1}^{d} \sum_{|\beta|=1}^{d+1-|\alpha|} \frac{\epsilon^{|\alpha|+|\beta|+d-2}}{\alpha!\beta!} (\partial^\alpha U_j)(z_s)\partial_z^\beta \mathbf{N}(x,z_s)(M^s)_{\alpha\beta}^j$$
$$+ O(\epsilon^{2d}) \ ,$$

where $(M^s)_{\alpha\beta}^j$ are the EMTs corresponding to B_s, $s = 1,\cdots,m$.

11.2 Further Results and Open Problems

Asymptotic formulae similar to those derived in this chapter can be easily obtained in the extreme cases: $\widetilde{\lambda}$ and $\widetilde{\mu}$ go to zero or $\widetilde{\mu}$ goes to infinity. To this end, it suffices to replace the elastic moment tensor by its limit. It can be shown that the remainder is uniform in $\widetilde{\lambda}$ and $\widetilde{\mu}$, as $\widetilde{\lambda}, \widetilde{\mu} \to 0$ and in $\widetilde{\mu}$, as $\widetilde{\mu} \to +\infty$.

A very interesting and quite challenging problem is to derive the leading-order term in the boundary perturbations of the displacement field when the elastic inclusion D is brought close to the boundary of the background medium Ω.

Imaging of Elastic Inclusions

Introduction

Most existing algorithms to solve inverse problems for the Lamé system are iterative and are therefore based on regularization techniques. See [154, 247]. This chapter develops efficient and robust direct (non-iterative) algorithms for reconstructing the location and certain features of unknown elastic inclusions.

One medical problem for which knowledge of internal elastic properties would be useful is tumor detection, particularly in the breast, liver, kidney, and prostate [62]. The elastic properties are very different for cancerous and normal tissues.

As in the previous chapter, assume that the elastic inclusion D in Ω is given by $D = \epsilon B + z$, where B is a bounded Lipschitz domain in $\mathbb{R}^d$. In this chapter, we propose a method to detect the elastic moment tensors and the center z of D from a finite number of boundary measurements. The reconstructed EMT will provide information on the size and some geometric features of the inclusion. Our approach is based on the asymptotic formula derived in the previous chapter.

12.1 Detection of EMTs

Given a traction $\mathbf{g} \in L^2_\Psi(\partial\Omega)$, let $\mathbf{H}[\mathbf{g}]$ be defined by

$$\mathbf{H}[\mathbf{g}](x) = -\mathcal{S}_\Omega(\mathbf{g})(x) + \mathcal{D}_\Omega(\mathbf{f})(x) \,, \quad x \in \mathbb{R}^d \setminus \partial\Omega, \quad \mathbf{f} := \mathbf{u}|_{\partial\Omega} \,, \qquad (12.1)$$

where $\mathbf{u}$ is the solution of (9.23) and $\mathcal{S}_\Omega$ and $\mathcal{D}_\Omega$ are the single and double layer potentials for the Lamé system on $\partial\Omega$.

Theorem 12.1 *For $x \in \mathbb{R}^d \setminus \overline{\Omega}$,*

$$\mathbf{H}[\mathbf{g}](x) = -\sum_{j=1}^{d}\sum_{|\alpha|=1}^{d}\sum_{|\beta|=1}^{d+1-|\alpha|} \frac{\epsilon^{|\alpha|+|\beta|+d-2}}{\alpha!\beta!}(\partial^{\alpha}U_j)(z)\partial^{\beta}\boldsymbol{\Gamma}(x-z)M_{\alpha\beta}^{j}$$
$$+ O(\frac{\epsilon^{2d}}{|x|^{d-1}}) \,, \tag{12.2}$$

where $\mathbf{U} = (U_1,\ldots,U_d)$ *is the background solution, i.e., the solution of (9.14);* $M_{\alpha\beta}^{j}$ *are the elastic moment tensors associated with* B; *and* $\boldsymbol{\Gamma}$ *is the Kelvin matrix of fundamental solutions corresponding to the Lamé parameters* (λ,μ).

Proof.   Since for any preassigned y in a fixed bounded set $|\nabla\boldsymbol{\Gamma}(x-y)| = O(|x|^{1-d})$ as $|x| \to +\infty$, substituting (11.13) into (12.1) yields

$$\mathbf{H}[\mathbf{g}](x) = -\mathcal{S}_{\Omega}(\mathbf{g})(x) + \mathcal{D}_{\Omega}(\mathbf{U}|_{\partial\Omega})(x)$$
$$-\sum_{j=1}^{d}\sum_{|\alpha|=1}^{d}\sum_{|\beta|=1}^{d+1-|\alpha|}\frac{\epsilon^{|\alpha|+|\beta|+d-2}}{\alpha!\beta!}(\partial^{\alpha}U_j)(z)\mathcal{D}_{\Omega}\big(\partial_z^{\beta}\mathbf{N}(\cdot,z)\big)(x)M_{\alpha\beta}^{j}$$
$$+ O(\frac{\epsilon^{2d}}{|x|^{d-1}}) \,.$$

But $\partial\mathbf{U}/\partial\nu = \mathbf{g}$ on $\partial\Omega$. Therefore, it follows from (9.8) that

$$-\mathcal{S}_{\Omega}(\mathbf{g})(x) + \mathcal{D}_{\Omega}(\mathbf{U}|_{\partial\Omega})(x) = 0 \quad \text{for } x \in \mathbb{R}^d \setminus \overline{\Omega} \,.$$

From (9.9) and (9.39), we now obtain

$$\mathcal{D}_{\Omega}\big(\mathbf{N}(\cdot,z)\big)|_{+}(x) = (-\frac{1}{2}I + \mathcal{K}_{\Omega})(\mathbf{N}(\cdot,z))(x) = \boldsymbol{\Gamma}(x-z) \,, \quad x \in \partial\Omega, \text{ modulo } \Psi \,.$$

By $\mathcal{D}_{\Omega}\big(\mathbf{N}(\cdot,z)\big)(x) = O(|x|^{1-d})$ and $\boldsymbol{\Gamma}(x-z) - \boldsymbol{\Gamma}(z) = O(|x|^{1-d})$ as $|x| \to +\infty$, we have the identity

$$\mathcal{D}_{\Omega}\big(\mathbf{N}(\cdot,z)\big)(x) = \boldsymbol{\Gamma}(x-z) - \boldsymbol{\Gamma}(z) \,, \quad x \in \mathbb{R}^d \setminus \overline{\Omega} \,,$$

from which we conclude that

$$\mathcal{D}_{\Omega}\big(\partial_z^{\beta}\mathbf{N}(\cdot,z)\big)(x) = \partial_z^{\beta}\mathcal{D}_{\Omega}\big(\mathbf{N}(\cdot,z)\big)(x) = \partial_z^{\beta}\boldsymbol{\Gamma}(x-z) \,, \quad |\beta| \geq 1 \,,$$

and hence (12.2) is immediate. This completes the proof. $\qquad\square$

If $\mathbf{g} = \partial\mathbf{U}/\partial\nu|_{\partial\Omega}$ where $\mathbf{U}$ is linear, then $\partial^{\alpha}\mathbf{U} = 0$ if $|\alpha| > 1$ and therefore,

$$\mathbf{H}[\mathbf{g}](x) = -\sum_{j=1}^{d}\sum_{|\alpha|=1}^{d}\sum_{|\beta|=1}^{d}\frac{\epsilon^{|\beta|+d-1}}{\beta!}(\partial^{\alpha}U_j)(z)\partial^{\beta}\boldsymbol{\Gamma}(x-z)M_{\alpha\beta}^{j} + O(\frac{\epsilon^{2d}}{|x|^{d-1}}) \,.$$

Since $\partial^{\beta}\boldsymbol{\Gamma}(x-z) = O(|x|^{-d+2-|\beta|})$ as $|x| \to +\infty$ if $|\beta| \geq 1$, we have

$$\mathbf{H}[\mathbf{g}](x) = -\epsilon^d \sum_{j=1}^{d} \sum_{|\alpha|=1} \sum_{|\beta|=1} (\partial^\alpha U_j)(z)\partial^\beta \mathbf{\Gamma}(x-z)M^j_{\alpha\beta} + O(\frac{\epsilon^{d+1}}{|x|^d})$$
$$+ O(\frac{\epsilon^{2d}}{|x|^{d-1}}) \, ,$$

or equivalently, for $k = 1, \ldots, d$,

$$H_k[\mathbf{g}](x) = -\epsilon^d \sum_{i,j,p,q=1}^{d} (\partial_i U_j)(z)\partial_p \Gamma_{kq}(x-z)m^{ij}_{pq} + O(\frac{\epsilon^{d+1}}{|x|^d}) \tag{12.3}$$
$$+ O(\frac{\epsilon^{2d}}{|x|^{d-1}}) \, .$$

Since $\partial_p \Gamma_{kq}(x-z) = \partial_p \Gamma_{kq}(x) + O(|x|^d)$, we obtain from (12.3) that

$$H_k[\mathbf{g}](x) = -\epsilon^d \sum_{i,j,p,q=1}^{d} (\partial_i U_j)(z)\partial_p \Gamma_{kq}(x)m^{ij}_{pq} + O(\frac{\epsilon^d}{|x|^d}) + O(\frac{\epsilon^{2d}}{|x|^{d-1}}) \, . \tag{12.4}$$

For a general $\mathbf{g}$, we have the following formula:

$$H_k[\mathbf{g}](x) = -\epsilon^d \sum_{i,j,p,q=1}^{d} (\partial_i U_j)(z)\partial_p \Gamma_{kq}(x-z)m^{ij}_{pq} + O(\frac{\epsilon^{d+1}}{|x|^{d-1}}) \, ,$$

from which the following expansion is obvious:

$$H_k[\mathbf{g}](x) = -\epsilon^d \sum_{i,j,p,q=1}^{d} (\partial_i U_j)(z)\partial_p \Gamma_{kq}(x)m^{ij}_{pq} + O(\frac{\epsilon^d}{|x|^d}) + O(\frac{\epsilon^{d+1}}{|x|^{d-1}}) \, . \tag{12.5}$$

Finally, (12.4) and (12.5) yield the following far-field relations.

Theorem 12.2 *If* $|x| = O(\epsilon^{-1})$, *then, for* $k = 1, \ldots, d$,

$$|x|^{d-1} H_k[\mathbf{g}](x) = -\epsilon^d |x|^{d-1} \sum_{i,j,p,q=1}^{d} (\partial_i U_j)(z)\partial_p \Gamma_{kq}(x)m^{ij}_{pq} \, . \tag{12.6}$$

Moreover, if $\mathbf{U}$ *is linear, then for all* x *such that* $|x| = O(\epsilon^{-d})$,

$$|x|^{d-1} H_k[\mathbf{g}](x) = -\epsilon^d |x|^{d-1} \sum_{i,j,p,q=1}^{d} (\partial_i U_j)(z)\partial_p \Gamma_{kq}(x)m^{ij}_{pq} \, . \tag{12.7}$$

Both identities hold modulo $O(\epsilon^{2d})$.

Theorem 12.3 (Reconstruction of EMT) *For $u, v = 1, \ldots, d$, let*

$$\mathbf{g}_{uv} := \frac{\partial}{\partial \nu}\left(\frac{x_u \mathbf{e}_v + x_v \mathbf{e}_u}{2}\right)\bigg|_{\partial\Omega},$$

and define

$$h_{kl}^{uv} := \lim_{t \to +\infty} t^{d-1} H_k[\mathbf{g}_{uv}](t\mathbf{e}_l), \quad k, l, u, v = 1, \ldots, d. \tag{12.8}$$

Then the entries m_{kl}^{uv}, $u, v, k, l = 1, \ldots, d$, of the EMT can be recovered, modulo $O(\epsilon^d)$, as follows: For $u, v, k, l = 1, \ldots, d$,

$$\epsilon^d m_{kl}^{uv} = \begin{cases} -\dfrac{2\omega_d \mu(\lambda + 2\mu)}{\lambda + (d-2)\mu}\left[\dfrac{\lambda + \mu}{\mu}\displaystyle\sum_{j=1}^{d} h_{jj}^{uv} + h_{kk}^{uv}\right] \\ \hspace{6cm} \text{if } k = l, \\ -\omega_d(\lambda + 2\mu)h_{kl}^{uv} \quad \text{if } k \neq l, \end{cases} \tag{12.9}$$

modulo $O(\epsilon^{2d})$, where $\omega_d = 2\pi$ if $d = 2$ and $\omega_d = 4\pi$ if $d = 3$.

Proof.   Easy computations show that

$$\partial_p \Gamma_{kq}(x) = \frac{A}{\omega_d}\frac{\delta_{kq} x_p}{|x|^d} - \frac{B}{\omega_d}\frac{\delta_{kp} x_q + \delta_{pq} x_k}{|x|^d} + \frac{dB}{\omega_d}\frac{x_k x_q x_p}{|x|^{d+2}}. \tag{12.10}$$

If $x = t\mathbf{e}_l$, $t \in \mathbb{R}$, $l = 1, \ldots, d$, then

$$\partial_p \Gamma_{kq}(t\mathbf{e}_l) = \frac{1}{\omega_d t^{d-1}}\left[A\delta_{kq}\delta_{pl} - B(\delta_{kp}\delta_{ql} + \delta_{kl}\delta_{pq}) + dB\delta_{kl}\delta_{ql}\delta_{pl}\right]$$

$$:= \frac{1}{\omega_d t^{d-1}} e_{klpq}. \tag{12.11}$$

The background solution $\mathbf{U}$ corresponding to $\mathbf{g}_{uv}$ is given by $\mathbf{U}(x) = (x_u \mathbf{e}_v + x_v \mathbf{e}_u)/2$ and hence

$$\partial_i U_j(z) = \frac{1}{2}(\delta_{iu}\delta_{jv} + \delta_{iv}\delta_{ju}). \tag{12.12}$$

Therefore the right-hand side of (12.7) is equal to

$$-\frac{\epsilon^d}{2\omega_d}\sum_{i,j,p,q=1}^{d}(\delta_{iu}\delta_{jv} + \delta_{iv}\delta_{ju})e_{klpq}m_{pq}^{ij} = -\frac{\epsilon^d}{\omega_d}\sum_{p,q=1}^{d} e_{klpq}m_{pq}^{uv}.$$

The last equality is valid because of the symmetry of the EMT, in particular, $m_{pq}^{uv} = m_{pq}^{vu}$. It then follows from (12.7) that, if $t = O(\epsilon^{-1})$, then, modulo $O(\epsilon^{2d})$,

$$
t^{d-1} H_k[\mathbf{g}_{uv}](t\mathbf{e}_l) = \begin{cases} -\dfrac{\epsilon^d}{\omega_d}\left[(A + (d-2)B)m_{kk}^{uv} - B\sum_{i \neq k} m_{ii}^{vu}\right] & \text{if } k = l\,, \\[2ex] -\dfrac{\epsilon^d}{\omega_d}(-B + A)m_{kl}^{uv} & \text{if } k \neq l\,. \end{cases}
$$

$$(12.13)$$

By solving (12.13) for m_{pq}^{ij}, we obtain (12.9). This completes the proof. $\qquad\square$

Once we determine the EMT, $\epsilon^d m_{pq}^{ij}$, associated with D, then we can estimate the size of D by Corollary 10.7.

Theorem 12.4 (Size estimation) *For $i \neq j$,*

$$
|D| \approx \left|\frac{\mu + \widetilde{\mu}}{\mu(\mu - \widetilde{\mu})}\right| |\epsilon^d m_{ij}^{ij}|
$$

if $\widetilde{\mu}$ is known. If $\widetilde{\mu}$ is unknown, then $|(\mu + \widetilde{\mu})/(\mu(\mu - \widetilde{\mu}))|$ is assumed to be $1/\mu$.

12.2 Representation of the EMTs by Ellipses

Suppose $d = 2$. As in the electrostatic case, the reconstructed EMT carries information about the inclusion other than the size. In order to visualize this information, we now describe a method that enables for finding out an ellipse that represents the reconstructed EMT in the two-dimensional case.

For an ellipse D centered at the origin, let $m_{pq}^{ij}(D)$ be the EMT associated with D. Let $\widehat{D}$ be the ellipse of the form

$$
\widehat{D} : \frac{x_1^2}{a^2} + \frac{x_2^2}{b^2} = 1
$$

such that

$$
D = R_\theta(\widehat{D})\,,
$$

for some θ. Then by Theorem 10.14, m_{pq}^{ij} are determined by θ, $|D|$, and m defined by (10.47).

Let M_{pq}^{ij}, $i,j,p,q = 1,2$, be the EMT determined by the method of the previous section. Our goal is to find an ellipse D so that

$$
m_{pq}^{ij}(D) = M_{pq}^{ij}, \quad i,j,p,q = 1,2\,. \tag{12.14}
$$

Observe that the collection of two-dimensional EMTs has six degrees of freedom, whereas the collection of ellipses has only three of them. So the equation (12.14) may not have a solution. Thus instead we seek an ellipse D so that $m_{pq}^{ij}(D)$ best fits M_{pq}^{ij} for $i,j,p,q = 1,2$.[1] We can achieve this goal by the following steps.

---

[1] It would be interesting and useful to find a class of domains that can represent the reconstructed EMT in a unique and canonical way.

Representation by Ellipses with Prior Knowledge of $(\widetilde{\lambda}, \widetilde{\mu})$: Suppose that the Lamé constants $(\widetilde{\lambda}, \widetilde{\mu})$ of the inclusion D are known.

Step 1: First we set a tolerance τ. If both $|M_{12}^{11} + M_{22}^{12}|$ and $|M_{11}^{11} - M_{22}^{22}|$ are smaller than τ, then represent the EMT by the disk of the size found out in the previous section. If either $|M_{12}^{11} + M_{22}^{12}|$ or $|M_{11}^{11} - M_{22}^{22}|$ is larger than τ, then first determine the angle of rotation θ by solving (10.42), namely,

$$\frac{M_{12}^{11} + M_{22}^{12}}{M_{11}^{11} - M_{22}^{22}} = \frac{1}{2}\tan 2\theta\,, \quad 0 \le \theta < \frac{\pi}{2}\,. \tag{12.15}$$

Step 2: We then compute $\widehat{M}_{pq}^{ij}$ by reversing the rotation by θ found in (12.15) using formula (10.37). Since it suffices to replace r_{ij} by $(-1)^{i+j}r_{ij}$ in (10.37), we get

$$\widehat{M}_{pq}^{ij} = \sum_{u,v=1}^{2}\sum_{k,l=1}^{2}(-1)^{i+j+u+v+k+l+p+q}r_{pu}r_{qv}r_{ik}r_{jl}M_{uv}^{kl}\,, \tag{12.16}$$

where

$$\begin{pmatrix} r_{11} & r_{12} \\ r_{21} & r_{22} \end{pmatrix} = \begin{pmatrix} \cos\theta & -\sin\theta \\ \sin\theta & \cos\theta \end{pmatrix}\,.$$

Step 3: The ideal next step would be to use (10.52) and (10.59) for finding $|D|$ and m that produce the entries $\widehat{m}_{pq}^{ij}$ that minimize

$$\left|\widehat{m}_{11}^{11} - \widehat{M}_{11}^{11}\right| + \left|\widehat{m}_{22}^{22} - \widehat{M}_{22}^{22}\right| + \left|\widehat{m}_{22}^{11} - \widehat{M}_{22}^{11}\right| + \left|\widehat{m}_{12}^{12} - \widehat{M}_{12}^{12}\right|\,. \tag{12.17}$$

But it is not so clear how to proceed to minimize (12.17) since $\widehat{m}_{pq}^{ij}$ is a non-linear function of m, defined by (10.47), and $|D|$. So we propose a different method to find $|D|$ and m.

The relation (10.40) suggests that $2(\widehat{m}_{22}^{11} + 2\widehat{m}_{12}^{12}) - (\widehat{m}_{11}^{11} + \widehat{m}_{22}^{22})$ carries information on the size of m, the ratio of the measure of the long to the short axes. On the other hand, (10.35) shows that m_{12}^{12} carries information on $|D|$. So, we solve

$$2(\widehat{m}_{22}^{11} + 2\widehat{m}_{12}^{12}) - (\widehat{m}_{11}^{11} + \widehat{m}_{22}^{22}) = 2(\widehat{M}_{22}^{11} + 2M_{12}^{12}) - (M_{11}^{11} + \widehat{M}_{22}^{22})$$
$$\widehat{m}_{12}^{12} = \widehat{M}_{12}^{12}\,,$$

$$\tag{12.18}$$

using (10.52) and (10.59). Numerical tests show that (12.18) may have multiple solutions. Among the solutions found by solving (12.18), we choose the one that minimizes (12.17).

Representation by Ellipses without Prior Knowledge of $(\widetilde{\lambda}, \widetilde{\mu})$: Suppose that the Lamé constants $(\widetilde{\lambda}, \widetilde{\mu})$ of the inclusion D are unknown. Then Step 1 and Step 2 are the same as before. Instead of Step 3, we use Step 3'.

Step 3′: If the reconstructed M_{pq}^{ij} is negative-definite on symmetric matrices, then $\widetilde{\mu} < \mu$ by Theorem 10.6. So, set $\widetilde{\lambda} = \widetilde{\mu} = 0$ and solve (12.18) for m and $|D|$ using (10.67). If the reconstructed M_{pq}^{ij} is positive-definite on symmetric matrices, then set $\widetilde{\mu} = +\infty$ and solve (12.18) for m and $|D|$ using (10.64). Among the solutions found by solving (12.18), we choose the one that minimizes (12.17).

12.3 Detection of the Location

Having found $\epsilon^d m_{kp}^{uv}$, we now proceed to find the location z of D. We propose two methods, one using only linear solutions and the other one using quadratic solutions.

Detection of the Location—Linear Method. In view of (12.3) and (12.12), we have

$$-\epsilon^d \sum_{p,q=1}^{d} \partial_p \Gamma_{kq}(x - z) m_{pq}^{uv} = H_k[\mathbf{g}_{uv}](x) + O(\frac{\epsilon^{d+1}}{|x|^d}) + O(\frac{\epsilon^{2d}}{|x|^{d-1}}) , \quad (12.19)$$

for $k, u, v = 1, \ldots, d$. Since $m_{pq}^{uv} = m_{qp}^{vu}$, $p, q, u, v = 1, \ldots, d$, we can symmetrize (12.19) to obtain

$$-\frac{\epsilon^d}{2} \sum_{p,q=1}^{d} \left[\partial_p \Gamma_{kq}(x - z) + \partial_q \Gamma_{kp}(x - z) \right] m_{pq}^{uv}$$
$$= H_k[\mathbf{g}_{uv}](x) + O(\frac{\epsilon^{d+1}}{|x|^d}) + O(\frac{\epsilon^{2d}}{|x|^{d-1}}) . \quad (12.20)$$

Let V be the space of $d \times d$ symmetric matrices, and define a linear transformation P on V by

$$P((a_{pq})) = (\sum_{p,q=1}^{d} a_{pq} \epsilon^d m_{pq}^{uv}) .$$

Then by Theorem 10.6, P is invertible on V. Let (n_{pq}^{ij}) be the matrix for P^{-1} on V, namely,

$$P^{-1}((a_{pq})) = (\sum_{p,q=1}^{d} a_{pq} n_{pq}^{ij}) , \quad (a_{pq}) \in V . \quad (12.21)$$

It then follows from (12.20) that

$$-\frac{1}{2} \left[\partial_p \Gamma_{kq}(x - z) + \partial_q \Gamma_{kp}(x - z) \right]$$
$$= \sum_{i,j=1}^{d} H_k[\mathbf{g}_{ij}](x) n_{ij}^{pq} + O(\frac{\epsilon}{|x|^d}) + O(\frac{\epsilon^d}{|x|^{d-1}}) , \quad k = 1, \ldots, d . \quad (12.22)$$

Observe from (12.10) that

$$\sum_{p=1}^{d} \partial_p \Gamma_{kp}(x - z) = \frac{(-B + A)}{\omega_d} \frac{x_k - z_k}{|x - z|^d} = \frac{1}{\omega_d(2\mu + \lambda)} \frac{x_k - z_k}{|x - z|^d} \,,$$

for $k = 1, \ldots, d$. Hence we obtain from (12.22) that

$$\frac{x_k - z_k}{|x - z|^d} = -\omega_d(2\mu + \lambda) \sum_{i,j=1}^{d} H_k[\mathbf{g}_{ij}](x) \sum_{p=1}^{d} n_{ij}^{pp} + O(\frac{\epsilon}{|x|^d})$$
$$+ O(\frac{\epsilon^d}{|x|^{d-1}}) \,. \tag{12.23}$$

Multiplying both sides of (12.23) by $|x|^{d-1}$, we arrive at the following formula. If $|x| = O(\epsilon^{-d+1})$, then

$$\frac{x_k - z_k}{|x - z|} = -\omega_d(2\mu + \lambda)|x|^{d-1} \sum_{i,j=1}^{d} H_k[\mathbf{g}_{ij}](x) \sum_{p=1}^{d} n_{ij}^{pp} + O(\epsilon^d) \,, \tag{12.24}$$

for $k = 1, \ldots, d$. Formula (12.24) says that we can recover $(x_k - z_k)/|x - z|$, $k = 1, \ldots, d$, from $H_k[\mathbf{g}_{ij}]$.

We now use an idea from Theorem 7.2 to recover the center z from $(x - z)/|x - z|$. Fix k and freeze x_l, $l \neq k$, so that $\sum_{l \neq k} |x_l| = O(\epsilon^{-d+1})$. Then consider

$$\omega_d(2\mu + \lambda)|x|^{d-1} \sum_{i,j=1}^{d} H_k[\mathbf{g}_{ij}](x) \sum_{p=1}^{d} n_{ij}^{pp}$$

as a function of x_k. In fact, for

$$x = x_k \mathbf{e}_k + \sum_{l \neq k} x_l \mathbf{e}_l \,,$$

define

$$\Phi_k(x_k) = \omega_d(2\mu + \lambda)|x|^{d-1} \sum_{i,j=1}^{d} H_k[\mathbf{g}_{ji}](x) \sum_{p=1}^{d} n_{ij}^{pp} \,. \tag{12.25}$$

We then find the unique zero of Φ_k, say z_k^*, and therefore, the point $(z_1^*, \ldots, z_d^*)$ is the center z within a precision of $O(\epsilon^d)$.

Detection of the Location—Quadratic Method. This method uses the relation (12.6). In view of (12.6) and (12.11), we get

$$t^{d-1} H_k[\mathbf{g}](t\mathbf{e}_l) = -\frac{1}{\omega_d} \sum_{i,j,p,q=1}^{d} (\partial_i U_j)(z) e_{klpq} \epsilon^d m_{pq}^{ij} \quad \text{modulo } O(\epsilon^{d+1}) \,. \tag{12.26}$$

By $m_{pq}^{ij} = m_{qp}^{ij}$, we obtain that

$$\sum_{i,j,p,q=1}^{d} (\partial_i U_j)(z) e_{klpq} \epsilon^d m_{pq}^{ij} = \frac{1}{2} \sum_{p,q=1}^{d} (e_{klpq} + e_{klqp}) \sum_{i,j=1}^{d} (\partial_i U_j)(z) \epsilon^d m_{pq}^{ij} \, .$$

Since $e_{klpq} + e_{klqp} = e_{lkpq} + e_{lkqp}$, we can define a linear transformation T on V by

$$T((a_{pq})) := \frac{1}{2} \left(\sum_{p,q=1}^{d} (e_{klpq} + e_{klqp}) a_{pq} \right) \, .$$

We claim that T is invertible. To prove it, suppose that $T((a_{pq}))_{kl} = 0$, $k, l = 1, \ldots, d$. If $k = l$, then

$$(A + (d-1)B)a_{kk} + \sum_{p \neq k} a_{pp} = 0 \, , \quad k = 1, \ldots, d \, .$$

In view of $A + (d-1)B \neq -1$, this implies $a_{kk} = 0$, $k = 1, \ldots, d$. On the other hand, if $k \neq l$, then

$$(-A + B)(a_{kl} + a_{lk}) = 0 \, ,$$

and hence $a_{kl} = 0$ since (a_{pq}) is symmetric. Therefore $(a_{pq})_{p,q=1}^{d} = 0$ and T is invertible on V.

It then follows from (12.26) that

$$-\sum_{i,j=1}^{d} (\partial_i U_j)(z) \epsilon^d m_{pq}^{ij} = \omega_d T^{-1}(t^{d-1} H_k[\mathbf{g}](t\mathbf{e}_l))_{pq} \quad \text{modulo } O(\epsilon^{d+1}) \, .$$

$$(12.27)$$

We then apply second-order homogeneous solutions for $\mathbf{U}$. In fact, in the two-dimensional case, take

$$\mathbf{U}(x) = (2x_1 x_2, x_1^2 - x_2^2) \, ,$$

and $\mathbf{g} = \partial \mathbf{U} / \partial \nu$. Then using (12.27), we can determine $(\partial_i U_j)(z)$, thus z, from the elastic moment tensor m_{pq}^{ij} and the limit value of $H_k[\mathbf{g}]$ as $t \to +\infty$. In the three-dimensional case, we apply two homogeneous polynomials:

$$\mathbf{U}(x) = (2x_1 x_2, x_1^2 - x_2^2, 0), \quad (2x_1 x_3, 0, x_1^2 - x_3^2) \, .$$

12.4 Numerical Results

In this section we summarize the algorithms described in detail in the previous sections and show some results of numerical experiments. The first algorithm is designed to identify a disk that represents the reconstructed EMT by using (10.7). We call this algorithm the *disk identification algorithm*. The second one is for finding an ellipse that can represent the reconstructed EMT by using the method described in Sect. 12.2. We call this algorithm the *ellipse identification algorithm*. It is worth emphasizing that both of these recovery methods are non-iterative direct algorithms. We only present them in two dimensions even though they work as well in the three-dimensional case. Details of the implementation of the proposed algorithms can be found in [174]. When comparing these two algorithms, it turns out that the ellipse reconstruction algorithm performs far better in estimating the size and orientation of the inclusion. But unlike the disk reconstruction algorithm, the ellipse reconstruction method requires Lamé constants not only for the background but also for the inclusion.

The proposed identification algorithms do not rely on a forward solver, whereas iterative algorithms require a sequence of forward solutions. Solutions of the elastostatic problem obtained by a second-order finite-difference forward solver are used only for the generation of numerical simulations. In Example 1, the effectiveness and stability of the algorithms for a disk inclusion are numerically demonstrated. The validity of the asymptotic expansions for the radius and the centers has been checked under various physical configurations in Example 2. Example 3 shows that the disk reconstruction algorithm provides fairly good disk approximations even for domains with non-circular inclusions. Example 4 shows that the ellipse recovery method gives perfect reconstruction results for elliptic inclusions and fairly good approximations for general domains in the sense that it provides correct estimations on both the major and the minor axes and the orientation.

Disk Reconstruction Procedure.

Step R: Compute $\epsilon^2 m_{kl}^{uv}$ using formulae (12.8),

$$h_{kl}^{uv} := \lim_{t \to +\infty} t H_k[\mathbf{g}_{uv}](t\mathbf{e}_l) ,$$

and m_{kl}^{uv} in (12.9) for $u \le v$, $k \le l$, $u \le k$, and $v \le l$,

$$\epsilon^2 m_{kl}^{uv} = \begin{cases} -\pi\mu \left[\dfrac{\lambda}{2\mu} \sum_{j=1}^{2} h_{jj}^{uv} + h_{kk}^{uv} \right] , & k = l , \\ -\pi(\lambda + \mu) h_{kl}^{uv} , & k \ne l . \end{cases}$$

Then the computed radius is given by

$$r_c = \sqrt{\frac{|m_{12}^{12}|}{\pi}} .$$

Step C1: Compute the matrix $(n_{ij}^{pq})_{i,j,p,q=1,2}$, defined in (12.21),

$$\left(\sum_{p,q=1}^{2} a_{pq} n_{pq}^{ij} \right) := P^{-1}((a_{pq})), \quad \text{where} \quad P((a_{pq})) = \left(\sum_{p,q=1}^{2} a_{pq} \epsilon^2 m_{pq}^{uv} \right) .$$

Then find the unique zero $z_k^*, k = 1, 2$, defined in (12.25),

$$\Phi_k(x_k) = 2\pi(\mu + \lambda)|x| \sum_{i,j=1}^{2} H_k[\mathbf{g}_{ji}](x) \sum_{p=1}^{2} n_{ij}^{pp} \, ,$$

by Newton's method with $H_k[\mathbf{g}_{ji}](x)$ and $(\partial/\partial x_k) H_k[\mathbf{g}_{ji}](x)$. In the iteration, the other coordinate x_{2-k} is frozen to a constant larger than $O(\epsilon^{-2})$ and we just choose x_{2-k} to be 10^3.

Step C2: Compute the center point z using (12.27):

$$- \sum_{i,j=1}^{2} (\partial_i U_j)(z)\epsilon^2 m_{pq}^{ij} = 2\pi T^{-1}(t H_k[\mathbf{g}](t\mathbf{e}_l))_{pq} \, ,$$

where

$$T(a_{pq}) := \frac{1}{2} \sum_{p,q=1}^{2} (e_{klpq} + e_{klqp})a_{pq} \, , \quad \mathbf{U}(x) = (2x_1 x_2, x_1^2 - x_2^2) \, .$$

Example 1: In [174], the following reconstruction procedure is implemented for two-dimensional domains using Matlab and its performance is tested using a circular inclusion. The disk is centered at $(0.4, 0.2)$ and is of radius $r = 0.2$. The Lamé constants of the disk are $(\widetilde{\lambda}, \widetilde{\mu}) = (9, 6)$ whereas the background Lamé constants are $(\lambda, \mu) = (6, 4)$. The functions $\mathbf{u}^{1,1}$, $\mathbf{u}^{1,2}$, $\mathbf{u}^{2,2}$, and $\mathbf{u}^{\mathsf{q}}$ denote the inhomogeneous solutions with the same boundary values of the corresponding homogeneous solutions, $\mathbf{U}^{1,1} = (2x, 0)$, $\mathbf{U}^{1,2} = (y, x)$, $\mathbf{U}^{2,2} = (0, y)$, and $\mathbf{U}^{\mathsf{q}} = (2xy, x^2 - y^2)$, respectively.

The following table summarizes a computational result of the algorithm using the forward solutions on a 128×128 mesh. The radius r^c is the computed radius in Step R, (x_1^c, y_1^c) is the center obtained by the linear method in Step C1, and (x_2^c, y_2^c) is the one obtained by the quadratic method in Step C2.

(λ, μ)	$(\widetilde{\lambda}, \widetilde{\mu})$	(x, y)	r	r^c	(x_1^c, y_1^c)	(x_2^c, y_2^c)
(6,4)	(9,6)	(0.4, 0.2)	0.25	0.3036	(0.4110, 0.1961)	(0.3983, 0.1985)

The left-hand diagram in Figure 12.1 shows the original disk as a solid curve; the dashed-dotted circle is the reconstructed disk by the linear disk reconstruction method, and the dashed circle is by the quadratic reconstruction method. In order to check the stability of the algorithm, we add random white noise to the Neumann and Dirichlet boundary data. Since computational results for radius and centers have some errors even without noise, we compare the difference between those with and without noise. We plot the absolute perturbation error of the reconstructed values with respect to the white random noise level measured in the root mean square sense. The right-hand plot

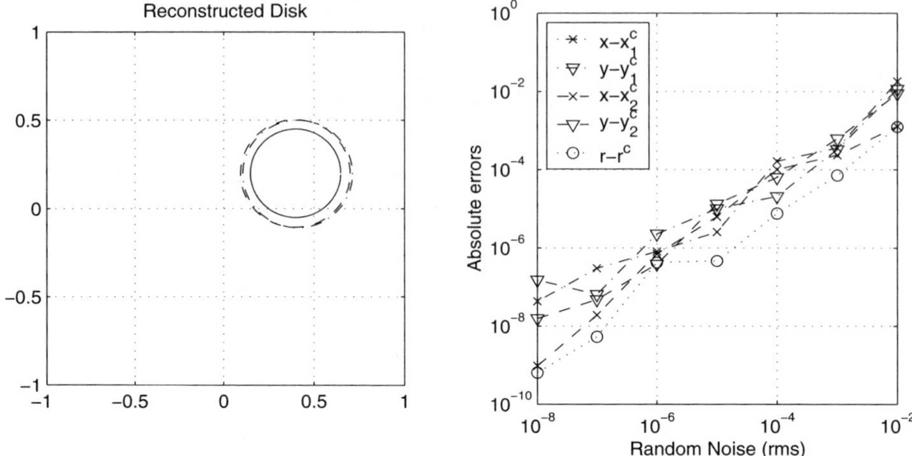

Fig. 12.1. The dashed-dotted circle represents the solution by the linear method and the dashed circle by the quadratic method. The right-hand plot shows the perturbation error due to the random boundary noise.

in Figure 12.1 demonstrates that the algorithm is linearly stable with respect to the random boundary noise.

Example 2: In this example, we test the disk identification algorithm with various configurations of disk inclusions and check the validity of the asymptotic expansions for the radius in the case where the inclusion has finite size much larger than 0. The following table and Figure 12.2 summarize the computational results for three different locations with two different Lamé parameter configurations. The linear and the quadratic methods compute the center quite well, but the radii of the top three cases are about 20% larger than the original disks and those of the bottom cases are about 30% smaller than the originals.

(λ,μ)	$(\widetilde{\lambda},\widetilde{\mu})$	(x,y)	r	r^c	(x_1^c, y_1^c)	(x_2^c, y_2^c)
(6,4)	(9.0,6.0)	(0.5, 0.1)	0.2	0.2474	(0.5198, 0.0967)	(0.4988, 0.1014)
(6,4)	(9.0,6.0)	(0.2, 0.2)	0.3	0.3638	(0.1999, 0.1999)	(0.1962, 0.1982)
(6,4)	(9.0,6.0)	(-0.3, -0.3)	0.5	0.5931	(-0.2974, -0.2972)	(-0.2947, -0.2981)
(6,4)	(7.0,4.5)	(0.5, 0.1)	0.2	0.1371	(0.5203, 0.0967)	(0.4995, 0.1009)
(6,4)	(7.0,4.5)	(0.2, 0.2)	0.3	0.2029	(0.2003, 0.2003)	(0.1969, 0.1977)
(6,4)	(7.0,4.5)	(-0.3, -0.3)	0.5	0.3366	(-0.3006, -0.3005)	(-0.2990, -0.2995)

In order to check the validity of the asymptotic expansion, we compute the radii by the disk reconstruction method for various combinations of radii and Lamé parameters while we keep fixed the center of the inclusion at $(0.4, 0.2)$.

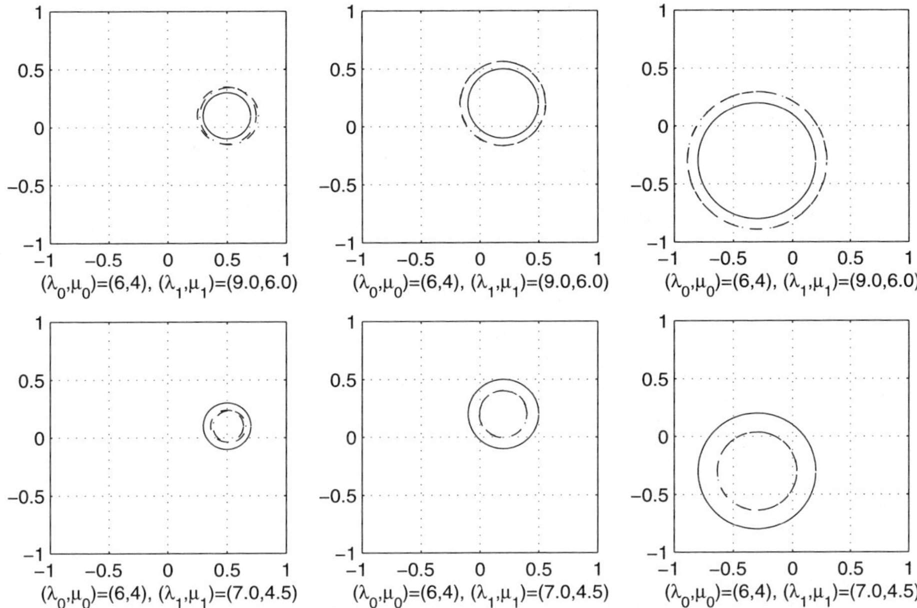

Fig. 12.2. Reconstruction results. Dashed-dotted circles by the linear method and dashed circles by the quadratic method. The three upper cases have stiff inclusions with $(\widetilde{\lambda}, \widetilde{\mu}) = (9,6)$, $(\lambda, \mu) = (6,4)$ and the three lower cases with $(\widetilde{\lambda}, \widetilde{\mu}) = (6,4)$, $(\lambda, \mu) = (9,6)$. We use the notation λ_0, μ_0 for λ, μ and λ_1, μ_1 for $\widetilde{\lambda}, \widetilde{\mu}$.

We use three different computational grids to check the computational accuracy of our forward and inverse solvers. In Figure 12.3, the dotted line is used for the results on 48×48, the dashed line on 64×64, and the solid line on the 128×128 grids; the computational results on the three different grids seem to be almost identical. The figure also shows that the computed radius is not identical but proportional to the original value. The ratio between the computed and the original radius is independent of the radius, which is strong evidence of a missing second-order asymptotic expansion term for the radius. It is worth noting that the asymptotic expansion of EMT in (12.9) is correct up to $O(\epsilon^{2d})$, which gives a valid expression for the radius up to second-order accuracy in the two-dimensional case.

Example 3 (General Domain Cases): We now test the disk reconstruction algorithm with non-circular shape inclusions even though the algorithm has been derived for circular inclusions. The computational results on the 64×64 grid show fairly good agreement with their circular approximations. It is also worth mentioning that $(\lambda_0, \mu_0) = (6,4)$, $(\lambda_1, \mu_1) = (9,6)$ gives about 20% larger results and $(\lambda_0, \mu_0) = (4,6)$, $(\lambda_1, \mu_1) = (6,9)$ about 50% larger than

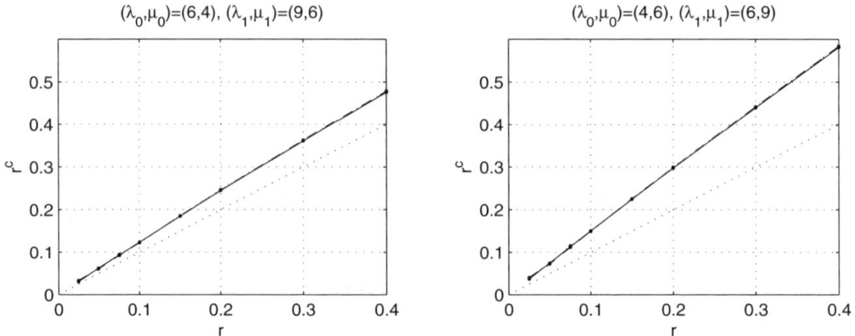

Fig. 12.3. Computed radius r^c on three different computational grids. The dotted line for 48×48, dashed line for 64×64, and solid line for 128×128 grid coincide well.

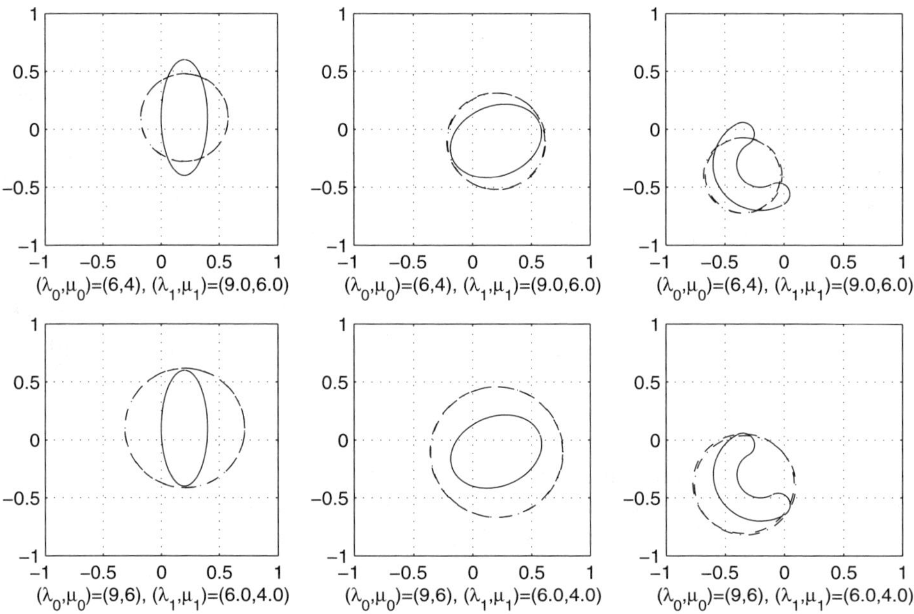

Fig. 12.4. Reconstruction of general shape inclusion.

originally, in disk cases shown in Figure 12.4; therefore, the computed results are bigger than the inclusions, especially for the three lower examples.

We now summarize the ellipse identification algorithm.

Ellipse Reconstruction Procedure. Let M^{ij}_{pq} be the reconstructed EMT. Given a tolerance τ, if both $|M^{11}_{12} + M^{12}_{22}|$ and $|M^{11}_{11} - M^{22}_{22}|$ are smaller than

τ, then find the disk of the size given in the previous subsection. If either $|M_{12}^{11} + M_{22}^{12}|$ or $|M_{11}^{11} - M_{22}^{22}|$ is larger than τ, then

(E1): Determine the angle of rotation θ by solving (12.15), namely

$$\frac{M_{12}^{11} + M_{22}^{12}}{M_{11}^{11} - M_{22}^{22}} = \frac{1}{2}\tan 2\theta\,, \quad 0 \le \theta < \frac{\pi}{2}\,.$$

(E2): Using the angle θ found in (E1), solve (12.16) to find $\widehat{M}_{pq}^{ij}$:

$$\widehat{M}_{pq}^{ij} = \sum_{u,v=1}^{2}\sum_{k,l=1}^{2}(-1)^{u+k+p+i}r_{pu}r_{vq}r_{ik}r_{lj}M_{uv}^{kl}\,,$$

where

$$\begin{pmatrix} r_{11} & r_{12} \\ r_{21} & r_{22} \end{pmatrix} = \begin{pmatrix} \cos\theta & -\sin\theta \\ \sin\theta & \cos\theta \end{pmatrix}\,.$$

(E3): Find $|D|$ and m by solving (12.18):

$$2(\widehat{m}_{22}^{11} + 2\widehat{m}_{12}^{12}) - (\widehat{m}_{11}^{11} + \widehat{m}_{22}^{22}) = 2(\widehat{M}_{22}^{11} + 2M_{12}^{12}) - (M_{11}^{11} + \widehat{M}_{22}^{22})\,,$$
$$\widehat{m}_{12}^{12} - \widehat{M}_{12}^{12}\,.$$

The relation between $|D|, m$ and $\widehat{m}_{pq}^{ij}$ is given by (10.49), (10.52), and (10.59) if the Lamé constants $(\widetilde{\lambda}, \widetilde{\mu})$ are known. Otherwise, it is given by (10.64) [resp. (10.67)] if the reconstructed EMT is negative-definite (resp. positive-definite).

(E4): Among the solutions in (E3), choose the one that minimizes the quantity given in (12.17):

$$\left|\widehat{m}_{11}^{11} - \widehat{M}_{11}^{11}\right| + \left|\widehat{m}_{22}^{22} - \widehat{M}_{22}^{22}\right| + \left|\widehat{m}_{22}^{11} - \widehat{M}_{22}^{11}\right| + \left|\widehat{m}_{12}^{12} - \widehat{M}_{12}^{12}\right|\,.$$

Example 4: In this example, we test the algorithm using the same domains as in Example 3. Figure 12.5 shows the reconstructed ellipses when their Lamé constants $(\widetilde{\lambda}, \widetilde{\mu})$ are known. It is not surprising that the ellipse recovery method gives perfect size information for disks and ellipses, as shown in the first diagram in Figure 12.5, since the information on the Lamé constants $(\widetilde{\lambda}, \widetilde{\mu})$ is used.

12.5 Further Results and Open Problems

As shown in Section 4.11.1, for each given polarization tensor associated with an arbitrary bounded Lipschitz domain and a constant isotropic conductivity, we can find a unique ellipse whose polarization tensor is the given one. In this

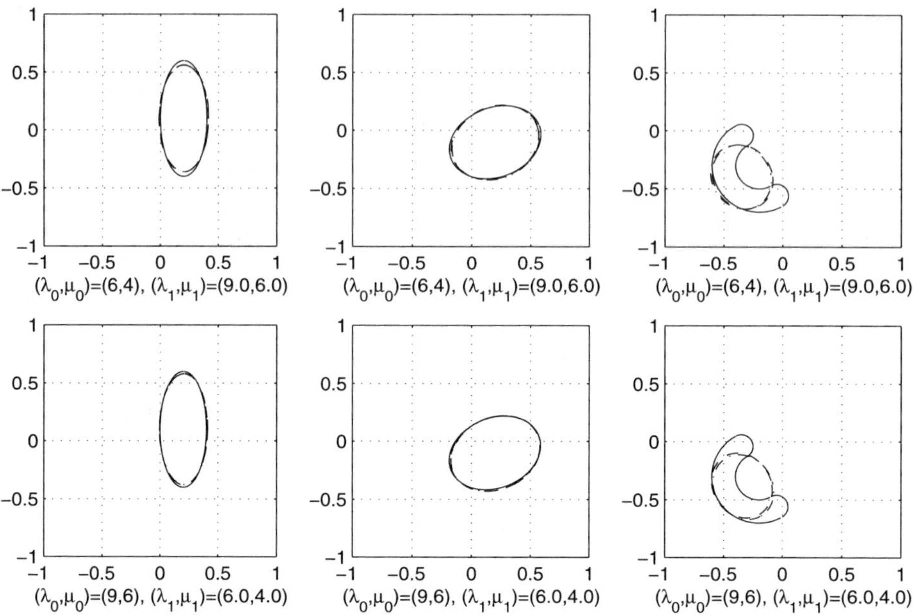

Fig. 12.5. Computed ellipses for various inclusions marked with solid curves. The centers of dotted ellipses are computed by the linear method and dashed-dotted ones by the quadratic method.

way, we can visualize the detected polarization tensor. It is important to have a class of fourth-order curves that can represent EMTs in a unique way. Once we have such a class, the detected EMT can be visualized by a curve in this class, not by an ellipse as done in the previous section.

The techniques discussed in this chapter can be extended to elastodynamics. In [27], we presented non-iterative algorithms for reconstructing small elastic inclusions from dynamic boundary measurements for a finite interval in time.

We mention another very interesting problem concerning the simultaneous characterization of the shape and the elastic parameters of a small inclusion from interior measurements of the displacement field. This imaging approach is termed Magnetic Resonance Elastography (MRE) and can be a very effective method for detecting tumors, particularly in breast, liver, kidney, and prostate [224]. We think that a promising direction for analyzing MRE data is to utilize the asymptotic formulae derived in the previous chapter together with the bounds satisfied by the first-order elastic moment tensor.

Effective Properties of Elastic Composites

Introduction

Let $Y =]-1/2, 1/2[^2$ denote the unit cell. Suppose that an inclusion D is embedded in Y and that the background material has elasticity properties defined by the tensor $C^0 = ((C^0)_{ij}^{kl})_{i,j,k,l=1,2}$, where

$$(C^0)_{ij}^{kl} := \lambda \delta_{ij} \delta_{kl} + \mu(\delta_{ik}\delta_{jl} + \delta_{il}\delta_{jk}) \,,$$

while the inclusion D has the tensor $\widetilde{C} = (\widetilde{C})_{i,j,k,l=1,2}$, where

$$(\widetilde{C})_{i,j,k,l=1,2} := \widetilde{\lambda} \delta_{ij}\delta_{kl} + \widetilde{\mu}(\delta_{ik}\delta_{jl} + \delta_{il}\delta_{jk}) \,.$$

Thus the periodic (with period 1 in each direction) elasticity tensor $C = (C_{ij}^{kl})_{i,j,k,l=1,2}$ for this two phase material is given by

$$C_{ij}^{kl} := \Big(\lambda + (\widetilde{\lambda} - \lambda)\chi(D)\Big)\delta_{ij}\delta_{kl} + \Big(\mu + (\widetilde{\mu} - \mu)\chi(D)\Big)(\delta_{ik}\delta_{jl} + \delta_{il}\delta_{jk}) \,, \quad (13.1)$$

where $\chi(D)$ is the characteristic function of D.

Let ϵ be a small parameter. Suppose that $D = \epsilon^{1+\beta}B$ for some $\beta > 0$. Here B is a reference Lipschitz bounded domain containing 0 whose volume $|B|$ is 1. Denote $\rho = \epsilon^{\beta}$ and $f = \rho^2$, the volume fraction of the elastic inclusion.

The periodic elasticity tensor $C(x/\epsilon)$ makes a highly oscillating elasticity tensor and represents the material properties of a dilute composite. We consider the problem of determining the effective elastic properties of the dilute composite with the elasticity tensor $C(x/\epsilon)$ as $\epsilon \to 0$.

Our aim in this chapter is to extend the formula (8.15) to elastic composites. We present a simple and general scheme to derive accurate asymptotic expansions of the elastic effective properties of dilute composite materials. The main result, which was proved in [33], is that the effective elasticity tensor C^* has the following high-order asymptotic expansion in terms of f:

$$C^* = C^0 + fM(I - fSM)^{-1} + O(f^3) \,. \quad (13.2)$$

Here M is the elastic moment tensor and $S = (S_{ij}^{kl})$ is a 4-tensor given by

$$\begin{cases} S_{11}^{11} = S_{22}^{22} = -a,\, S_{22}^{11} = S_{11}^{22} = -c\,, \\ S_{12}^{12} = S_{21}^{12} = S_{21}^{21} = S_{12}^{21} = -\dfrac{b+c}{2}\,, \end{cases} \tag{13.3}$$

and its other entries are zero, where a and c are defined by (9.64), and b is given by (9.63).

The formula (13.2) is valid for general shaped Lipschitz inclusions with arbitrary phase moduli. Moreover, it exhibits an interesting feature of the effective elasticity tensor of composite materials that consists of the presence of the distortion factor S. A mere comparison of (13.2) with (8.15) shows that the presence of the factor S in (13.2) is somewhat unexpected.

13.1 Derivation of the Effective Elastic Properties

We now derive the asymptotic expansion of the effective elasticity tensor C^* as the volume fraction $f = \rho^2$ goes to zero.

Let $\mathbf{w}_k^l = (w_{kp}^l)_{p=1,2}$ be the solution of (9.70). The effective elasticity tensor $C^* = ((C^*)_{kl}^{ij})$ is defined by (see, for example, [97])

$$(C^*)_{kl}^{ij} = \int_Y (C\mathcal{E}(\mathbf{w}_k^l))_{ij}\, dx\,.$$

We note that, if $\mathbf{u} \in W^{1,2}(Y)$ and $\mathcal{L}_{\lambda,\mu}\mathbf{u} = 0$ in Y, then for all $\mathbf{v} \in W^{1,2}(Y)$,

$$\int_{\partial Y} \mathbf{v}\cdot\frac{\partial\mathbf{u}}{\partial\nu}\,d\sigma = \int_Y C\mathcal{E}(\mathbf{u}):\mathcal{E}(\mathbf{v})\,dx\,, \tag{13.4}$$

which can be seen from the divergence theorem. Since

$$\mathcal{E}(x_k\mathbf{e}_l)_{ij} = (\delta_{ki}\delta_{lj} + \delta_{kj}\delta_{li})/2\,,$$

we have

$$\int_Y (C\mathcal{E}(\mathbf{w}_k^l))_{ij}\,dx = \int_Y C\mathcal{E}(\mathbf{w}_k^l):\mathcal{E}(x_i\mathbf{e}_j)\,dx\,,$$

and hence we obtain from (13.4) that

$$(C^*)_{kl}^{ij} = \int_{\partial Y} x_i\mathbf{e}_j\cdot\frac{\partial\mathbf{w}_k^l}{\partial\nu}\,d\sigma,\quad i,j,k,l = 1,2\,. \tag{13.5}$$

Let (φ_k^l, ψ_k^l) be as in Lemma 9.22. It follows from (13.5) and (9.71) that

$$(C^*)_{ij}^{kl} = \int_{\partial Y} x_i\mathbf{e}_j\cdot\frac{\partial(x_k\mathbf{e}_l)}{\partial\nu}(x)\,d\sigma(x) + \int_{\partial Y} x_i\mathbf{e}_j\cdot\frac{\partial(\mathcal{G}_D\psi_k^l)}{\partial\nu}(x)\,d\sigma$$

$$= (C^0)_{ij}^{kl} + \int_{\partial Y} x_i\mathbf{e}_j\cdot\frac{\partial(\mathcal{G}_D\psi_k^l)}{\partial\nu}(x)\,d\sigma\,.$$

Observe that $\mathcal{L}_{\lambda,\mu}\mathcal{G}_D\psi_k^l = 0$ in D as well as in $Y \setminus \overline{D}$. Thus, using the periodicity of $\mathcal{G}_D\psi_k^l$, together with the divergence theorem and the jump formula (9.69), we obtain

$$\int_{\partial Y} x_i \mathbf{e}_j \cdot \frac{\partial(\mathcal{G}_D\psi_k^l)}{\partial\nu}\, d\sigma = \int_{\partial D} x_i \mathbf{e}_j \cdot \frac{\partial(\mathcal{G}_D\psi_k^l)}{\partial\nu}\Big|_+ d\sigma - \int_{\partial D} \frac{\partial(x_i\mathbf{e}_j)}{\partial\nu} \cdot \mathcal{G}_D\psi_k^l\, d\sigma$$

$$= \int_{\partial D} x_i \mathbf{e}_j \cdot \frac{\partial(\mathcal{G}_D\psi_k^l)}{\partial\nu}\Big|_+ d\sigma - \int_{\partial D} x_i \mathbf{e}_j \cdot \frac{\partial(\mathcal{G}_D\psi_k^l)}{\partial\nu}\Big|_- d\sigma$$

$$= \int_{\partial D} x_i \mathbf{e}_j \cdot \psi_k^l(x)\, d\sigma \ .$$

Recalling that $D = \rho B$, we let

$$\widetilde{\varphi}_k^l(x) = \varphi_k^l(\rho x) \quad \text{and} \quad \widetilde{\psi}_k^l(x) = \psi_k^l(\rho x), \quad x \in \partial B \ .$$

Then we have

$$C^* = C^0 + fP \ , \tag{13.6}$$

where $P = (P_{ij}^{kl})$ is defined by

$$P_{ij}^{kl} = \int_{\partial B} x_i \mathbf{e}_j \cdot \psi_k^l\, d\sigma \ . \tag{13.7}$$

Observe that the pair $(\widetilde{\varphi}_k^l, \widetilde{\psi}_k^l) \in L^2(\partial B) \times L^2(\partial B)$ is the unique solution of

$$\begin{cases} \widetilde{\mathcal{S}}_B\widetilde{\varphi}_k^l\big|_- - (\mathcal{S}_B + \mathcal{R}_B)\widetilde{\psi}_k^l\big|_+ = x_k\mathbf{e}_l\big|_{\partial B} + C \ , \\ \dfrac{\partial}{\partial\widetilde{\nu}}\widetilde{\mathcal{S}}_B\widetilde{\varphi}_k^l\Big|_- - \dfrac{\partial}{\partial\nu}(\mathcal{S}_B + \mathcal{R}_B)\widetilde{\psi}_k^l\Big|_+ = \dfrac{\partial(x_k\mathbf{e}_l)}{\partial\nu}\Big|_{\partial B} \ , \end{cases} \tag{13.8}$$

for some constant C and $\widetilde{\psi}_k^l \in L_\Psi^2(\partial B)$.

Let $(\mathbf{f}_k^l, \mathbf{g}_k^l)$ be the solution of (9.13) with D replaced by B. It then follows from (13.8) that

$$\begin{cases} \widetilde{\mathcal{S}}_B(\widetilde{\varphi}_k^l - \mathbf{f}_k^l)\big|_- - \mathcal{S}_B(\widetilde{\psi}_k^l - \mathbf{g}_k^l)\big|_+ = \mathcal{R}_B\widetilde{\psi}_k^l + C \\ \dfrac{\partial}{\partial\nu}\widetilde{\mathcal{S}}_B(\widetilde{\varphi}_k^l - \mathbf{f}_k^l)\big|_- - \dfrac{\partial}{\partial\nu}\mathcal{S}_B(\widetilde{\psi}_k^l - \mathbf{g}_k^l)\big|_+ = \dfrac{\partial}{\partial\nu}\mathcal{R}_B\widetilde{\psi}_k^l \end{cases} \quad \text{on } \partial B \ , \tag{13.9}$$

where

$$\mathcal{R}_B\psi(x) := \int_{\partial B} \mathbf{R}(\rho(x - y))\psi(y)\, d\sigma(y) \ .$$

By (9.62),

$$\mathbf{R}(\rho(x - y)) = \mathbf{R}(0) - \rho^2 \begin{pmatrix} ax_1y_1 + bx_2y_2 & cx_1y_2 + cx_2y_1 \\ cx_1y_2 + cx_2y_1 & bx_1y_1 + ax_2y_2 \end{pmatrix}$$

$$+ \rho^2(Q_1(x) + Q_2(y)) + O(\rho^4) \ ,$$

where $Q_1(x)$ and $Q_2(x)$ are 2×2 matrices whose components are homogeneous polynomials of degree 2 in x and y, respectively. Let $X_{ij} = x_i \mathbf{e}_j$ and $Y_{ij} = y_i \mathbf{e}_j$, $i, j = 1, 2$, for convenience. Then we can write

$$
\begin{pmatrix}
ax_1y_1 + bx_2y_2 & cx_1y_2 + cx_2y_1 \\
cx_1y_2 + cx_2y_1 & bx_1y_1 + ax_2y_2
\end{pmatrix}
$$

$$
= X_{11} \otimes (aY_{11} + cY_{22}) + X_{12} \otimes (bY_{12} + cY_{21}) + X_{21} \otimes (cY_{12} + bY_{21})
$$

$$
+ X_{22} \otimes (cY_{11} + aY_{22}) .
$$

Since $P_{ij}^{kl} = \int_{\partial B} Y_{ij} \cdot \widetilde{\psi}_k^l \, d\sigma$ and $\int_{\partial B} \widetilde{\psi}_k^l \, d\sigma = 0$, we get for $x \in \partial B$

$$
\mathcal{R}_B \widetilde{\psi}_k^l(x) = \int_{\partial D} \mathbf{R}(\rho(x - y)) \widetilde{\psi}_k^l(y) \, d\sigma(y)
$$

$$
= -\rho^2 X_{11}(aP_{11}^{kl} + cP_{22}^{kl}) - \rho^2 X_{12}(bP_{12}^{kl} + cP_{21}^{kl})
$$

$$
- \rho^2 X_{21}(cP_{12}^{kl} + bP_{21}^{kl}) - \rho^2 X_{22}(cP_{11}^{kl} + aP_{22}^{kl}) + C + O(\rho^4) ,
$$

for some constant C. The term $\partial(\mathcal{R}_B \widetilde{\psi}_k^l)/\partial\nu$ also has the same expression with X_{ij} replaced by $\partial X_{ij}/\partial\nu$.

It is proved in Lemma 9.14 that, if $(\mathbf{f}, \mathbf{g})$ is the solution of

$$
\begin{cases}
\widetilde{\mathcal{S}}_B \mathbf{f}|_- - \mathcal{S}_B \mathbf{g}|_+ = C \\
\dfrac{\partial}{\partial\nu} \widetilde{\mathcal{S}}_B \mathbf{f}|_- - \dfrac{\partial}{\partial\nu} \mathcal{S}_B \mathbf{g}|_+ = 0
\end{cases}
\qquad \text{on } \partial D ,
$$

then $\mathbf{g} = 0$. Therefore it follows from (13.9) and the linearity of the integral equation that

$$
\widetilde{\psi}_k^l - \mathbf{g}_k^l = -\rho^2 \mathbf{g}_1^1(aP_{11}^{kl} + cP_{22}^{kl}) - \rho^2 \mathbf{g}_1^2(bP_{12}^{kl} + cP_{21}^{kl}) - \rho^2 \mathbf{g}_2^1(cP_{12}^{kl} + bP_{21}^{kl})
$$

$$
- \rho^2 \mathbf{g}_2^2(cP_{11}^{kl} + aP_{22}^{kl}) + O(\rho^4) .
$$

By substituting this formula into (13.7), we get

$$
P_{ij}^{kl} = m_{ij}^{kl} - f\left[m_{ij}^{11}(aP_{11}^{kl} + cP_{22}^{kl}) + m_{ij}^{12}(bP_{12}^{kl} + cP_{21}^{kl}) + m_{ij}^{21}(cP_{12}^{kl} + bP_{21}^{kl}) \right.
$$

$$
\left. + m_{ij}^{22}(cP_{11}^{kl} + aP_{22}^{kl}) \right] + O(f^2) .
$$

Since $m_{ij}^{12} = m_{ij}^{21}$, we can rewrite this in the following form:

$$
P_{ij}^{kl} = m_{ij}^{kl} - f\left[m_{ij}^{11}(aP_{11}^{kl} + cP_{22}^{kl}) + \frac{b+c}{2} m_{ij}^{12}(P_{12}^{kl} + P_{21}^{kl}) \right.
$$

$$
\left. + \frac{b+c}{2} m_{ij}^{21}(P_{12}^{kl} + P_{21}^{kl}) + m_{ij}^{22}(cP_{11}^{kl} + aP_{22}^{kl}) \right] + O(f^2) . \tag{13.10}
$$

Define the (anisotropic) 4-tensor $S = (S_{ij}^{kl})$ by (13.3) and the other entries as zero. Thus, (13.10) now takes the form

$$P = M + fPSM + O(f^2) \, ,$$

where M is the EMT associated with B.

Finally, from (13.6), the following theorem is straightforward.

Theorem 13.1 *Let S be the tensor defined by (13.3). The following asymptotic expansion for the effective elasticity tensor C^* holds:*

$$C^* = C^0 + fM(I - fSM)^{-1} + O(f^3) \, , \tag{13.11}$$

where M is the EMT associated with B.

Note that, if $\widetilde{\mu} = \mu$, then according to Francfort and Tartar [127] the effective elasticity tensor C^* is isotropic, which is consistent with the expansion (13.11) since in this case, as may be shown by a direct computation, the tensor SM is isotropic.

13.2 Further Results and Open Problems

Following the arguments developed in this chapter, we can derive further terms in the asymptotic expansion of C^* by inserting more terms in the Taylor expansion of **R** and using higher order elastic moment tensors. It would be interesting to obtain similar formulae for anisotropic elastic composites.

The approach presented in this chapter is also expected to have a great potential for rigorously deriving accurate approximations for the effective viscosity of a suspension of general shaped obstacles suspended in a viscous fluid. We refer to Einstein [118] and Batchelor and Green [56] for approximations corresponding to a suspension of hard spheres in a viscous fluid. Einstein's method consisted of calculating the energy dissipated by the flow around the spherical particles, and associating that with the work done in moving the particles relative to the fluid. It would be very interesting to evaluate the effective viscosity of arbitrary shaped particles. Another challenging problem is to compute the viscous dissipation rate due to particles approaching each other. The analysis of this problem requires delicate estimates analogous to those presented in Chapter 6.

A

Appendices

Introduction

We conclude the book with three appendices. The first of these recalls a few basic facts about compactness, which is needed for our study of the layer potentials in Chapter 2. The second states for the sake of completeness the celebrated theorem of Coifman, McIntosh, and Meyer[98]. The third establishes the continuity method, which is useful for the proof of Theorem 2.21.

A.1 Compact Operators

Let X be a Banach space. A bounded linear operator T is compact, if whenever $\{x_j\}$ is a bounded sequence in X, the sequence $\{Tx_j\}$ has a convergent subsequence. The operator T is said to be of finite rank if $\mathrm{Range}(T)$ is finite-dimensional. Clearly every operator of finite rank is compact.

We now provide some basic results on compact operators.

Lemma A.1 *The set of compact operators on X is a closed two-sided ideal in the algebra of bounded operators on X with the norm topology.*

Lemma A.2 *If T is a bounded operator on the Banach space X and there is a sequence $\{T_N\}_{N \in \mathbb{N}}$ of operators of finite rank such that $||T_N - T|| \to 0$, then T is compact.*

Lemma A.3 *The operator T is compact on the Banach space X if and only if the dual operator T^* is compact on the dual space X^*.*

We also recall the main structure theorem for compact operators.

Theorem A.4 (Fredholm alternative) *Let T be a compact operator on the Hilbert space X (which we identify with its dual). For each $\lambda \in \mathbb{C}$, let $V_\lambda = \{x \in X : Tx = \lambda x\}$ and $V_{\bar\lambda} = \{x \in X : T^*x = \lambda x\}$.*

Then

(i) *The set of $\lambda \in \mathbb{C}$ for which $V_\lambda \neq \{0\}$ is finite or countable, and in the latter case, its only accumulation point is zero. Moreover, $dim(V_\lambda) < +\infty$ for all $\lambda \neq 0$.*

(ii) *If $\lambda \neq 0$, $dim(V_\lambda) = dim(V_{\bar{\lambda}})$.*

(iii) *If $\lambda \neq 0$, the range of $\lambda I - T$ is closed.*

Corollary A.5 *Suppose $\lambda \neq 0$. Then*

(i) *The equation $(\lambda I - T)x = y$ has a solution if and only if $y \perp V_{\bar{\lambda}}$.*

(ii) *$(\lambda I - T)$ is surjective if and only if it is injective.*

To conclude this appendix, we recall the concept of a Fredholm operator acting between Banach spaces X and Y. We say that a bounded linear operator $T : X \to Y$ is Fredholm if the subspace Range(T) is closed in Y and the subspaces Ker(T) and $Y/$Range(T) are finite-dimensional. In this case, the index of T is the integer defined by

$$\text{index } (T) = \dim \text{Ker}(T) - \dim(Y/\text{Range}(T)) \, .$$

The next theorem encapsulates the main conclusion of Fredholm's original theory.

Theorem A.6 *If $T = I + K$, where $K : X \to X$ is compact, then $T : X \to X$ is Fredholm with index zero.*

The last theorem shows that the index is stable under compact perturbations.

Theorem A.7 *If $T : X \to Y$ is Fredholm and $K : X \to Y$ is compact, then their sum $T + K : X \to Y$ is Fredholm, and index $(T + K) =$ index (T).*

A.2 Theorem of Coifman, McIntosh, and Meyer

The proof of Theorem 2.17 is based on the following celebrated theorem of Coifman, McIntosh, and Meyer [98].

Theorem A.8 *Let A, φ be Lipschitz functions on $\mathbb{R}^{d-1}$. The singular integral operator with the integral kernel*

$$\frac{A(x') - A(y')}{(|x' - y'|^2 + (\varphi(x') - \varphi(y'))^2)^{\frac{d}{2}}}$$

is bounded on $L^2(\mathbb{R}^{d-1})$.

Theorem A.8 was proved by reducing to one dimension using the method of rotation of Calderón[77], and then by using the following general theorem obtained in the same paper.

Theorem A.9 *Let K be a compact convex subset in the complex plane, U be an open set containing K, and $F : U \to \mathbb{C}$ be a holomorphic function. Let A and B be Lipschitz functions on $\mathbb{R}$ such that*

$$\frac{A(x) - A(y)}{x - y} \in K \ .$$

Then the principal value operator defined by the kernel

$$\frac{B(x) - B(y)}{(x - y)^2} F\left(\frac{A(x) - A(y)}{x - y} \right)$$

is bounded on $L^2(\mathbb{R})$.

The L^2-boundedness of the operators $\mathcal{K}_D$ and $\mathcal{K}_D^*$ in Theorem 2.17 follows immediately from Theorem A.8. In order to keep the technicalities to a minimum, we suppose that $d \geq 3$, and the domain D is given by a Lipschitz graph, namely, $D = \{(x', x_d) : x_d = \varphi(x')\}$, where $\varphi : \mathbb{R}^{d-1} \to \mathbb{R}$ is a Lipschitz function. If $x = (x', x_d), y = (y', y_d)$, then $\mathcal{K}_D$ is the principle value operator with the kernel

$$\frac{1}{\omega_d} \frac{\varphi(y') - \varphi(x') - \langle y' - x', \nabla\varphi(y') \rangle}{(|x' - y'|^2 + (\varphi(x') - \varphi(y'))^2)^{\frac{d}{2}}} \ ,$$

and $\mathcal{K}_D^*$ is the principle value operator with the kernel

$$\frac{1}{\omega_d} \frac{(\varphi(x') - \varphi(y') - \langle x' - y', \nabla\varphi(x') \rangle)\sqrt{1 + |\nabla\varphi(y')|^2}}{(|x' - y'|^2 + (\varphi(x') - \varphi(y'))^2)^{\frac{d}{2}} \sqrt{1 + |\nabla\varphi(x')|^2}} \ .$$

From Theorem A.8 [with first $A(x') = x'$, then $A(x') = \varphi(x')$] and the boundedness of $\nabla\varphi(x')$, we conclude that $\mathcal{K}_D$ is a bounded operator on $L^2(\partial D)$.

The integral kernel for the same operator $\mathcal{K}_D$ for the Lamé system involves terms defined by

$$\frac{(x'_j - y'_j)^2 (x'_k - y'_k)}{|x' - y'|^{d+2}} \ .$$

The L^2-boundedness of such operators can be proved in a similar way using the method of rotation and Theorem A.9.

A.3 Continuity Method

Theorem A.10 *For $0 \leq t \leq 1$, suppose that the family of operators $A_t : L^2(\mathbb{R}^{d-1}) \to L^2(\mathbb{R}^{d-1})$ satisfy*

(i) $||A_t \phi||_{L^2(\mathbb{R}^{d-1})} \geq C||\phi||_{L^2(\mathbb{R}^{d-1})}$, *where C is independent of t,*
(ii) $t \mapsto A_t$ *is continuous in norm,*
(iii) $A_0 : L^2(\mathbb{R}^{d-1}) \to L^2(\mathbb{R}^{d-1})$ *is invertible.*

Then, $A_1 : L^2(\mathbb{R}^{d-1}) \to L^2(\mathbb{R}^{d-1})$ is invertible.

We provide a brief proof for the sake of the reader. Let

$$T := \left\{ t \in [0,1] : A_t \text{ is invertible on } L^2(\mathbb{R}^{d-1}) \right\}.$$

Then T is non-empty by (iii). We can infer from (ii) that T is an open subset of $[0,1]$. To prove that T is closed, choose a sequence t_j, $j = 1, 2, \ldots$, from T and assume that t_j converges to t_0 as $j \to +\infty$. For a given $g \in L^2(\mathbb{R}^{d-1})$, let f_j be such that $A_{t_j} f_j = g$. Then by (i) there is a subsequence of f_j, which is still denoted by f_j, converging weakly to, say, f_0. We claim that $A_{t_0} f_0 = g$. In fact, if $h \in L^2(\mathbb{R}^{d-1})$, then

$$\langle A_{t_0} f_0 - g, h \rangle = \langle A_{t_0}(f_0 - f_j)g, h \rangle + \langle (A_{t_0} - A_{t_j})f_j, h \rangle$$

$$= \langle (f_0 - f_j)g, A_{t_0}^* h \rangle + \langle (A_{t_0} - A_{t_j})f_j, h \rangle \to 0 \quad \text{as } j \to +\infty .$$

References

1. G. Alessandrini, Stable determination of conductivity by boundary measurements, Applicable Anal., 27 (1988), 153–172.
2. ——————, Remark on a paper of Bellout and Friedman, Boll. Unione. Mat. Ita., 7 (1989), 243–250.
3. ——————, Singular solutions of elliptic equations and the determination of conductivity by boundary measurements, J. Diff. Equat., 84 (1990), 252–272.
4. ——————, Examples of instability in inverse boundary value problems, Inverse Problems, 13 (1997), 887–897.
5. G. Alessandrini, V. Isakov, and J. Powell, Local uniqueness in the inverse conductivity problem with one measurement, Trans. Amer. Math. Soc., 347 (1995), 3031–3041.
6. G. Alessandrini, A. Morassi, and E. Rosset, Detecting an inclusion in an elastic body by boundary measurements, SIAM J. Math. Anal., 33 (2002), 1247–1268.
7. ——————, Detecting cavities by electrostatic boundary measurements, Inverse Problems, 18 (2002), 1333–1353.
8. ——————, Size estimates in *Inverse Problems: Theory and Applications*, 1–33, Contemp. Math., 333, Amer. Math. Soc., Providence, RI, 2003.
9. G. Alessandrini and E. Rosset, The inverse conductivity problem with one measurement: bounds on the size of the unknown object, SIAM J. Appl. Math., 58 (1998), 1060–1071.
10. G. Alessandrini, E. Rosset, and J.K. Seo, Optimal size estimates for the inverse conductivity problem with one measurement, Proc. Amer. Math. Soc., 128 (2000), 53–64.
11. G. Allaire, *Shape Optimization by the Homogenization Method*, Springer-Verlag, New York, 2002.
12. C. Alves and H. Ammari, Boundary integral formulae for the reconstruction of imperfections of small diameter in an elastic medium, SIAM J. Appl. Math., 62 (2002), 94–106.
13. H. Ammari, M. Asch, and H. Kang, Boundary voltage perturbations caused by small conductivity inhomogeneities nearly touching the boundary, Adv. Appl. Math., 35 (2005), 368–391.
14. H. Ammari, E. Beretta, and E. Francini, Reconstruction of thin conductivity imperfections, Applicable Anal., 83 (2004), 63–78.

15. ——————————-, Reconstruction of thin conductivity imperfections II: The case of multiple segments, Applicable Anal., 85 (2006), 87–105.

16. H. Ammari, Y. Capdeboscq, H. Kang, E. Kim, and M. Lim, Numerical attainability by simply connected domains of optimal bounds for the polarization tensors, Euro. J. Appl. Math., 17 (2006), 201–219.

17. H. Ammari, P. Garapon, H. Kang, and H. Lee, A method of biological tissues elasticity reconstruction using magnetic resonance elastography measurements, preprint, 2007.

18. H. Ammari, E. Iakovleva, H. Kang, and K. Kim, Direct algorithms for thermal imaging of small inclusions, Multiscale Model. Simul., 4 (2005), 1116–1136.

19. H. Ammari, E. Iakovleva, and D. Lesselier, A MUSIC algorithm for locating small inclusions buried in a half-space from the scattering amplitude at a fixed frequency, Multiscale Model. Simul., 3 (2005), 597–628.

20. ——————————, Two numerical methods for recovering small electromagnetic inclusions from scattering amplitude at a fixed frequency, SIAM J. Sci. Comput., 27 (2005), 130–158.

21. H. Ammari, E. Iakovleva, and S. Moskow, Recovery of small inhomogeneities from the scattering amplitude at a fixed frequency, SIAM J. Math. Anal., 34 (2003), 882–900.

22. H. Ammari and H. Kang, High-order terms in the asymptotic expansions of the steady-state voltage potentials in the presence of conductivity inhomogeneities of small diameter, SIAM J. Math. Anal., 34 (2003), 1152–1166.

23. ——————————, Properties of generalized polarization tensors, Multiscale Model. Simul., 1 (2003), 335–348.

24. ——————————, A new method for reconstructing electromagnetic inhomogeneities of small volume, Inverse Problems, 19 (2003), 63–71.

25. ——————————, Boundary layer techniques for solving the Helmholtz equation in the presence of small inhomogeneities, J. Math. Anal. Appl., 296 (2004), 190–208.

26. ——————————, *Reconstruction of Small Inhomogeneities from Boundary Measurements*, Lecture Notes in Mathematics, Volume 1846, Springer-Verlag, Berlin, 2004.

27. ——————————, Reconstruction of elastic inclusions of small volume via dynamic measurements, Appl. Math. Opt., 54 (2006), 223–235.

28. H. Ammari, H. Kang, and K. Kim, Polarization tensors and effective properties of anisotropic composite materials, J. Differ. Equat., 215 (2005), 401–428.

29. H. Ammari, H. Kang, E. Kim, and M. Lim, Reconstruction of closely spaced small inclusions, SIAM J. Numer. Anal., 42 (2005), 2408–2428.

30. H. Ammari, H. Kang, and H. Lee, A boundary integral method for computing elastic moment tensors for ellipses and ellipsoids, J. Comp. Math., 25 (2007), 2–12.

31. H. Ammari, H. Kang, H. Lee, J. Lee, and M. Lim, Optimal bounds on the gradient of solutions to conductivity problems, preprint, 2005.

32. H. Ammari, H. Kang, and M. Lim, Gradient estimates for solutions to the conductivity problem, Math. Ann., 332 (2005), 277–286.

33. ——————————, Effective parameters of elastic composites, Indiana Univ. J. Math., 55 (2006), 903–922.

34. ——————————, Polarization tensors and their applications, to appear in *Proceedings of the second International Conference on Inverse Problems: recent*

developments and numerical approaches, Shanghai, 2004, Journal of Physics: Conference Series, 12 (2005), 13–22.

35. H. Ammari, H. Kang, M. Lim, and H. Zribi, Layer potential techniques in spectral analysis. Part I: complete asymptotic expansions for eigenvalues of the Laplacian in domains with small inclusions, preprint, 2005.

36. H. Ammari, H. Kang, G. Nakamura, and K. Tanuma, Complete asymptotic expansions of solutions of the system of elastostatics in the presence of an inclusion of small diameter and detection of an inclusion, J. Elasticity, 67 (2002), 97–129.

37. H. Ammari, H. Kang, S. Soussi, and H. Zribi, Layer potential techniques in spectral analysis. Part II: sensitivity analysis of spectral properties of high contrast band-gap materials, Multiscale Model. Simul., 5 (2006), 646–663.

38. H. Ammari, H. Kang, and K. Touibi, Boundary layer techniques for deriving the effective properties of composite materials, Asymp. Anal., 41 (2005), 119–140.

39. H. Ammari and A. Khelifi, Electromagnetic scattering by small dielectric inhomogeneities, J. Math. Pures Appl., 82 (2003), 749–842.

40. H. Ammari, O. Kwon, J.K. Seo, and E.J. Woo, Anomaly detection in T-scan trans-admittance imaging system, SIAM J. Appl. Math., 65 (2004), 252–266.

41. H. Ammari and S. Moskow, Asymptotic expansions for eigenvalues in the presence of small inhomogeneities, Math. Meth. Appl. Sci., 26 (2003), 67–75.

42. H. Ammari, S. Moskow, and M.S. Vogelius, Boundary integral formulas for the reconstruction of electromagnetic imperfections of small diameter, ESAIM: Cont. Opt. Calc. Var., 9 (2003), 49–66.

43. H. Ammari and J.K. Seo, An accurate formula for the reconstruction of conductivity inhomogeneities, Adv. Appl. Math., 30 (2003), 679–705.

44. H. Ammari and G. Uhlmann, Reconstruction of the potential from partial Cauchy data for the Schrödinger equation, Indiana Univ. Math. J., 53 (2004), 169–184.

45. H. Ammari, M.S. Vogelius, and D. Volkov, Asymptotic formulas for perturbations in the electromagnetic fields due to the presence of imperfections of small diameter II. The full Maxwell equations, J. Math. Pures Appl., 80 (2001), 769–814.

46. H. Ammari and D. Volkov, Correction of order three for the expansion of two dimensional electromagnetic fields perturbed by the presence of inhomogeneities of small diameter, J. Comput. Phys., 189 (2003), 371–389.

47. D.H. Armitage and S.J. Gardiner, *Classical Potential Theory*, Springer Monographs in Mathematics, Springer-Verlag, Berlin, 2001.

48. K. Asami, T. Hanai, and N. Koizumi, Dielectric approach to suspensions of ellipsoidal particles covered with a shell in particular reference to biological cells, Japanese J. Appl. Physics, 19 (1980), 359–365.

49. M. Assenheimer, O. Laver-Moskovitz, D. Malonek, D. Manor, U. Nahliel, R. Nitzan, and A. Saad, The T-scan technology: Electrical impedance as a diagnostic tool for breast cancer detection, Physiol. Meas., 22 (2001), 1–8.

50. K. Astala and L. Païvärinta, Calderon's inverse conductivity problem in the plane, Ann. Math., 163 (2006), 265–299.

51. I. Babuška, B. Andersson, P. Smith, and K. Levin, Damage analysis of fiber composites. I. Statistical analysis on fiber scale, Comput. Methods Appl. Mech. Engrg., 172 (1999), 27–77.

52. A. El Badia and T. Ha-Duong, An inverse source problem in potential analysis, Inverse Problems, 16 (2000), 651–663.

53. C. Bandle, *Isoperimetric Inequalities and Applications*, Monogr. Stud. Math. 7, Pitman, Boston, MA, 1980.

54. D.C. Barber and B.H. Brown, Applied potential tomography, J. Phys. Sci. Instrum., 17 (1984), 723–733.

55. B. Barcelo, E. Fabes, and J.K. Seo, The inverse conductivity problem with one measurement, uniqueness for convex polyhedra, Proc. Amer. Math. Soc., 122 (1994), 183–189.

56. G.K. Batchelor and J.T. Green, The determination of the bulk stress is suspension of spherical particles to order c^2, J. Fluid. Mech., 56 (1972), 401-427.

57. H. Bellout and A. Friedman, Identification problems in potential theory, Arch. Rational Mech. Anal., 101 (1988), 143–160.

58. H. Bellout, A. Friedman, and V. Isakov, Stability for an inverse problem in potential theory, Trans. Amer. Math. Soc., 332 (1992), 271–296.

59. F. Ben Hassen and E. Bonnetier, Asymptotic formulas for the voltage potential in a composite medium containing close or touching disks of small diameter, Multiscale Model. Simul., 4 (2005), 250–277.

60. ——————, Asymptotics of the voltage potential in a composite medium that contains misplaced inclusions, Proc. Roy. Soc. Edinburgh Sect. A, 136 (2006), 669–700.

61. A. Bensoussan, J.L. Lions, and G. Papanicolaou, *Asymptotic Analysis of Periodic Structures*, North Holland, 1978.

62. J. Bercoff, S. Chaffai, M. Tanter, L. Sandrin, S. Catheline, M. Fink, J.L. Gennisson, and M. Meunier, In vivo breast tumor detection using transient elastography, Ultrasound Med. Bio., 29 (2003), 1387–1396.

63. E. Beretta and E. Francini, Asymptotic formulas for perturbations in the electromagnetic fields due to the presence of thin inhomogeneities in *Inverse Problems: Theory and Applications*, 49–63, Contemp. Math., 333, Amer. Math. Soc., Providence, RI, 2003.

64. E. Beretta, E. Francini, and M.S. Vogelius, Asymptotic formulas for steady state voltage potentials in the presence of thin inhomogeneities. A rigorous error analysis, J. Math. Pures Appl., 82 (2003), 1277–1301.

65. E. Beretta, A. Mukherjee, and M.S. Vogelius, Asymptotic formuli for steady state voltage potentials in the presence of conductivity imperfections of small area, Z. Angew. Math. Phys., 52 (2001), 543–572.

66. J. Bergh and J. Löfström, *Interpolation Spaces. An Introduction*, Grundlehren der Mathematischen Wissenschaften, 223, Springer-Verlag, Berlin-New York, 1976.

67. J. Blitz, *Electrical and Magnetic Methods of Nondestructive Testing*, IOP Publishing, Adam Hilger, 1991.

68. C.L. Berman and L. Greengard, A renormalization method for the evaluation of lattice sums, J. Math. Phys., 35 (1994), 6036–6048.

69. E. Bonnetier and M. Vogelius, An elliptic regurality result for a composite medium with touching fibers of circular cross-section, SIAM J. Math. Anal., 31 (2000), 651–677.

70. L. Borcea, Electrical impedance tomography, Inverse Problems, 18 (2002), 99–136.

71. M. Brühl, Explicit characterization of inclusions in electrical impedance tomography, SIAM J. Math. Anal., 32 (2001), 1327–1341.

72. M. Brühl and M. Hanke, Numerical implementation of two noniterative methods for locating inclusions by impedance tomography, Inverse Problems, 16 (2000), 1029–1042.

73. M. Brühl, M. Hanke, and M.S. Vogelius, A direct impedance tomography algorithm for locating small inhomogeneities, Numer. Math., 93 (2003), 635–654.

74. K. Bryan, Numerical recovery of certain discontinuous electrical conductivities, Inverse Problems, 7 (1991), 827–840.

75. K. Bryan and M.S. Vogelius, A computational algorithm to determine crack locations from electrostatic boundary measurements. The case of multiple cracks, Int. J. Engng. Sci, 32 (1994), 579–603.

76. B. Budiansky and G.F. Carrier, High shear stresses in stiff fiber composites, J. Appl. Mech., 51 (1984), 733–735.

77. A.P. Calderón, Cauchy integrals on Lipschitz curves and related operators, Proc. Nat. Acad. Sci. U.S.A., 74 (1977), 1324–1327.

78. —————, On an inverse boundary value problem, Seminar on Numerical Analysis and its Applications to Continuum Physics, Soc. Brasileira de Matemática, Rio de Janeiro, 1980, 65–73.

79. Y. Capdeboscq and H. Kang, Improved Hashin-Shtrikman bounds for elastic moment tensors and an application, preprint, 2007.

80. —————, Improved Hashin-Shtrikman bounds for thick domains, Inverse problems, multi-scale analysis and effective medium theory, 69-74, Contemp. Math., 408, Amer. Math. Soc., Providence, RI, 2006.

81. Y. Capdeboscq and M.S. Vogelius, A general representation formula for the boundary voltage perturbations caused by internal conductivity inhomogeneities of low volume fraction, Math. Modelling Num. Anal., 37 (2003), 159–173.

82. —————, Optimal asymptotic estimates for the volume of internal inhomogeneities in terms of multiple boundary measurements, Math. Modelling Num. Anal., 37 (2003), 227–240.

83. —————, A review of some recent work on impedance imaging for inhomogeneities of low volume fraction, Proceedings of the Pan-American Advanced Studies Institute on PDEs, Inverse Problems and Nonlinear Analysis, January 2003, 69–87, Contemp. Math., 362, Amer. Math. Soc., Providence, RI, 2005.

84. D.J. Cedio-Fengya, S. Moskow, and M.S. Vogelius, Identification of conductivity imperfections of small diameter by boundary measurements: Continuous dependence and computational reconstruction, Inverse Problems, 14 (1998), 553–595.

85. D.H. Chambers and J.G. Berryman, Time-reversal analysis for scatterer characterization, Phys. Rev. Lett., 92 (2004), 023902-1–023902-4.

86. A. Charalambopoulos, G. Dassios, and M. Hadjinicolaou, An analytic solution for the low-frequency scattering by two soft spheres, SIAM J. Appl. Math., 58 (1998), 370–386.

87. M. Cheney, The linear sampling method and the MUSIC algorithm, Inverse Problems, 17 (2001), 591–595.

88. M. Cheney and D. Isaacson, Distinguishability in impedance imaging, IEEE Trans. Biomed. Engr., 39 (1992), 852–860.

89. M. Cheney, D. Isaacson, and J.C. Newell, Electrical impedance tomography, SIAM Rev., 41 (1999), 85–101.

90. M. Cheney, D. Isaacson, J.C. Newell, S. Simske, and J. Goble, NOSER: an algorithm for solving the inverse conductivity problem, Int. J. Imag. Syst. Technol., 22 (1990), 66–75.

91. H. Cheng and L. Greengard, A method of images for the evaluation of electrostatic fields in systems of closely spaced conducting cylinders, SIAM J. Appl. Math., 58 (1998), 122–141.

92. V.A. Cherepenin, A. Karpov, A. Korjenevsky, V. Kornienko, A. Mazaletskaya, D. Mazourov, and D. Meister, A 3D electrical impedance tomography (EIT) system for breast cancer detection, Physiol. Meas., 22 (2001), 9–18.

93. V.A. Cherepenin, A. Y. Karpov, A. V. Korjenevsky, V. N. Kornienko, Y. S. Kultiasov, M. B. Ochapkin, O. V. Trochanova, and J. D. Meister, Three-dimensional EIT imaging of breast tissues: system design and clinical testing, IEEE Trans. Med. Imag., 21 (2002), 662–667.

94. A. Cherkaev, *Variational Methods for Structural Optimization*, Appl. Math. Sciences 140, Springer, New York, 2000.

95. T.C. Choy, *Effective Medium Theory. Principles and Applications*, International Series of Monographs on Physics, 102, Oxford Science Publications, New York, 1999.

96. P.G. Ciarlet, *Mathematical Elasticity*, Vol. I, Norh-Holland, Amsterdam (1988).

97. D. Cioranescu and P. Donato, *An Introduction to Homegenization*, Oxford Lecture Series in Mathematics and its Application 17, Oxford University Press, 1999.

98. R.R. Coifman, A. McIntosh, and Y. Meyer, L'intégrale de Cauchy définit un opérateur borné sur L^2 pour les courbes lipschitziennes, Ann. Math., 116 (1982), 361–387.

99. R.E. Collin, *Field Theory of Guided Waves*, Second Edition, IEEE Press, New York, 1991.

100. D. Colton and A. Kirsch, A simple method for solving inverse scattering problems in the resonance region, Inverse Problems, 12 (1996), 383–393.

101. D. Colton and R. Kress, *Integral Equation Methods in Scattering Theory*, John Wiley, New York, 1983.

102. —————, *Inverse Acoustic and Electromagnetic Scattering Theory*, Applied Math. Sciences 93, Springer-Verlag, New York, 1992.

103. M. Costabel, Boundary integral operators on Lipschitz domains: elementary results, SIAM J. Math. Anal., 19 (1988), 613–626.

104. B.E. Dahlberg, C.E. Kenig, and G. Verchota, Boundary value problem for the systems of elastostatics in Lipschitz domains, Duke Math. Jour., 57 (1988), 795–818.

105. G. Dassios, Low-frequency moments in inverse scattering theory, J. Math. Phys., 31 (1990), 1691–1692.

106. G. Dassios and R.E. Kleinman, On Kelvin inversion and low-frequency scattering, SIAM Rev., 31 (1989), 565–585.

107. —————, *Low Frequency Scattering*, Oxford Science Publications, The Clarendon Press, Oxford University Press, New York, 2000.

108. I. Daubechies, *Ten Lectures on Wavelets*, SIAM, Philadelphia, 1992.

109. G. David and J.-L. Journé, A boundedness criterion for generalized Calderón-Zygmund operators, Ann. Math., 120 (1984), 371–397.

110. A.J. Devaney, Super-resolution processing of multi-static data using reversal and MUSIC, to appear in J. Acoust. Soc. Am. (2003).

111. A. Dienstfrey, F. Hang, and J. Huang, Lattice sums and the two-dimensional, periodic Green's function for the Helmholtz equation, Proc. Royal Soc. London A, 457 (2001), 67–85.

112. D.C. Dobson and F. Santosa, An image-enhancement technique for electrical impedance tomography, Inverse Problems, 10 (1994), 317–334.

113. ——————, Resolution and stability analysis of an inverse problem in electrical impedance tomography: dependence of the input current patterns, SIAM J. Appl. Math., 54 (1994), 1542–1560.

114. J.F. Douglas and A. Friedman, Coping with complex boundaries, IMA Series on Mathematics and its Applications Vol. 67, 166–185, Springer, New York, 1995.

115. J.F. Douglas and E.J. Garboczi, Intrinsic viscosity and polarizability of particles having a wide range of shapes, Adv. Chem. Phys., 91 (1995), 85–153.

116. V. Druskin, The unique solution of the inverse problem of electrical surveying and electrical well-logging for piecewise-continuous conductivity, Izvestiya, Earth Physics, 18 (1982), 51–53.

117. M.R. Eggleston, R.J. Schwabe, D. Isaacson, and L.F. Coffin, The application of electric current computed tomography to defect imaging in metals, in *Review of Progress in Quantitative NDE*, D.O. Thompson and D.E. Chimenti, eds., Plenum, New York, 1989.

118. A. Einstein, Eine neue Bestimmung der Moleküldimensionen, Ann. Phys., 19 (1906), 289–306.

119. I. Ekeland and R. Temam, *Convex analysis and variational problems*, North Holland, 1976.

120. L. Escauriaza, E.B. Fabes, and G. Verchota, On a regularity theorem for weak solutions to transmission problems with internal Lipschitz boundaries, Proc. Amer. Math. Soc., 115 (1992), 1069–1076.

121. L. Escauriaza and J.K. Seo, Regularity properties of solutions to transmission problems, Trans. Amer. Math. Soc., 338 (1) (1993), 405–430.

122. E.B. Fabes, M. Jodeit, and N.M. Riviére, Potential techniques for boundary value problems on $\mathcal{C}^1$ domains, Acta Math., 141 (1978), 165–186.

123. E. Fabes, H. Kang, and J.K. Seo, Inverse conductivity problem with one measurement: Error estimates and approximate identification for perturbed disks, SIAM J. Math. Anal., 30 (1999), 699–720.

124. E. Fabes, C. Kenig, and G. Verchota, The Dirichlet problem for the Stokes system on Lipschitz domains, Duke Math. J., 57 (1988), 769–793.

125. E. Fabes, M. Sand, and J.K. Seo, The spectral radius of the classical layer potentials on convex domains, The IMA volumes in Mathematics and its Applications, 42 (1992), 129–137.

126. G.B. Folland, *Introduction to Partial Differential Equations*, Princeton University Press, Princeton, NJ, 1976.

127. G. Francfort and L. Tartar, Comportement effectif d'un mélange de matériaux élastiques isotropes ayant le même module de cisaillement, C. R. Acad. Sci. Sér. I. Math., 312 (1991), 301–307.

128. H. Fricke, The Maxwell-Wagner dispersion in a suspension of ellipsoids, J. Phys. Chem., 57 (1953), 934–937.

129. A. Friedman, Detection of mines by electric measurements, SIAM J. Appl. Math., 47 (1987), 201–212.

130. A. Friedman and B. Gustafsson, Identification of the conductivity coefficient in an elliptic equation, SIAM J. Math. Anal., 18 (1987), 777–787.

131. A. Friedman and V. Isakov, On the uniqueness in the inverse conductivity problem with one measurement, Indiana Univ. Math. J., 38 (1989), 553–580.

132. A. Friedman and M.S. Vogelius, Identification of small inhomogeneities of extreme conductivity by boundary measurements: a theorem on continuous dependence, Arch. Rat. Mech. Anal., 105 (1989), 299–326.

133. L.F. Fuks, M. Cheney, D. Isaacson, D.G. Gisser, and J.C. Newell, Detection and imaging of electric conductivity and permittivity at low frequencies, IEEE Trans. Biomed. Engr., 3 (1991), 1106–1110.

134. E.J. Garboczi and J.F. Douglas, Intrinsic conductivity of objects having arbitrary shape and conductivity, Physical Review E, 53 (1996), 6169–6180.

135. S.J. Gardiner, *Harmonic Approximation*, London Mathematical Society, Lecture Note Series 221, Cambridge Univ. Press, Cambridge, 1995.

136. N. Garofalo and F. Lin, Monotonicity properties of variational integrals, A_p weights and unique continuation, Indiana Univ. Math. J., 35 (1986), 245–268.

137. S. Garreau, Ph. Guillaume, and M. Masmoudi, The topological asymptotic for PDE systems: the elasticity case, SIAM J. Control Optim., 39 (2001), 1756–1778.

138. D. Gilbarg and N.S. Trudinger, *Elliptic Partial Differential Equations of Second Order*, Grundlehren der Mathematischen Wissenschaften, 224, Springer-Verlag, Berlin-New York, 1977.

139. D. Gisser, D. Isaacson, and J.C. Newell, Electric current tomography and eigenvalues, SIAM J. Appl. Math., 50 (1990), 1623–1634.

140. L. Greengard and M. Moura, On the numerical evaluation of electrostatic fields in composite materials, Acta Numerica (1994), 379–410.

141. L. Greengard and J.Y. Lee, Electrostatics and heat conduction in high contrast composite materials, J. Comput. Phys., 211 (2006), 64–76.

142. Ph. Guillaume and K. Sid Idris, The topological asymptotic expansion for the Dirichlet problem, SIAM J. Control Optim., 41 (2003), 1042–1072.

143. Q. Han and F. Lin, *Elliptic Partial Differential Equations*, Courant Lecture Notes in Mathematics, 1, New York University, Courant Institute of Mathematical Sciences, New York, Amer. Math. Soc., Providence, RI, 1997.

144. P. Hähner, An inverse problem in electrostatics, Inverse Problems, 15 (1999), 961–975.

145. Z. Hashin and S. Shtrickman, A variational approach to the theory of effective magnetic permeability of multiphase materials, J. Appl. Phys., 33 (1962), 3125–3131.

146. Z. Hashin, Analysis of composite materials—A survey, J. Appl. Mech., 50 (1983), 481–505.

147. Z. Hashin and P.J.M. Monteiro, An inverse method to determine the elastic properties of the interphase between the aggregate and the cement paste, Cement and Concrete Research, 32 (2002), 1291–1300.

148. H. Hasimoto, On the periodic fundamental solutions of the Stokes equations and their application to viscous flow past a cubic array of spheres, J. Fluid Dynamics, 5 (1959), 317–328.

149. J. Helsing, An integral equation method for electrostatics of periodic composites, J. Mech. Phys. Solids, 43 (1995), 815–828.

150. G.C. Herman, Transmission of elastic waves through solids containing small-scale heterogeneities, Geophys. J. Int., 145 (2001), 436–446.

151. E. Hille, *Analytic Function Theory, Volume II*, Blaisdell, 1962.

152. B. Hofmann, Approximation of the inverse electrical impedance tomography by an inverse transmission problem, Inverse Problems, 14 (1998), 1171–1187.

153. D. Holder, *Clinical and Physiological Applications of Electrical Impedance Tomography*, UCL Press, London, 1993.

154. S.C. Hsieh and T. Mura, Nondestructive cavity identification in structures, Internat. J. Solids Structures, 30 (1993), 1579–1587.

155. E. Iakovleva, Inverse Scattering from Small Inhomogeneities, Ph.D. thesis, Ecole Polytechnique, 2004.

156. M. Ikehata, Enclosing a polygonal cavity in a two-dimensional bounded domain from Cauchy data, Inverse Problems, 15 (1999), 1231–1241.

157. —————, Reconstruction of the support function for inclusion from boundary measurements, J. Inverse Ill-Posed Probl., 8 (2000), 367–378.

158. —————, On reconstruction in the inverse conductivity problem with one measurement, Inverse Problems, 16 (2000), 785–793.

159. —————, Reconstruction of inclusion from boundary measurements, J. Inverse Ill-Posed Probl., 10 (2002), 37–65.

160. M. Ikehata and T. Ohe, A numerical method for finding the convex hull of polygonal cavities using the enclosure method, Inverse Problems, 18 (2002), 111–124.

161. M. Ikehata and S. Siltanen, Numerical method for finding the convex hull of an inclusion in conductivity from boundary measurements, Inverse Problems, 16 (2000), 1043–1052.

162. D. Isaacson, Distinguishability of conductivities by electric current computed tomography, IEEE Trans. Medical Imag., 5 (1986), 91–95.

163. D. Isaacson and M. Cheney, Effects of measurements precision and finite numbers of electrodes on linear impedance imaging algorithms, SIAM J. Appl. Math., 51 (1991), 1705–1731.

164. D. Isaacson and E.L. Isaacson, Comments on Calderón's paper: "On an inverse boundary value problem," Math. Compt., 52 (1989), 553–559.

165. V. Isakov, On uniqueness of recovery of a discontinuous conductivity coefficient, Comm. Pure Appl. Math., 41 (1988), 865–877.

166. —————, *Inverse Source Problems*, Math. Surveys and Monograph Series Vol. 34, AMS, Providence, RI, 1990.

167. —————, *Inverse Problems for Partial Differential Equations*, Springer-Verlag, New York, 1998.

168. V. Isakov and J. Powell, On the inverse conductivity problem with one measurement, Inverse Problems, 6 (1990), 311–318.

169. V. Isakov and A. Sever, Numerical implementation of an integral equation method for the inverse conductivity problem, Inverse Problems, 12 (1996), 939–953.

170. V. Isakov and S.F. Wu, On theory and application of the Helmholtz equation least squares method in inverse acoustics, Inverse Problems, 18 (2002), 1147–1159.

171. D.J. Jefferey, Conduction through a random suspension of spheres, Proc. R. Soc. London Ser. A, 335 (1973), 355–367.

172. D.S. Jerison and C. Kenig, The Neumann problem in Lipschitz domains, Bull. Amer. Math. Soc., 4 (1981), 203–207.

173. V.V. Jikov, S.M. Kozlov, and O.A. Oleinik, *Homogenization of Differential Operators and Integral Functionals*, Springer-Verlag, Berlin, 1994.

174. H. Kang, E. Kim, and J. Lee, Identification of Elastic Inclusions and Elastic Moment Tensors by Boundary Measurements, Inverse Problems, 19 (2003), 703–724.

175. H. Kang, E. Kim, and K. Kim, Anisotropic polarization tensors and determination of an anisotropic inclusion, SIAM J. Appl. Math., 65 (2003), 1276–1291.

176. H. Kang and K. Kim, Anisotropic polarization tensors for ellipses and ellipsoids, J. Comp. Math., 25 (2007), 157–168.

177. H. Kang and H. Lee, Identification of simple poles via boundary measurements and an application to EIT, Inverse Problems, 20 (2004), 1853–1863.

178. H. Kang and G.W. Milton, On conjectures of Pólya-Szegö and Eshelby, Inverse problems, multi-scale analysis and effective medium theory, 75-80, Contemp. Math., 408, Amer. Math. Soc., Providence, RI, 2006.

179. —————————-, Solutions to the conjectures of Polya-Szegö and Eshelby, preprint, 2006.

180. H. Kang and J.K. Seo, Layer potential technique for the inverse conductivity problem, Inverse Problems, 12 (1996), 267–278.

181. —————————, Identification of domains with near-extreme conductivity: Global stability and error estimates, Inverse Problems, 15 (1999), 851–867.

182. —————————, Inverse conductivity problem with one measurement: Uniqueness of balls in R^3, SIAM J. Appl. Math., 59 (1999), 1533–1539.

183. —————————, Recent progress in the inverse conductivity problem with single measurement, in Inverse Problems and Related Fields, CRC Press, Boca Raton, FL, 2000, 69–80.

184. H. Kang, J.K. Seo, and D. Sheen, The inverse conductivity problem with one measurement: stability and estimation of size, SIAM J. Math. Anal., 28 (1997), 1389–1405.

185. —————————, Numerical identification of discontinuous conductivity coefficients, Inverse Problems, 13 (1997), 113–123.

186. T. Kato, *Perturbation Theory for Linear Operators*, Springer-Verlag, New York, 1980.

187. J.B. Keller, Stresses in narrow regions, Trans. ASME J. Appl. Mech., 60 (1993), 1054–1056.

188. —————————, Removing small features from computational domains, J. Comput. Phys., 113 (1994), 148–150.

189. O.D. Kellogg, *Foundations of Potential Theory*, Dover, New York, 1953.

190. C.E. Kenig, *Harmonic Analysis Techniques for Second Order Elliptic Boundary Value Problems*, Regional Conference Series in Mathematics, Amer. Math. Soc., Providence, RI, 1994.

191. A. Kirsch, *An Introduction to the Mathematical Theory of Inverse Problems*, Applied Mathematical Sciences 120, Springer-Verlag, New York, 1996.

192. —————————, Characterization of the shape of the scattering obstacle using the spectral data of the far field operator, Inverse Problems, 14 (1998), 1489–1512.

193. —————————, The MUSIC algorithm and the factorization method in inverse scattering theory for inhomogeneous media, Inverse Problems, 18 (2002), 1025–1040.

194. R.E. Kleinman and P.M. van den Berg, A modified gradient method for two-dimensional problems in tomography, J. Comput. Appl. Math., 42 (1992), 17–35.

195. R.E. Kleinman and T.B.A. Senior, Rayleigh scattering in *Low and High Frequency Asymptotics*, 1–70, edited by V.K. Varadan and V.V. Varadan, North-Holland, 1986.

196. R.V. Kohn and A. McKenny, Numerical implementation of a variational method for electrical impedance tomography, Inverse Problems, 6 (1990), 389–414.

197. R.V. Kohn and G.W. Milton, On bounding the effective conductivity of anisotropic composites, in *Homogenization and Effective Moduli of Materials and Media*, eds. J.L. Ericksen, D. Kinderlehrer, R.V. Kohn, and J.L. Lions, IMA Volumes in Mathematics and its Applications, 1, 97–125, Springer-Verlag, 1986.

198. R.V. Kohn and M.S. Vogelius, Determining conductivity by boundary measurements, Comm. Pure Appl. Math., 37 (1984), 289–298.

199. —————, Determining conductivity by boundary measurements, interior results, II, Comm. Pure Appl. Math., 38 (1985), 643–667.

200. —————, Relaxation of a variational method for impedance computed tomography, Comm. Pure Appl. Math., 40 (1987), 745–777.

201. S.M. Kozlov, Geometric aspects of averaging, Usp. Mat. Nauk., 44 (1989), 79–120.

202. —————, On the domain of variations of added masses, polarization and effective characteristics of composites, J. Appl. Math. Mech., 56 (1992), 102–107.

203. R. Kress, On the low wave number asymptotics for the two-dimensional exterior problem for the reduced wave equation, Math. Meth. Appl. Sci., 9 (1987), 335–341.

204. —————, *Linear Integral Equations*. Second edition. Applied Mathematical Sciences, 82. Springer-Verlag, New York, 1999.

205. P. Kuchment, The mathematics of photonic crystals, in *Mathematical Modelling in Optical Science*, eds. Bao, Cowsar and Masters, 207–272, Frontiers in Appl. Math. 22, SIAM, Philadelphia, PA, 2001.

206. V.D. Kupradze, *Potential Methods in the Theory of Elasticity*, Daniel Davey & Co., New York, 1965.

207. O. Kwon and J.K. Seo, Total size estimation and identification of multiple anomalies in the inverse electrical impedance tomography, Inverse Problems, 17 (2001), 59–75.

208. O. Kwon, J.K. Seo, and J.R. Yoon, A real-time algorithm for the location search of discontinuous conductivities with one measurement, Comm. Pure Appl. Math., 55 (2002), 1–29.

209. O. Kwon, J.R. Yoon, J.K. Seo, E.J. Woo, and Y.G. Cho, Estimation of anomaly location and size using impedance tomography, IEEE Trans. Biomed. Engr., 50 (2003), 89–96.

210. N.S. Landkof, *Foundations of Modern Potential Theory*, Springer, New York, 1972.

211. P.D. Lax and A.N. Milgram, Parabolic equations, Ann. Math. Stud., 33 (1954), 167–190.

212. N.N. Lebedev, I.P. Shalskyaya, and Y.S. Uflyand, *Worked Problems in Applied Mathematics*, Dover, New York, 1965.

213. S.K. Lehman and A.J. Devaney, Transmission mode time-reversal super-resolution imaging, J. Acoust. Soc. Am., 113 (2003), 2742–2753.

214. D. Lesnic, A numerical investigation of the inverse potential conductivity problem in a circular inclusion, Inverse Probl. Engr., 9 (2001), 1–17.

215. T. Lévy and E. Sánchez-Palencia, Einstein-like approximation for homogenization with small concentration. II. Navier-Stokes equation, Nonlinear Anal., 9 (1985), 1255–1268.

216. T. Lewiński and Sokolowski, Energy change due to the appearance of cavities in elastic solids, International J. Solids Structures, 40 (2003), 1765–1803.

217. Y.Y. Li and L. Nirenberg, Estimates for elliptic systems from composite material, Comm. Pure Appl. Math. LVI (2003), 892–925.

218. Y.Y. Li and M. Vogelius, Gradient estimates for solutions to divergence form elliptic equations with discontinuous coefficients, Arch. Rational Mech. Anal., 153 (2000), 91–151.

219. M. Lim, Symmetry of an boundary integral operator and a characterization of balls, Illinois Jour. Math., 45 (2001), 537–543.

220. —————, Reconstruction of Inhomogeneities via Boundary Measurements, Ph.D. thesis, Seoul National University, 2003.

221. C.M. Linton, The Green's function for the two-dimensional Helmholtz equation in periodic domains, J. Eng. Math., 33 (1998), 377–402.

222. R. Lipton, Inequalities for electric and elastic polarization tensors with applications to random composites, J. Mech. Phys. Solids, 41 (1993), 809–833.

223. K.A. Lurie and A.V. Cherkayev, Exact estimates of conductivity of composites formed by two isotropically conducting media taken in prescribed proportion, Proc. Roy. Soc. Edinburgh, 99 A (1984), 71–87.

224. A. Manduca, T.E. Oliphant, M.A. Dresner, J.L. Mahowald, S.A. Kruse, E. Amromin, J.P. Felmlee, J.F. Greenleaf, and R.L. Ehman, Magnetic resonance elastography: non-invasive mapping of tissue elasticity, Medical Image Analysis, 5 (2001), 237–254.

225. M.L. Mansfield, J.F. Douglas, and E.J. Garboczi, Intrinsic viscosity and electrical polarizability of arbitrary shaped objects, Physical Review E, 64 (2001), 061401.

226. E. Martensen, Eine Integralgleichung für die legarithmische Gleichgewichtsbelegung und die Krümung der Randkurve eines ebenen Gebiets, Z. Angew Math. Mech., 72 (1992), T596-T599.

227. T.D. Mast, A. Nachman, and R.C. Waag, Focusing and imagining using eigenfunctions of the scattering operator, J. Acoust. Soc. Am., 102 (1997), 715–725.

228. V.G. Maz'ya and S.A. Nazarov, The asymptotic behavior of energy integrals under small perturbations of the boundary near corner points and conical points (in Russian). Trudy Moskovsk. Matem. Obshch. Vol. 50, English Translation: Trans. Moscow Math. Soc. (1988), 77–127.

229. V.G. Maz'ya, S.A. Nazarov, and B.A. Plamenevskii, *Asymptotic Theory of Elliptic Boundary Value Problems in Singularly Perturbed Domains*, Vol. 1, Operator Theory: Advances and Applications, 111, Birkhäuser Verlag, Basel, 2000.

230. —————, *Asymptotic Theory of Elliptic Boundary Value Problems in Singularly Perturbed Domains*, Vol. 2, Operator Theory: Advances and Applications, 112, Birkhäuser Verlag, Basel, 2000.

231. W. McLean, *Strongly Elliptic Systems and Boundary Integral Equations*, Cambridge University Press, Cambridge, 2000.

232. R.C. McPhedran and A.B. Movchan, The Rayleigh multipole method for linear elasticity, J. Mech. Phys. Solids, 42 (1994), 711–727.

233. K. Miller, Stabilized numerical analytic prolongation with poles, SIAM J. Appl. Math., 18 (1970), 346–363.

234. O. Mendez and W. Reichel, Electrostatic characterization of spheres, Forum Math., 12 (2000), 223–245.

235. G.W. Milton, On characterizing the set of possible effective tensors of composites: the variational methods and the translation methods, Commun. Pure Appl. Math., 43 (1990), 63–125.

236. ——————, The Theory of Composites, Cambridge Monographs on Applied and Computational Mathematics, Cambridge University Press, 2001.

237. D. Mitrea and M. Mitrea, Uniqueness for inverse conductivity and transmission problems in the class of Lipschitz domains, Commun. Part. Diff. Eqns, 23 (1998), 1419–1448.

238. D. Mitrea, M. Mitrea, and J. Pipher, Vector potential theory on nonsmooth domains in $\mathbb{R}^3$ and applications to electromagnetic scattering, J. Fourier Anal. Appl., 3 (1997), 131–192.

239. P. Moon and D.E. Spencer, Field Theory Handbook, Springer-Verlag, Berlin, 1961.

240. C.B. Morrey, Multiple Integrals in the Calculus of Variations, Springer-Verlag, New York, 1966.

241. A.B. Movchan, Integral characteristics of elastic inclusions and cavities in the two-dimensional theory of elasticity, European J. Appl. Math., 3 (1992), 21–30.

242. A.B. Movchan and N.V. Movchan, Mathematical Modelling of Solids with Nonregular Boundaries, CRC Press, Boca Raton, 1995.

243. A.B. Movchan, N.V. Movchan, and C.G. Poulton, Asymptotic Models of Fields in Dilute and Densely Packed Composites, Imperial College Press, London, 2002.

244. A.B. Movchan, N.A. Nicorovici, and R.C. McPhedran, Green's tensors and lattice sums for elastostatics and elastodynamics, Proc. Royal Soc. London A, 453 (1997), 643–662.

245. A.B. Movchan and S.K. Serkov, The Pólya-Szegö matrices in asymptotic models of dilute composite, European J. Appl. Math., 8 (1997), 595–621.

246. J. Mueller, D. Isaacson, and J. Newell, A reconstruction algorithm for electrical impedance tomography data collected on rectangular electrode arrays, IEEE Trans. Biomed. Engr., 46 (1999), 1379–1386.

247. T. Mura and T. Koya, Variational Methods in Mechanics, The Clarendon Press, Oxford University Press, New York, 1992.

248. F. Murat and L. Tartar, Optimality conditions and homogenization, Research Notes in Mathematics, 127, 1–8, Pitman, London, 1985.

249. N.I. Muskhelishvili, Some Basic Problems of the Mathematical Theory of Elasticity, English translation, Noordhoff International Publishing, Leyden, 1977.

250. A. Nachman, Reconstructions from boundary measurements, Ann. Math., 128 (1988), 531–587.

251. ——————, Global uniqueness for a two-dimensional inverse boundary value problem, Ann. Math., 142 (1996), 71–96.

252. G. Nakamura and G. Uhlmann, Identification of Lamé parameters by boundary observations, American J. Math., 115 (1993), 1161–1187.

253. S.A. Nazarov and J. Sokolowski, Asymptotic analysis of shape functionals, J. Math. Pures Appl., 82 (2003), 125–196.

254. J. Nečas, Les Méthodes Directes en Théorie des Équations Elliptiques, Academia, Prague, 1967.

255. J.C. Nédélec, Acoustic and Electromagnetic Equations. Integral Representations for Harmonic Problems, Springer-Verlag, New-York, 2001.

256. N.A. Nicorovici, R.C. McPhedran, and L.C. Botten, Photonic band gaps for arrays of perfectly conducting cylinders, Phys. Review E, 52 (1995), 1135–1145.

257. T. Ohe and K. Ohnaka, A precise estimation method for locations in an inverse logarithmic potential for point mass models, Appl. Math. Modelling, 18 (1994), 446–452.

258. —————, Determination of locations of point-like masses in an inverse source problem of the Poisson equation, J. Comput. Appl. Math., 54 (1994), 251–261.

259. S. Ozawa, Singular variation of domains and eigenvalues of the Laplacian, Duke Math. J., 48 (1981), 767–778.

260. —————, Spectra of domains with small spherical Neumann boundary, J. Fac. Sci. Univ. Tokyo, Sect IA, 30 (1983), 259–277.

261. G.C. Papanicolaou, Diffusion in random media, in *Surveys in Applied Mathematics, Volume 1*, 205–253, eds. J.P. Keller, D.W. McLaughlin, and G.C. Papanicolaou, Plenum Press, New York, 1995.

262. M. Pavlin, T. Slivnik, and D. Miklavčič, Effective conductivity of cell suspensions, IEEE Trans. Biomedical Eng., 49 (2002), 77–80.

263. L. Payne, Isoperimetric inequalities and their applications, SIAM Rev., 9 (1967), 453–488.

264. L. Payne and G. Philippin, On some maximum principles involving harmonic functions and their derivatives, SIAM J. Math Anal., 10 (1979), 96–104.

265. —————, Isoperimetric inequalities for polarization and virtual mass, J. Anal. Math., 47 (1986), 255–267.

266. L. Payne and H. Weinberger, New bounds in harmonic and biharmonic problems, J. Math. Phys., 33 (1954), 291–307.

267. I.G. Petrovsky, *Lectures on Partial Differential Equations*, Dover, New York, 1954.

268. G. Philippin, On a free boundary value problem in electrostatics, Math. Meth. Appl. Sci., 12 (1990), 387–392.

269. C.G. Poulton, L.C. Botten, R.C. McPhedran, and A.B. Movchan, Source-neutral Green's functions for periodic problems in electrostatics, and their equivalents in electromagnetism, Proc. Royal Soc. London A, 455 (1999), 1107–1123.

270. C.G. Poulton, A.B. Movchan, R.C. McPhedran, N.C. Nicorovici, and Y.A. Antipov, Eigenvalue problems for doubly periodic elastic structures and phononic band gaps, Proc. R. Soc. Lond. A, 456 (2000), 2543–2559.

271. G. Pólya and G. Szegö, *Isoperimetric Inequalities in Mathematical Physics*, Annals of Mathematical Studies Number 27, Princeton University Press, Princeton, NJ, 1951.

272. W. Reichel, Radial symmetry for an electrostatic, a capillarity and some fully nonlinear overdetermined problem on exterior domains, Z. Anal. Anwendungen, 15 (1996), 619–635.

273. —————, Radial symmetry for elliptic boundary-value problems on exterior domains, Arch. Rational Mech. Anal., 137 (1997), 381–394.

274. F. Rellich, Darstelling der eigenwerte von $\Delta u = \lambda u$ durch ein randintegral, Math Z., 46 (1940), 635–646.

275. B. Samet, S. Amstutz, and M. Masmoudi, The topological asymptotic for the Helmholtz equation, SIAM J. Control Optim., 42 (2004), 1523–1544.

276. E. Sánchez-Palencia, Einstein-like approximation for homogenization with small concentration. I. Elliptic problems, Nonlinear Anal., 9 (1985), 1243–1254.

277. A.S. Sangani, Conductivity of n-dimensional composites containing hyperspherical inclusion, SIAM J. Appl. Math., 50 (1990), 64–73.

278. A.S. Sangani and A. Acrivos, The effective conductivity of a periodic array of spheres, Proc. Roy. Soc. London A, 386 (1983), 263.

279. F. Santosa and M.S. Vogelius, A backprojection algorithm for electrical impedance imaging, SIAM J. Appl. Math., 50 (1990), 216–243.

280. M. Schiffer and G. Szegö, Virtual mass and polarization, Trans. Amer. Math. Soc., 67 (1949), 130–205.

281. J.K. Seo, A uniqueness result on inverse conductivity problem with two measurements, J. Fourier Anal. Appl., 2 (1996), 227–235.

282. J.K. Seo, O. Kwon, H. Ammari, and E.J. Woo, Mathematical framework and anomaly estimation algorithm for breast cancer detection using TS2000 configuration, IEEE Trans. Biomedical Engineering, 51 (2004), 1898–1906.

283. S. Siltanen, J. Mueller, and D. Isaacson, An implementation of the reconstruction algorithm of A. Nachman for the 2D inverse conductivity problem, Inverse Problems, 16 (2000), 681–699.

284. E. Somersalo, M. Cheney, D. Isaacson, and E. Isaacson, Layer-stripping: a direct numerical method for impedance imaging, Inverse Problems, 7 (1991), 899–926.

285. J. Sylvester and G. Uhlmann, A global uniqueness theorem for an inverse boundary value problem, Ann. Math., 125 (1987), 153–169.

286. ——————, The Dirichlet to Neumann map and applications, Inverse Problems in Partial Differential Equations, SIAM, Philadelphia (1990), 197–221.

287. J. Tausch and J. White, Capacitance extraction of 3-D conductor systems in dielectric media with high-permittivity ratios, IEEE Trans. Microwave Theory Tech., 47, 18–26.

288. J. Tausch, J. Wang, and J. White, Improved integral formulations for fast 3-D method of moment solvers, IEEE Trans. Comput. Aided Design, 20, 1398–1405.

289. C.W. Therrien, *Discrete Random Signals and Statistical Signal Processing*, Englewood Cliffs, NJ, Prentice-Hall, 1992.

290. C.F. Tolmasky and A. Wiegmann, Recovery of small perturbations of an interface for an elliptic inverse problem via linearization, Inverse Problems, 15 (1999), 465–487.

291. S.T. Torquato, *Random Heterogeneous Materials: Microstructure and Macroscopic Properties*, Springer-Verlag, New York, 2002.

292. ——————, Modeling of physical properties of composite materials, Internal J. Solids Struc., 37 (2000), 411–422.

293. R. Torres and G. Welland, The Helmholtz equation and transmission problems with Lipschitz interfaces, Indiana Univ. Math. J., 42 (1993), 1457–1485.

294. D.S. Tuch, V.J. Wedeen, A.M. Dale, J.S. George, and J.W. Belliveau, Conductivity tensor of the humain brain using diffusion tensor MRI, Proc. Nat. Acad. Sci., 98 (2001), 11697–11701.

295. G. Uhlmann, Inverse boundary value problems for partial differential equations, Proceedings of the International Congress of Mathematicians, Berlin (1998), Documenta Mathematica Vol. III, 77–86.

296. ——————, Developments in inverse problems since Calderón's foundational paper, Chapter 19 in *"Harmonic Analysis and Partial Differential Equations"*, 295–345, eds. M. Christ, C. Kenig, and C. Sadosky, University of Chicago Press, 1999.

297. M. Vauhkonen, D. Vadasz, P.A. Karjalainen, E. Somersalo, and J.P. Kaipio, Tikhonov regularization and prior information in electrical impedance tomography, IEEE Trans. Med. Imag., 17 (1998), 285–293.

298. G.C. Verchota, Layer potentials and boundary value problems for Laplace's equation in Lipschitz domains, J. Funct. Anal., 59 (1984), 572–611.

299. M.S. Vogelius and D. Volkov, Asymptotic formulas for perturbations in the electromagnetic fields due to the presence of inhomogeneities, Math. Model. Numer. Anal., 34 (2000), 723–748.

300. D. Volkov, An Inverse Problem for the Time Harmonic Maxwell Equations, Ph.D. thesis, Rutgers University, New Brunswick, NJ, 2001.

301. ——————, Numerical methods for locating small dielectric inhomogeneities, Wave Motion, 38 (2003), 189–206.

302. J.L. Walsh, The approximation of harmonic functions by harmonic polynomials and by harmonic rational functions, Bull. Amer. Math. Soc., (2), 35 (1929), 499–544.

303. E.J. Woo, P. Hua, J.G. Webster, and W.J. Tompkins, Measuring lung resistivity using electrical impedance tomography, IEEE Trans. Biomed. Engr., 39 (1992), 756–760.

304. E.J. Woo, J.G. Webster, and W.J. Tompkins, A robust image reconstruction algorithm and its parallel implementation in electrical impedance tomography, IEEE Trans. Med. Imag., 12 (1993), 137–146.

305. K. Yamatani, T. Ohe, and K. Ohnaka, An identification method of electric current dipoles in spherically symmetric conductor, J. Comput. Appl. Math., 143 (2002), 189–200.

306. T. Yorkey, J. Webster, and W. Tompkins, Comparing reconstruction algorithms for electrical impedance tomography, IEEE Trans. Biomed. Engr., 34 (1987), 843–852.

307. X. Zheng, M.G. Forest, R. Lipton, R. Zhou, and Q. Wang, Exact scaling laws for electrical conductivity properties of nematic polymer nanocomposite monodomains, Adv. Funct. Mater., 15 (2005), 627–638.

308. J.M. Ziman, *Principles of the Theory of Solids*, Cambridge University Press, 1972.

309. R.W. Zimmerman, Elastic moduli of a solid containing spherical inclusions, Mech. Materials, 12 (1991), 17–24.

310. ——————, Effective conductivity of a low-dimensional medium containing elliptical inhomogeneities, Proc. R. Soc. Lond. A, 452 (1996), 1713–1727.

311. M. Zuzovski and H. Brenner, Effective conductivity of composite materials composed of cubic arrangements of spherical particles embedded in an isotropic matrix, ZAMP, 28 (1977), 979–992.

312. *Light Scattering from Microstructures*, edited by F. Moreno and F. Gonzalez, Lecture Notes in Physics, vol. 534, Springer-Verlag 2000.

Index

A-harmonic function, 64–66, 123, 126

anisotropic conductivity, 52
asymptotic formula, 129, 140, 261, 269

bispherical coordinate system, 160

Calderón method, 161, 174
capacity, 39, 89
Cauchy integral formula, 172
Cauchy principal value, 24
cell problem, 197
closely spaced inclusions, 106, 140
compact operators, 18, 291
complex representation, 225
conjecture of Pólya–Szegö, 102
continuity method, 30, 293

decomposition theorem, 45, 129
detection, 167, 169, 275, 276
dipole, 15
dipole approximation, 129, 130
Dirac delta function, 15
Dirichlet-to-Neumann map, 70, 90
displacement field, 212
divergence theorem, 12, 212

effective conductivity, 199
effective elasticity tensor, 289
eigenvalues of EMTs, 246
elastic moment tensors, 225, 237, 265, 269
energy identities, 50
equivalent ellipse, 118

far field, 77, 271
Fourier transform algorithm, 174
Fredholm alternative, 26
fundamental solution, 14, 51, 212

Green's formula, 13
Green's function, 44, 139, 224
Green's identity, 15, 213

harmonic conjugate, 10, 172
harmonic functions, 10
harmonic polynomial, 11, 84, 86, 89, 92–94, 96, 103–105, 108, 186, 188, 203
Hashin–Shtrikman bounds, 101, 259
Hashin-Shtrikman variational technique, 98
Hasimoto's method, 197
heat equation, 144
Helmholtz equation, 66, 144, 192
high-contrast material, 37
homogeneous harmonic polynomial, 56
homogeneous polynomial, 84
homogenization, 195

imaging, 269
impedance imaging, 161
injectivity, 25
inverse Fourier transform, 175
invertibility, 25, 37
isoperimetric inequalities, 5, 76, 97

jump formulae, 20, 24, 51

Kelvin matrix, 212
Korn's inequality, 215, 222

Lamé constants, 211
Lamé system, 211
lattice sum, 53
Lax–Milgram lemma, 14
layer potentials, 14, 51, 211
least-squares algorithm, 173
linear sampling method, 162, 176
Lipschitz character, 7
Lipschitz domain, 7
logarithmic capacity, 39

maximum principle, 11, 44, 74, 134
Maxwell's equations, 66, 144
Maxwell–Garnett formula, 3, 196
mean value property, 10, 115
moment estimation, 185
monotonicity, 103, 127
MUSIC algorithm, 176, 193

near-boundary inclusion, 150
Neumann function, 39, 43, 130, 264

partial Neumann-to-Dirichlet map, 177
periodic Green's function, 53, 59, 230
Poincaré's inequality, 10
Poisson summation formula, 53, 59
Poisson's kernel, 44
polarization tensor of Pólya–Szegö, 77
polarization tensors, 75, 130
polarization tensors of ellipses, 81
positivity of EMTs, 241
positivity of the GPTs, 91

projection algorithm, 163

quadratic algorithm, 169, 276

random noise, 176, 189, 190, 279, 280
real holomorphic polynomial, 61
reflection with respect to a disk, 112, 147, 148
Rellich identity, 27, 28, 132, 222
representation by ellipses, 118
Runge approximation, 11, 71

Shannon's sampling theorem, 175
singular kernel, 24
size estimations, 164, 166
source point, 15
stability, 171
Stokes's formula, 13
strain tensor, 212
symmetry of EMTs, 241
symmetry of the GPTs, 91

Taylor's formula, 43, 54, 77
transmission problem, 7, 218, 220

unique continuation property, 11, 91, 184
uniqueness, 48, 67, 90

variational algorithm, 174
variational characterization, 95
variational principle, 98

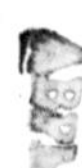

Applied Mathematical Sciences

(continued from page ii)

61. *Sattinger/Weaver:* Lie Groups and Algebras with Applications to Physics, Geometry, and Mechanics.
62. *LaSalle:* The Stability and Control of Discrete Processes.
63. *Grasman:* Asymptotic Methods of Relaxation Oscillations and Applications.
64. *Hsu:* Cell-to-Cell Mapping: A Method of Global Analysis for Nonlinear Systems.
65. *Rand/Armbruster:* Perturbation Methods, Bifurcation Theory and Computer Algebra.
66. *Hlavácek/Haslinger/Necasl/Lovísek:* Solution of Variational Inequalities in Mechanics.
67. *Cercignani:* The Boltzmann Equation and Its Application.
68. *Temam:* Infinite Dimensional Dynamical Systems in Mechanics and Physics, 2nd ed.
69. *Golubitsky/Stewart/Schaeffer:* Singularities and Groups in Bifurcation Theory, Vol. II.
70. *Constantin/Foias/Nicolaenko/Temam:* Integral Manifolds and Inertial Manifolds for Dissipative Partial Differential Equations.
71. *Catlin:* Estimation, Control, and The Discrete Kalman Filter.
72. *Lochak/Meunier:* Multiphase Averaging for Classical Systems.
73. *Wiggins:* Global Bifurcations and Chaos.
74. Mawhin/Willem: Critical Point Theory and Hamiltonian Systems.
75. *Abraham/Marsden/Ratiu:* Manifolds, Tensor Analysis, and Applications, 2nd ed.
76. *Lagerstrom:* Matched Asymptotic Expansions: Ideas and Techniques.
77. *Aldous:* Probability Approximations via the Poisson Clumping Heuristic.
78. *Dacorogna:* Direct Methods in the Calculus of Variations.
79. *Hernández-Lerma:* Adaptive Markov Processes.
80. *Lawden:* Elliptic Functions and Applications.
81. *Bluman/Kumei:* Symmetries and Differential Equations.
82. *Kress:* Linear Integral Equations, 2nd ed.
83. *Bebernes/Eberly:* Mathematical Problems from Combustion Theory.
84. *Joseph:* Fluid Dynamics of Viscoelastic Fluids.
85. *Yang:* Wave Packets and Their Bifurcations in Geophysical Fluid Dynamics.
86. *Dendrinos/Sonis:* Chaos and Socio-Spatial Dynamics.
87. *Weder:* Spectral and Scattering Theory for wave Propagation in Perturbed Stratified Media.
88. *Bogaevski/Povzner:* Algebraic Methods in Nonlinear Perturbation Theory.
89. *O'Malley:* Singular Perturbation Methods for Ordinary Differential Equations.
90. *Meyer/Hall:* Introduction to Hamiltonian Dynamical Systems and the N-body Problem.

91. *Straughan:* The Energy Method, Stability, and Nonlinear Convection, 2nd ed.
92. *Naber:* The Geometry of Minkowski Spacetime.
93. *Colton/Kress:* Inverse Acoustic and Electromagnetic Scattering Theory, 2nd ed.
94. *Hoppensteadt:* Analysis and Simulation of Chaotic Systems.
95. *Hackbusch:* Iterative Solution of Large Sparse Systems of Equations.
96. *Marchioro/Pulvirenti:* Mathematical Theory of Incompressible Nonviscous Fluids.
97. *Lasota/Mackey:* Chaos, Fractals, and Noise: Stochastic Aspects of Dynamics, 2nd ed.
98. *de Boor/Höllig/Riemenschneider:* Box Splines.
99. *Hale/Lunel:* Introduction to Functional Differential Equations.
100. *Sirovich (ed):* Trends and Perspectives in Applied Mathematics.
101. *Nusse/Yorke:* Dynamics: Numerical Explorations, 2nd ed.
102. *Chossat/Iooss:* The Couette-Taylor Problem.
103. *Chorin:* Vorticity and Turbulence.
104. *Farkas:* Periodic Motions.
105. *Wiggins:* Normally Hyperbolic Invariant Manifolds in Dynamical Systems.
106. *Cercignani/Ilner/Pulvirenti:* The Mathematical Theory of Dilute Gases.
107. *Antman:* Nonlinear Problems of Elasticity, 2nd ed.
108. *Zeidler:* Applied Functional Analysis: Applications to Mathematical Physics.
109. *Zeidler:* Applied Functional Analysis: Main Principles and Their Applications.
110. *Diekman/van Gils/Verduyn Lunel/Walther:* Delay Equations: Functional-, Complex-, and Nonlinear Analysis.
111. *Visintin:* Differential Models of Hysteresis.
112. *Kuznetsov:* Elements of Applied Bifurcation Theory, 3rd ed.
113. *Hislop/Sigal:* Introduction to Spectral Theory.
114. *Kevorkian/Cole:* Multiple Scale and Singular Perturbation Methods.
115. *Taylor:* Partial Differential Equations I, Basic Theory.
116. *Taylor:* Partial Differential Equations II, Qualitative Studies of Linear Equations.
117. *Taylor:* Partial Differential Equations III, Nonlinear Equations.
118. *Godlewski/Raviart:* Numerical Approximation of Hyperbolic Systems of Conservation Laws.
119. *Wu:* Theory and Applications of Partial Functional Differential Equations.
120. *Kirsch:* An Introduction to the Mathematical Theory of Inverse Problems.
121. *Brokate/Sprekels:* Hysteresis and Phase Transitions.
122. *Gliklikh:* Global Analysis in Mathematical Physics: Geometric and Stochastic Methods.

(continued on next page)

Applied Mathematical Sciences

(continued from previous page)

123. *Khoi Le/Schmitt:* Global Bifurcation in Variational Inequalities: Applications to Obstacle and Unilateral Problems.
124. *Polak:* Optimization: Algorithms and Consistent Approximations.
125. *Arnold/Khesin:* Topological Methods in Hydrodynamics.
126. *Hoppensteadt/Izhikevich:* Weakly Connected Neural Networks.
127. *Isakov:* Inverse Problems for Partial Differential Equations, 2nd ed.
128. *Li/Wiggins:* Invariant Manifolds and Fibrations for Perturbed Nonlinear Schrödinger Equations.
129. *Müller:* Analysis of Spherical Symmetries in Euclidean Spaces.
130. *Feintuch:* Robust Control Theory in Hilbert Space.
131. *Ericksen:* Introduction to the Thermodynamics of Solids, Revised Edition.
132. *Ihlenburg:* Finite Element Analysis of Acoustic Scattering.
133. *Vorovich:* Nonlinear Theory of Shallow Shells.
134. *Vein/Dale:* Determinants and Their Applications in Mathematical Physics.
135. *Drew/Passman:* Theory of Multicomponent Fluids.
136. *Cioranescu/Saint Jean Paulin:* Homogenization of Reticulated Structures.
137. *Gurtin:* Configurational Forces as Basic Concepts of Continuum Physics.
138. *Haller:* Chaos Near Resonance.
139. *Sulem/Sulem:* The Nonlinear Schrödinger Equation: Self-Focusing and Wave Collapse.
140. *Cherkaev:* Variational Methods for Structural Optimization.
141. *Naber:* Topology, Geometry, and Gauge Fields: Interactions.
142. *Schmid/Henningson:* Stability and Transition in Shear Flows.
143. *Sell/You:* Dynamics of Evolutionary Equations.
144. *Nédélec:* Acoustic and Electromagnetic Equations: Integral Representations for Harmonic Problems.
145. *Newton:* The N-Vortex Problem: Analytical Techniques.
146. *Allaire:* Shape Optimization by the Homogenization Method.
147. *Aubert/Kornprobst:* Mathematical Problems in Image Processing: Partial Differential Equations and the Calculus of Variations.
148. *Peyret:* Spectral Methods for Incompressible Viscous Flow.
149. *Ikeda/Murota:* Imperfect Bifurcation in Structures and Materials.
150. *Skorokhod/Hoppensteadt/Salehi:* Random Perturbation Methods with Applications in Science and Engineering.
151. *Bensoussan/Frehse:* Regularity Results for Nonlinear Elliptic Systems and Applications.
152. *Holden/Risebro:* Front Tracking for Hyperbolic Conservation Laws.
153. *Osher/Fedkiw:* Level Set Methods and Dynamic Implicit Surfaces.
154. *Bluman/Anco:* Symmetries and Integration Methods for Differential Equations.
155. *Chalmond:* Modeling and Inverse Problems in Image Analysis.
156. *Kielhöfer:* Bifurcation Theory: An Introduction with Applications to PDEs.
157. *Kaczynski/Mischaikow/Mrozek:* Computational Homology.
158. *Oertel:* Prandtl–Essentials of Fluid Mechanics, 10th Revised Edition.
159. *Ern:* Theory and Practice of Finite Elements.
160. *Kaipio:* Statistical and Computational Inverse Problems.
161. *Ting:* Viscous Vortical Flows II.
162. *Ammari/Kang:* Polarization and Moment Tensors: With Applications to Inverse Problems and Effective Medium Theory.

Printed in the United States of America.